Osteoarthritis

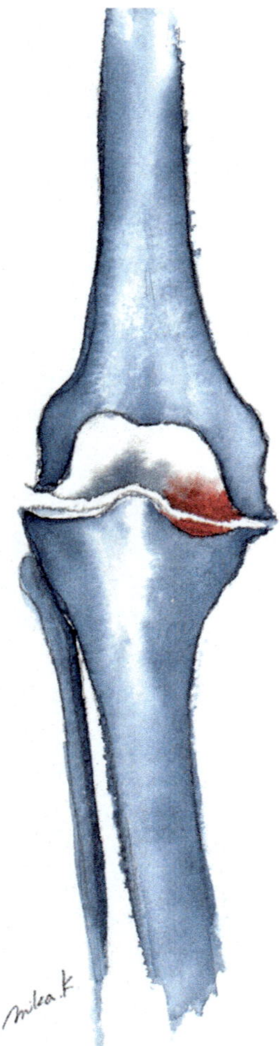

Osteoarthritic Knee Joint
Painted by Artist: Mika Katsuta (Japan)

Mohit Kapoor • Nizar N. Mahomed
Editors

Osteoarthritis

Pathogenesis, Diagnosis, Available Treatments, Drug Safety, Regenerative and Precision Medicine

Adis

Editors
Mohit Kapoor
Division of Genetics and Development
Toronto Western Research Institute
University Health Network
and Department of Surgery
University of Toronto
Toronto, Ontario
Canada

Nizar N. Mahomed
Division of Orthopaedics
Toronto Western Hospital
Toronto, Ontario
Canada

ISBN 978-3-319-19559-9 ISBN 978-3-319-19560-5 (eBook)
DOI 10.1007/978-3-319-19560-5

Library of Congress Control Number: 2015945968

Springer Cham Heidelberg New York Dordrecht London

Printed on acid-free paper

Adis is a brand of Springer
Springer International Publishing AG Switzerland is part of Springer Science+Business Media (www.springer.com)

Preface

Designed as a comprehensive resource, this book is a collaborative effort by leading clinicians and scientists in the field of osteoarthritis. This book consists of 13 chapters that explore the destruction of joints such as the knee, hip, shoulder, elbow, ankle, hand, wrist, and spine. Through the analysis of imaging modalities, joint conservation techniques, biomarkers, treatment options, and safety profiles of available treatments, this book aims to present the most current and cutting-edge research in the field of osteoarthritis. Finally, this book goes beyond to introduce regenerative approaches for treatment and the need for precision medicine in osteoarthritis. The production of this book has been an enjoyable experience, and we would like to thank the authors and everybody involved in creating this book.

Toronto, ON, Canada

Mohit Kapoor
Nizar N. Mahomed

Acknowledgement

The editors would like to thank each contributor of this book for their tremendous work, time and effort, without whom this book would not have been possible. Our special thanks to Helal Endisha (book coordinator) for her endless hours of work and commitment to this book. We also would like to thank Bandna Pal for her administrative assistance.

We also would like to acknowledge the support and help of members of the Arthritis Program at the University Health Network as well as the excellent team at Springer.

Finally, we would like to dedicate this book to our parents, our wives and children.

Contents

Chapter 1
Pathogenesis of Osteoarthritis

Mohit Kapoor

Key Points

- Osteoarthritis (OA) is one of the most chronic health disorders in the western world and becomes particularly common with advanced age. The joints most commonly affected by OA include the knees, hips, ankle, elbow, shoulder, hand, wrist and spine.
- Risk factors that may increase the risk of developing OA are age, gender, joint injury or overuse caused by physical labour or sports, obesity, and joint alignment etc.
- Symptoms of OA may appear well after disease onset. Such symptoms include joint pain, limitation of motion, stiffness after inactivity, tenderness, crepitus, and joint enlargement.
- While previously characterized as a disease of progressive articular cartilage degradation, OA pathophysiology involves all of the tissues that form the synovial joint which are the subchondral and metaphyseal bone, synovium, ligaments, joint capsules, and the muscles acting across the joint. Subchondral bone remodelling, osteophyte formation, synovial inflammation, ligamentous laxity (loose ligaments), and the weakening of periarticular muscles exemplify several joint structure alterations observed.

M. Kapoor, PhD
Division of Genetics and Development, The Toronto Western Research Institute,
The University Health Network (UHN), 60 Leonard Avenue, Toronto, ON, Canada M5T 2S8

Department of Surgery, University of Toronto, Toronto, ON, Canada

Division of Orthopaedics, Toronto Western Hospital, Toronto, ON, Canada
e-mail: mkapoor@uhnresearch.ca

M. Kapoor, N.N. Mahomed (eds.), *Osteoarthritis: Pathogenesis, Diagnosis, Available Treatments, Drug Safety, Regenerative and Precision Medicine*,
DOI 10.1007/978-3-319-19560-5_1

- Chondrocytes, the only cell types present in the articular cartilage, are responsible for maintaining an equilibrium between the anabolic and catabolic activities in the extracellular matrix (ECM).
- The trigger of OA is unclear; however, it may begin with tissue damage from mechanical injury, infiltration of inflammatory mediators from the synovium into the cartilage, or defects in cartilage metabolism/homeostasis. Chondrocytes attempt to repair cartilage damage/degradation by increasing the production of ECM macromolecules. As degeneration continues, catabolic mechanisms overpower the anabolic capabilities of chondrocytes, and the homeostatic balance is tipped resulting in progressed cartilage breakdown.

Introduction

Osteoarthritis (OA) is a debilitating disease that involves all structures of the affected joint. It is one of the most common chronic health disorders in the western world; with a higher prevalence among the ageing population [1, 2]. The National Arthritis Data Workshop reported a rise in OA prevalence with an estimated 27 million US adults in 2005 having clinical OA of their hand, knee, or hip joint, an increase from 21 million in 1995 [3]. For a disease with such a strong age-related association, such an increase is likely with the ageing population. The incidence of OA was also seen to rise hand in hand with the escalation of obesity in the population. Obese women have nearly four times the risk of knee OA as compared with nonobese women; for obese men, the risk is nearly five times greater [4]. Hence, obesity has been established as a major risk factor for the development and progression of OA. Other risk factors include sex, race and ethnicity, genetics, nutrition, smoking, and injuries/trauma to the joint [1, 5–13]. If an individual has the genetic predisposition to develop OA, they may not develop it unless they have experienced insult to the joint or are accompanied by one or more of the other risk factors. The relative significance of certain risk factors may differ from joint to joint, for early versus end-stage OA, for development as opposed to progression of disease, and for radiographic versus symptomatic disease. Before describing the pathogenesis of the joint structure during OA, it is important to understand the nature and function of the joint structure under normal conditions. In this chapter, we discuss the composition of the joint, the interplay of the joint components to maintain homeostasis, and the disruption of the homeostatic mechanisms that drive the development of OA.

Articular Cartilage: Structure, Function, and Composition

While OA is characterized as a progressive loss of articular cartilage, joint degeneration involves all of the tissues that form the synovial joint which are the subchondral and metaphyseal bone, synovium, ligaments, joint capsules, and the muscles acting across the joint [14]. Subchondral bone remodelling, osteophyte formation, synovial inflammation, ligamentous laxity (loose ligaments), and the weakening of periarticular muscles occur as a result of an imbalance in the equilibrium between the breakdown and repair of joint tissue [15]. Consequently, the affected individual experiences joint pain, stiffness, and limitation of movement. Without treatment, these symptoms slowly evolve to whole joint failure with pain and disability.

The primary functions of articular cartilage are to lubricate the surface of synovial joints allowing for painless, low-friction movement of the opposing joint surfaces and to facilitate the distribution of loads, thereby minimizing stress on the underlying subchondral bone [14].

Articular cartilage lacks blood vessels, nerves, and lymphatic vessels. Instead, it consists primarily of extracellular matrix (ECM) with sparsely distributed, highly specialized cells called chondrocytes [16]. The chondrocyte is the only cell type residing in the articular cartilage. The articular cartilage ECM is composed of tissue fluid and a framework of structural macromolecules (collagens, proteoglycans, and non-collagenous proteins and glycoproteins) synthesized by chondrocytes. Each chondrocyte is responsible for the establishment and maintenance of a specialized microenvironment in its surrounding area [17]. The interaction between the tissue fluid and the macromolecular framework helps retain water within the ECM, which is crucial to maintain its unique mechanical properties of stiffness and flexibility. The tissue fluid is 80 % of the wet weight of articular cartilage. It is essentially water but also contains gases, small proteins, metabolites, and a high concentration of cations to balance the negatively charged proteoglycans. About 30 % of the water exists within the intrafibrillar space within the collagen and appears to exist as a gel, while a small percentage is contained in the intracellular space. The rest is contained in the pore space of the matrix. In addition to providing lubrication, the flow of water through the cartilage and across the articular surface helps to transport and distribute nutrients to the chondrocytes.

Among the structural macromolecules of the ECM, collagen is the most abundant, contributing to about 60 % of the dry weight of articular cartilage. Specifically, type II collagen represents 90–95 % of the collagen in the ECM. Additional distinct collagen types I, IV, V, VI, IX, X, and XI contribute a minor proportion and serve to form and stabilize the type II collagen fibril network that intertwines with proteoglycan aggregates. The organization of this tight meshwork that extends throughout the tissue provides the tensile stiffness, cohesiveness, and strength of articular cartilage [18, 19].

The second-largest group of macromolecules in the ECM are proteoglycans. There are two major classes of proteoglycans: large aggregating molecules (aggrecans) and smaller proteoglycans (decorin, biglycan, and fibromodulin) [20]. Aggrecans interact with hyaluronic acid (also known as hyaluronan or HA) and link proteins to form large proteoglycan aggregates. This aggregation helps anchor proteoglycans within the matrix and provides the cartilage with its osmotic properties, which is essential to its role in resisting compressive loads [21–23]. Unlike aggrecans, the small nonaggregating proteoglycans do not contribute directly to the mechanical behaviour of articular cartilage. Decorin and fibromodulin are involved in fibrillogenesis and interfibril interactions via their interactions with type II collagen fibrils. Biglycan is localized in the immediate surroundings of chondrocytes and may interact with type VI collagen [16, 24, 25].

The structural macromolecules and chondrocytes are organized in a highly ordered structure to form the articular cartilage. The composition, organization, cell morphology, and mechanical properties of the matrix vary between zones of the cartilage. Within each zone, matrix composition, organization, and function also vary with the distance from the chondrocyte – giving rise to the pericellular region, the territorial region, and the interterritorial region. The four zones from the articular surface to the subchondral bone are defined as the superficial zone, the transitional zone, the middle (radial or deep) zone, and the calcified cartilage zone [14, 19].

The superficial zone is in contact with the synovial fluid and is the thinnest articular cartilage zone. It contains a relatively high number of flattened chondrocytes as well as mostly type II and type IX collagen tightly packed and aligned parallel to the articular surface. This zone is important for the protection and maintenance of the deeper zones. Additionally, the densely packed collagen fibrils lying parallel to the joint surface give the cartilage its tensile stiffness and enable the cartilage to resist the sheer, tensile, and compressive forces generated during joint use [26].

With 40–60 % of the total cartilage volume, proteoglycans, and thicker collagen fibrils, the transitional zone is the first line of resistance to compressive forces. The transitional zone also provides an anatomic bridge between the superficial and deep zones. The collagen fibrils have the largest diameter and are arranged in a perpendicular fashion. Also, the deep zone contains the highest proteoglycan content and the lowest water concentration. These properties render the deep zone responsible for providing the greatest resistance to compressive forces [14, 19].

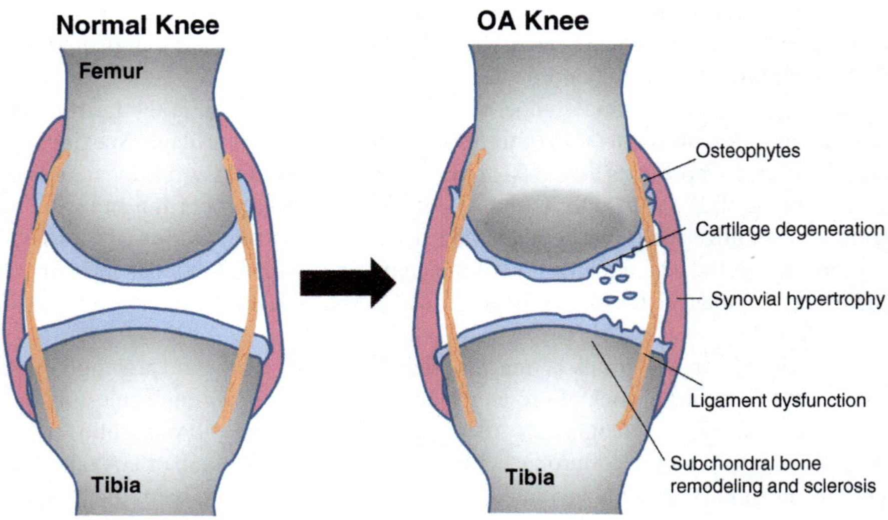

Fig. 1.1 Schematic of normal vs. osteoarthritic knee joint. OA is accompanied by considerable cartilage degradation, the generation of wear particles, thickening of synovium, subchondral bone alterations, and the growth of osteophytes at the margins of the joint

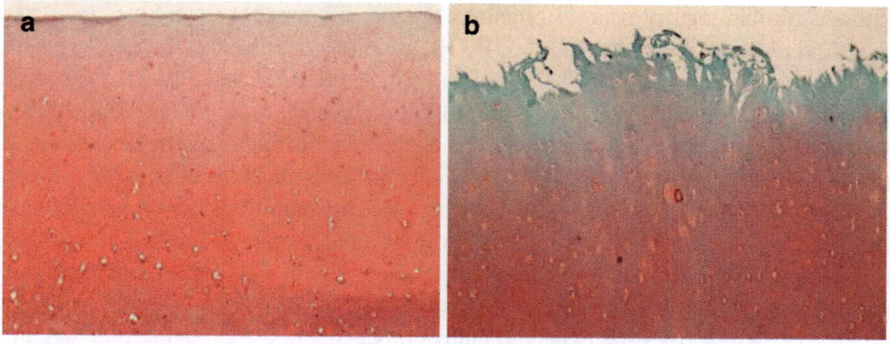

Fig. 1.2 Safranin-O staining of (**a**) normal and (**b**) OA human knee joint cartilage showing cartilage degradation and loss of proteoglycan

Finally, the 'tidemark', a dynamic structure that appears as a basophilic line in histological sections, separates the deep zone from the calcified cartilage. The calcified cartilage zone functions to secure the cartilage to the bone, by anchoring the collagen fibrils of the deep zone to the subchondral bone [27]. Additionally, calcified cartilage is permeable to small-molecule transport and plays an important role in the biochemical interaction between non-calcified cartilage and subchondral bone (Figs. 1.1 and 1.2) [28, 29].

Synovium

As mentioned in the beginning of this chapter, the characterization of OA not only involves the destruction of articular cartilage but also involves the integrity of multiple joint tissues [30]. Synovial joints include a joint cavity filled with synovial fluid, which is surrounded by articular cartilage and a fibrous capsule, including the inner lining synovium. The synovial fluid is in direct physical contact with the cartilage and synovium and exhibits biomechanical, metabolic, and regulatory functions [31, 32]. This physicality allows the synovial fluid to interact with and mediate interactions between synovial joint tissues. By providing boundary lubrication, the synovial fluid reduces friction and helps to protect and maintain the integrity of articular cartilage surfaces [32]. Two important molecules secreted by synovial lining cells and cells within the synovial joint space are the lubricant hyaluronan (HA) and proteoglycan 4 (PRG4, also known as lubricin and superficial zone protein (SZP)). HA contributes to the viscosity of synovial fluid and provides outflow buffering (the maintenance of synovial fluid volume by coupling between draining and input rates), while the mucinous glycoproteins, SZP and lubricin, mediate boundary lubrication of articular cartilage [33–36].

Cytokines and growth factors present in synovial fluid are important regulatory factors for cells within the synovium as well as chondrocytes in the cartilage [31]. According to their predominant tissue-specific effects, cytokines can be classified as either proinflammatory or anti-inflammatory. Proinflammatory cytokines in synovial fluid include interleukin (IL)-1α, IL-1β, tumour necrosis factor-α (TNF-α), leukaemia inhibitory factor (LIF), IL-6, IL-8, IL-17, and IL-18 [37–40]. Anti-inflammatory cytokines in synovial fluid include IL-4, IL-10, and IL-13 [38]. Growth factors found in synovial fluid include transforming growth factor beta 1 (TGF-β1) and insulin growth factor (IGF-1) and have anabolic effects [41]. Most cytokines and growth factors are at relatively low concentrations in normal synovial fluid and are significantly elevated in joint injury and disease [31, 42]. Later in this chapter, we will discuss the role played by these cytokines in OA pathogenesis and acceleration of joint destruction.

Proteolytic enzymes mediate degradative processes in the synovial joint and are carefully regulated [43]. Matrix-degrading enzymes, such as matrix metalloproteinases (MMPs), are a group of Zn^{2+}-dependent extracellular enzymes that function in normal and pathological tissue remodelling [44]. MMPs are capable of degrading all of the components of the ECM. Depending on their substrate and domain structure, MMPs are classified into collagenases (MMP-1, MMP-8, MMP-13), gelatinases, stromelysins (MMP-3), and membrane-type MMPs [45]. MMPs are present in normal synovial fluid; however, their levels are elevated in joint injury and disease as evidenced by increased mRNA levels in tissue and elevated levels of proMMPs in synovial fluid [46–48]. MMPs are secreted primarily from chondrocytes as zymogens, or proMMPs, with propeptide domains that are cleaved during extracellular activation [49]. Similarly, requiring subsequent activation are disintegrin and metalloproteinase with thrombospondin motifs (ADAMTS) proteinases that degrade aggrecan [50–54]. Tissue inhibitors of metalloproteinases (TIMPs) and inhibitors of proteinases that activate proMMPs are also present. Thus, changes in the levels and activities of matrix-degrading enzymes, and their corresponding inhibitors and activators, alter anabolic and catabolic homeostasis in joint injury and disease [55, 56].

Synovial fluid is an ultrafiltrate of blood plasma and is relatively acellular compared to whole blood, containing less than 200 leukocytes per mm^3 compared to 3,540–9,060 per mm^3 in whole blood [57, 58]. Also present are lymphocytes, macrophages, and shed lining cells [59–61]. The synovium, or synovial membrane, is a vascularized, thin sheet of connective tissue with fibroblast-like (type B) cells and macrophage-like (type A) cells within an ECM composed predominantly of HA, collagen, and proteoglycans [31]. Molecular sieving by the synovial membrane matrix is size dependent, with lubricant molecules HA and PRG4 retained within the synovial joint, while low-molecular-weight species, such as metabolic substrates and by-products, cytokines, and growth factors, are not [62–64].

Subchondral Bone

For many years, OA was characterized as a primary disorder of articular cartilage; however, the discovery of the contribution of other joint tissues to the pathophysiology of OA has changed the definition of OA. Subchondral bone remodelling is commonly associated with articular cartilage defects and subchondral sclerosis, along with progressive cartilage degradation, that are heavily involved in the pathogenesis of the disease [65, 66].

Subchondral bone refers to the bony lamella lying distal to calcified cartilage [67, 68]. The subchondral bone can be separated into the subchondral bone plate and subchondral trabecular bone [69]. The subchondral bone plate is rather porous and lies immediately beneath the calcified cartilage. It contains channels that provide a direct link between articular cartilage and subchondral trabecular bone [70]. Arterial and venous vessels penetrate through the channels and send tiny branches into calcified cartilage [67, 71]. Supporting trabeculae arise from the subchondral bone plate and make up the subchondral trabecular bone together with deeper bone structure [72]. Subchondral trabecular bone is more porous and metabolically more active than the subchondral bone plate, containing blood vessels, sensory nerves, and bone marrow. It has shock-absorbing as well as supportive functions and may also be important for cartilage nutrient supply and metabolism [68]. Subchondral bone is a very dynamic structure and is uniquely adapted to the mechanical forces imposed across the joint [68, 72]. Accordingly, mechanical stress modifies the contour and shape of subchondral bone by means of bone modelling and remodelling [73–75]. Similar to the 'tidemark', which separates the two dissimilar cartilage regions, there is also a sharp borderline between calcified cartilage and subchondral bone, called the 'cement line' [68]. Evidently, close contact exists between the deeper layer of non-calcified cartilage, the tidemark, calcified cartilage, the cement line, and subchondral bone – forming a closely composited functional unit called the 'osteochondral junction' [76]. The biomechanical and biochemical cross-talk across this region seems to play a role in maintenance and degeneration of the joint [77]. As we shall see, alterations of any of these components will modulate the properties and functions of other parts of the osteochondral junction.

Infrapatellar Fat Pad

One of the most commonly affected joints by OA is the knee [78, 79]. The presence of the infrapatellar fat pad (IFP), or Hoffa's fat pad, differentiates the knee joint from other articular joints [80]. The IFP is composed of a fibrous scaffold, on which fat tissue is embedded. Located underneath the patella, between the patellar tendon, femoral condyle, and tibial plateau, this intracapsular and extrasynovial adipose structure is in close contact with the articular cartilage, bone, and synovium [81–83]. Besides its role in facilitating the distribution of synovial fluid and absorbing forces through the knee joint, not much is known about how the IFP contributes to knee function [84]. Notably, earlier studies have shown that the IFP is preserved under extreme starvation conditions despite subcutaneous adipose tissue elimination [85, 86]. This suggests critical physiological importance for the presence of this fat depot in the knee.

The IFP contains large numbers of adipocytes, fibroblasts, macrophages, leukocytes, and other immune cells capable of producing inflammatory cytokines [84, 87, 88]. The presence of these cells indicates possible protective and/or damaging roles of adipose tissue in the inflammatory reactions in OA. Nociceptive nerve fibres are also present in the IFP. Substance P-positive nerves innervating the IFP, indicating that they are peptidergic C-fibres, are increased in the IFP of patients with chronic anterior knee pain [89, 90]. Hence, anterior knee pain, which is the most common symptom experienced by patients with knee OA, is thought to be associated with pathology of the IFP.

Cellular changes in the IFP during knee OA involves the infiltration of immune cells in the IFP, which contributes to disease progression by stimulating the production of numerous inflammatory mediators [85, 91]. Inflammatory cytokines may act to alter the sensitivity of the nerve fibres, lowering the threshold of the joint nociceptors, thus inducing and worsening pain [92]. The numbers of neutrophils, eosinophils, basophils, and monocytes were seen to be elevated in the IFPs from patients with knee OA [93]. Neutrophils produce cytokines such as IL-1, IL-8, and MMP-8, which contribute to cartilage breakdown and necrosis of adipose tissue [84, 93, 94]. Eosinophils and basophils release histamine, which increases the production of matrix-degrading enzymes and pro-inflammatory mediators in synovial fibroblasts and cartilage [95]. Lymphocytes have also been found in the IFP expressing Th1 cytokines, which can either degrade cartilage directly or activate macrophages through cell-cell interaction, to produce cartilage degrading mediators [96, 97]. Thus, inflammatory cells within the IFP may influence the inflammatory and destructive responses in knee OA.

While immune cells in the adipose tissue are responsible for the production and release of most inflammatory mediators, adipocytes are responsible for the secretion of the adipokines, such as leptin and adiponectin [87, 98, 99]. In OA cartilage, leptin stimulates IL-1β production, increases the effect of pro-inflammatory cytokines, and induces the expression of MMPs [100–103]. Leptin also contributes to inflammatory responses by facilitating the activation of macrophages, neutrophils, dendritic cells, natural killer cells, and T helper 1 (Th1) cells [104]. While adiponectin is known to act as a protective adipokine against obesity and vascular diseases [105], it is suggested to act as a pro-inflammatory agent in joint diseases, such as knee OA [106, 107]. Adiponectin induces MMP-1 and IL-6 production in synovial fibroblasts, which have adiponectin receptors [108]. These receptors are also present in normal or OA chondrocytes, since adiponectin-treated chondrocytes produce IL-6, MMP-3, MMP-9, and monocyte chemoattractant protein 1 (MCP1) [99, 107].

Alteration of Joint Homeostasis During OA

Chondrocytes are responsible for the development, maintenance, and repair of the ECM via degradative enzymes, MMPs (collagenase, gelatinase, and stromelysin), and cathepsins B and D [14]. As post-mitotic cells, chondrocytes have a low rate of replication resulting in a limited ability for articular cartilage to maintain and repair itself

[109]. Maintenance of the articular surface requires turnover of the matrix macromolecules, as well as alteration in the matrix macromolecular framework in response to joint use [14]. Although chondrocytes have low mitotic activity, they are still metabolically active. Their metabolic activity can be altered by changes in their surrounding mechanical as well as chemical environment [19]. While ECM protects chondrocytes from the potentially damaging biomechanical forces, it is the job of chondrocytes to sustain a homeostasis of ECM metabolism by sensing changes in matrix composition and then responding by degrading or synthesizing appropriate types and amounts of macromolecules. With age, the capacity of chondrocytes to synthesize certain proteoglycans, their proliferative capacity, and their response to anabolic stimuli including growth factors decrease [109]. As a result, the ability of chondrocytes to maintain and restore articular cartilage decreases, resulting in an increase in the risk of development and progression of articular cartilage degradation.

It is well established that the risk of developing OA increases dramatically with age; however, age is not the sole determinant of developing the disease [2, 5]. Genetic, environmental, metabolic, and biochemical factors or a combination of the above may lead to more severe outcomes [5]. Furthermore, inactivity of the joint may lead to accelerated cartilage degradation [110]. The progressive loss of articular cartilage is accompanied by alterations of the underlying subchondral bone, which include bone remodelling, sclerosis, and in many cases the presence of subchondral bone cysts and osteophytes [111]. The concomitant, albeit moderate inflammation observed in the synovial tissue introduces a clinical impact of synovitis to the initiation and/or progression of OA [112]. It is this inflammatory response that puts the '-itis' in osteoarthritis, previously known as osteoarthrosis [113]. Together, these structural changes combine forces to result in the symptoms: joint pain, restriction of motion, crepitus with motion, joint effusions, and deformity – as experienced by the affected individual [114].

The pathophysiological process of OA can be divided into three overlapping stages [115, 116]:

1. ECM network damage/alteration at a molecular level
2. Chondrocyte response to tissue damage
3. Failure to restore cartilage and progressive loss of tissue due to a decline of chondrocyte synthetic response

The early changes in joint degeneration are seen microscopically as localized fibrillation or disruption of the articular cartilage superficial zone [117, 118]. As the degeneration continues, the roughened and irregular articular surface forms clefts, and the fibrillation extends deeper throughout the cartilage zones until the fissures reach subchondral bone [119]. The superficial tips of the fibrillated cartilage eventually tear, decreasing the cartilage thickness and releasing free fragments into the joint space. When the products of cartilage breakdown come in contact with the synovium, synovial cells are activated and produce catabolic and pro-inflammatory mediators that can activate chondrocytes to produce MMPs, which result in further cartilage breakdown and an unforgiving vicious cycle ensues [120, 121].

Once cartilage degradation has initiated, synovial cells phagocytose the breakdown products released into the synovial fluid resulting in hypertrophy and hyperplasia of synoviocytes, accompanied by inflammatory cell infiltration of the tissue by mononuclear cells such as lymphocytes and macrophages [122]. On account of its association with an increased degree of inflammatory cell infiltration of the synovial tissue, an increased concentration of systemic high-sensitivity C-reactive protein (hsCRP) can be used as a predictor of rapid disease progression in early knee OA. hsCRP levels are also associated with level of pain, clinical severity, and disability [123–126]. Another molecule that shows distinct alterations in the initial stages of OA is cartilage oligomeric matrix protein (COMP) [127, 128]. In normal adult cartilage, COMP is primarily found some distance from articular cartilage chondrocytes, i.e. the interterritorial region. This protein plays a role in early stages of fibril formation to promote fibrillogenesis of collagens I and II, as well as cross bridging of the matrix collagen fibre network [129, 130]. However, during early OA, there is a characteristic change in the distribution pattern. A severe loss of COMP is observed from the interterritorial matrix through degradation accompanied by a new accumulation of the protein close to the cells, as a result of new synthesis [131]. Hence, altered distribution of COMP provides a distinct and characteristic hallmark of impaired cartilage during the early osteoarthritic process.

The involvement of the synovium in early OA can be seen histologically by changes that occur in the osteoarthritic synovial membrane in areas adjacent to sites of chondropathy [122]. However, the underlying molecular mechanisms during early OA are almost impossible to examine, since the disease is usually not diagnosed until the pronounced alterations lead to pain and radiographically detectable changes. For this reason, animal models of OA have been developed to help us examine the underlying biochemical and molecular processes leading to the histologically visible alterations [132–134].

ECM fragments, such as fibronectin and collagen type II fragments, may activate the innate immune response via pattern recognition receptors, which include membrane-associated Toll- like receptors (TLRs) [135, 136]. This is the first level of nonspecific immune system activation. TLRs are typically activated by microbial ligands during an infection, activating the immune system to elicit an appropriate response [136]. However, they can also be activated by pathogen-associated molecular patterns (PAMPs) and endogenous damage-associated molecular patterns (DAMPs) occurring during cellular stress and ECM damage [137]. Therefore, this innate immune response has been regarded as a predominant feature in various noninfectious diseases where tissue injury and/or defective repair takes place. In this context, the disruption of matrix homeostasis that occurs in an osteoarthritic joint mirrors a chronic injury. There are ten functional mammalian TLR homologues (TLR-1 to TLR-10). Some are constitutively expressed by many cells including macrophages and can be induced or up-regulated on other cell types [136]. Previous studies have shown that there is up-regulated expression of TLR-2 and TLR-4 in articular chondrocytes of OA lesional cartilage compared to non-OA and nonlesional cartilage [138]. Furthermore, TLR-2 and TLR-4 ligands such as small-molecular-weight species of HA [139–141], fibronectin isoforms [142], tenascin C [143, 144], and biglycan [24, 145, 146] were found in high concentration in OA synovial fluid. TLR-2 and TLR-4 signals then mediate catabolic responses by increasing MMP-3 and MMP-13 production, which result in cartilage degradation and the release of matrix components, which again activate TLRs to elicit further catabolic responses and hence, a self-perpetuating loop of cell activation [146, 147]. In the synovial membrane, TLR activation stimulates NF-κB activation and the subsequent production of chemokines (e.g. IL-8) and cytokines (e.g. IL-1β, IL-6, and TNF-α), which activate and promote cellular infiltration of macrophages, granulocytes, and lymphocytes [148]. As a result, the tightly regulated anabolic and catabolic processes responsible for the maintenance of cartilage homeostasis are disturbed due to the stimulation of inflammatory mechanisms and the release of cytokines. Therefore, TLR activation has been shown to have serious implications in promoting synovitis in OA [112].

In addition to the appearance of cartilage fibrillation microscopically, the matrix macromolecular framework is destabilized at the molecular and macromolecular level. Proteolytic degradation of proteoglycans, most pronounced in the superficial region, during early OA decreases the chain length of the proteoglycan, thus inhibiting the formation of macromolecular complexes and decreasing proteoglycan aggregation [149]. The breakdown of proteoglycan architecture, along with an increase in water content, leads to a more permeable matrix and reduces the compressive stiffness of the tissue [150, 151]. Taken together, these alterations may increase the vulnerability of the tissue to further mechanical damage.

Alterations of the subchondral bone accompany the degeneration of articular cartilage; however, whether these changes are a driving force or a consequence of articular cartilage breakdown still remains unclear [152, 153]. At early stages of OA, there is elevated bone remodelling, particularly in the areas underlying the regions of articular cartilage damage. Bone loss is also observed, notably in the subchondral bone plate resulting in reduced thickness of the subchondral bone plate and increased porosity [69, 154]. Further down in the subchondral trabecular bone, increased trabecular separation and deterioration and decreased bone volume fraction and trabecular thickness are detected in animal models of OA [68]. These subchondral bone changes cause alterations in joint shape and load transmission that may propagate further cartilage loss. Microdamage of calcified cartilage and subchondral bone is widely detected in osteoarthritic joints in the form of short interstitial cracks or microcracks [155]. Microcracks act as an initiator of the bone remodelling process, as well as provide a means of communication of catabolic agents across the osteochondral junction, i.e. between cartilage and subchondral bone [65, 68].

Depending on the type and location of joint affected, the growth of osteophytes is observed as another alteration that changes the structure of the subchondral bone during OA. These fibrous, cartilaginous, and bony protrusions may be marginal, capsular, or central with characteristic patterns of formation. Intraosseous lesions, termed subchondral bone cysts (SBCs), are also reported in patients with OA [156]. SBCs are composed of fibroconnective tissue that initially contain fluid but ossify with time; they present as well-defined lucent areas with sclerotic rims on radiographic images. The presence of osteophytes and SBCs can restrict motion and contribute to pain with joint movement [156].

As ECM degeneration continues and the chondrocytes' biomechanical environment is altered, mediators are released that stimulate the chondrocytes to elicit a cellular repair response. This response consists of a boost of anabolic and proliferative activity, primarily in the upper cartilage zones, in an attempt to restore the homeostatic matrix environment [149]. Suggestive of a tissue repair response, type II collagen deposition increases in the deeper cartilage zones [157]. The mechanism of chondrocyte stimulation is unclear; however, it may be that the chondrocytes in these areas have better access to the anabolic and mitogenic growth factors from the synovial fluid due to fissuring or loosening of the macromolecular framework [158]. Anabolic cytokines such as TGF-β, IGF-I, fibroblast growth factors (FGF-2, FGF-4, and FGF-8), and bone morphogenetic proteins (BMPs) have an important role in stimulating the synthesis of ECM macromolecules (e.g. type II, VI, IX, XI collagen) [38, 159–161]. In addition, an increased expression of type I collagen, a main component of fibrous cartilage, is seen, which modifies the composition of the ECM and accordingly its properties [157]. Unlike normal chondrocytes, OA chondrocytes have up-regulated proliferative activity in response to cartilage damage [162]. In fact, the presence of clones of proliferating cells, or clusters, surrounding newly synthesized matrix molecules is one of the characteristic hallmarks of the chondrocytic repair response to cartilage degeneration [14].

Chondrocytes in such clusters have been shown to produce alkaline phosphatase, annexin II, annexin V, and type X collagen [163]. These molecules are normally expressed in hypertrophic and mineralizing growth plate cartilage, suggesting that the osteoarthritic chondrocytes are undergoing terminal differentiation [164, 165]. Particularly, they express transcription factors Sox9 and Runx2, which play a role in differentiation and hypertrophy, respectively. Sox9 controls the differentiation of mesenchymal stem cells (MSCs) into chondrocytes, whereas hypertrophic differentiation of chondrocytes depends on the expression of Runx2 and the inhibition of Sox9 expression [166–169]. Hence, during OA, chondrocytes are believed to re-establish the process of endochondral ossification, a physiological process during embryonic development whereby cartilage is replaced by bone to form long bones [170]. The hypertrophic chondrocytes produce type X collagen (typically found in the calcified cartilage zone and the hypertrophic zone of growth plate), which is involved in cartilage mineralization [171, 172]. Thus, mineralization followed by chondrocyte replacement with bone tissue and ossification takes place. As a result, subchondral bone architecture is altered and cartilage thickness is decreased. Thinning of the cartilage adds insult to injury since it is now even more prone to damage. This process could explain the duplication and advancement of the tidemark, which is reflective of progressive calcification of the cartilage [173, 174]. Furthermore, an increased expression of vascular endothelial growth factor (VEGF) is associated with an increase in cartilage damage. This may contribute to the characteristically higher vasculature within the subchondral bone. The vascular channels containing blood vessels, sensory nerves, osteoblasts, and osteoclasts reach the non-calcified cartilage and enable molecular interactions between cartilage and bone leading to cartilage degradation [164, 175–177]. Hence, subchondral bone plate vascularity is associated with the severity of OA cartilage damage, as well as pain [178].

Characteristic microarchitectural subchondral bone changes can be detected in the late stage of OA. Thickening of the subchondral bone plate is observed, as well as increased trabecular thickness, decreased trabecular separation and bone marrow spacing, and transformation of the trabeculae from rod-like to platelike [65, 179]. By this stage, the subchondral bone is described as sclerotic. Subchondral sclerosis is considered a characterizing feature of progressive OA [65].

Moving on to the third stage of cartilage degeneration, the biosynthetic anabolic activity of the chondrocytes is unable to keep pace with the degradative catabolic activity and homeostasis is lost [180]. At this point, the chondrocytic repair response cannot reverse the damage made to the cartilage. With increasing age and progression of disease, catabolic mechanisms continue to degrade articular cartilage; however, there is a decline in the chondrocytic anabolic and proliferative response [109]. An increase in type II collagen synthesis is insufficient to compensate its proteolysis. Furthermore, this increase in anabolic activity tends to occur in areas distinct from those of proteolysis [180]. Expression levels of inhibitors such as tissue inhibitor of metalloproteinases (TIMP)-1 are reduced and chondrocytes tend to exhibit an age-related decline in their response to anabolic cytokines, which shifts cartilage tissue homeostasis toward tissue destruction and eventual cell death [109]. Reduced cellularity, whether by apoptosis, autophagy-associated cell death, or senescence, correlates strongly with age and severity of OA [181].

Cell Death

It is difficult to establish the exact cause of cell death in OA due to the fact that primary OA seemingly develops over many years, with cells dying with advancing age and progressiveness of disease [182, 183]. As you may know by now, chondrocytes are responsible for mediating cartilage homeostasis. As degeneration continues, changes in the chondrocyte biomechanical environment alter the physical and biochemical signals that regulate cell response propagating cell death and tissue degeneration [184]. Cell death in the form of apoptosis is highly controlled and distinct from pathologic cell death or necrosis, which occurs as a result of cellular damage, hypoxia, or exposure to toxins [185]. Apoptosis can be initiated by intrinsic signals (e.g. mitochondria dependent) or extrinsic signals through cell surface death receptors followed by the sequential activation of a proteolytic cascade of enzymes called caspases [183, 186–188]. Effector caspases (e.g. caspases 1, 3, 6, and 7) then cleave target proteins such as poly adenosine diphosphate ribose polymerase (important for DNA repair), I-CAD (inhibitor of caspase-activated DNAse), and cytoskeletal proteins [189]. As a result, the apoptotic cell displays the characteristic morphological features including chromatin condensation, membrane blebbing, and the formation of rigid apoptotic bodies, which prevent leakage of intracellular contents into the local microenvironment [190].

Extracellular death ligands, Fas ligand (FasL/CD95L) and TNF-α, initiate extrinsic pathways through their respective cell surface death receptors, Fas and TNF-α receptor [187]. Fas (CD95) is expressed on the cell surface of cultured chondrocytes from normal and OA donors [191]. When activated by agonistic antibody, it leads to apoptotic cell death in cultured chondrocytes. However, in tissue where chondrocytes reside in their ECM, antibody to Fas fails to induce cell death. This may be due to the barrier created by the ECM that prevents antibody interaction with the chondrocytes. Moreover, chondrocytes in the ECM may be protected from Fas-dependent apoptosis through survival signals generated by the interaction of cell membrane receptors (e.g. integrins) with their respective ECM ligands (e.g. laminin, fibronectin, and collagen types II and IV) [192]. However, in the case of OA, a loosened, if not degraded, ECM may expose Fas receptors and activate the Fas/FasL system to induce apoptosis [182, 193]. Due to the lack of macrophages in cartilage tissue, apoptotic bodies cannot be phagocytosed [194]. Additionally, chondrocytes do not make cell-cell contacts; therefore, neighbouring cells are unable to phagocytose apoptotic bodies either. As a result, apoptotic bodies in cartilage tend to release their contents, which include proteases, into the ECM causing serious damage [195].

The cytotoxic free radical nitric oxide (NO) mediates apoptosis through a mitochondria-dependent mechanism [196]. NO is present in normal and young cartilage, but it is produced in higher levels by the synovium and cartilage during OA [197]. Studies have shown that enhanced NO and reactive oxygen species (ROS) expression in OA chondrocytes is induced by up-regulated pro-inflammatory cytokine production (i.e. IL-1β and TNF-α) in osteoarthritic cartilage [198, 199]. These cytokines, through the production of NO, have been demonstrated to cause mitochondrial dysfunction by inducing mitochondrial DNA (mtDNA) damage, decreasing energy production, and decreasing mitochondrial transcription [188]. The mitochondria is a prime target for oxidative damage, since it is the predominant site for intracellular ROS production [200]. ROS production in the chondrocyte not only damages mitochondrial lipids, proteins, and nucleic acids but also leads to mitochondrial permeability transition (MPT) [188]. A combination of these events results in the mitochondrial pathway of apoptosis. Since chondrocytes are the only source of ECM component synthesis in articular cartilage, and there is no renewal of chondrocyte population, apoptotic cell death has been demonstrated to play a major role in the degeneration of osteoarthritic cartilage. In contrast, it has also been shown that apoptosis occurs at a very low rate in osteoarthritic cartilage [201]. According to this study, the low population of apoptotic cells has a lesser impact than previously described on the pathology of OA. The highest numbers of apoptotic chondrocytes as evidenced by empty lacunae were located in the calcified cartilage layer [202]. The greatly reduced number of living chondrocytes in this cartilage zone may have significance in the later stages of OA, when this zone becomes considerably larger and represents a higher proportion of the articular cartilage [160]. Since apoptotic cells are not efficiently removed from the cartilage, the products of cell death such as pyrophosphate and precipitated calcium may contribute to cartilage degradation.

Autophagy

In order for articular cartilage to function normally, it is important for the joint tissue to maintain its structure, which is governed by the presence of an appropriate number of cells with normal biosynthetic function. Post-mitotic tissue such as cartilage has a very minimal rate of cell replication, and cellular constituents cannot be continuously renewed [203]. Instead, cells such as chondrocytes depend on autophagy as a principal mechanism to remove damaged and dysfunctional organelles and macromolecules [204].

Autophagy is a lysosomal degradation pathway that is essential for survival, differentiation, development, and, of particular importance, homeostasis [205]. Inducers of autophagy include nutrient and energy deprivation, ROS, or hypoxia [204]. In response to a particular cue, an isolation membrane is formed around the contents to be degraded, which combines with a lysosome to form an autophagosome, the characteristic hallmark of autophagy [205]. The autophagy machinery is orchestrated by the Atg genes, first identified in yeast, with corresponding homologues identified in higher eukaryotes. Among the Atg genes, Atg1, Atg6, Atg8 (ULK1, Beclin 1, and LC3 in mammals, respectively), and Atg5 are four major regulators of the autophagy pathway [206]. ULK1 is a serine/threonine kinase that functions as an intermediate in the transduction of proautophagic signals to autophagosome formation [207]. Beclin 1 forms a complex with type II phosphatidylinositol 3-kinase (PI3K) and Vps34 allowing nucleation of the autophagic vesicle [208]. LC3 is present in two forms: LC3-I is located in the cytoplasm, while LC3-II is bound to the autophagosome membrane. During autophagy, LC3-I undergoes lipidation to be converted to LC3-II, resulting in the association of LC3-II with autophagy vesicles [209]. The enclosed contents are degraded when the autophagosome fuses with the lysosome and the constituents are released and reused.

Autophagy is constitutively active and maintains homeostatic functions in articular cartilage. It does so by removing aggregate-prone or misfolded proteins and dysfunctional organelles, including mitochondria, peroxisomes, and ribosomes [204]. As mentioned previously, the up-regulated expression of proinflammatory cytokines in osteoarthritic tissue results in mitochondrial dysfunction and excessive ROS production [186]. By preventing the accumulation of defective mitochondria, autophagy protects the tissue from a loss of homeostasis and cartilage damage and dysfunction [204].

The correlation between the loss of autophagy and ageing has been well established and believed to be mainly related to the failure of lysosomal hydrolases, resulting in an increase of toxic protein products and slow clearance of autophagosomes in the ageing tissues [210]. ULK1, Beclin 1, and LC3 have been shown to be expressed in normal human articular cartilage, suggesting activation of autophagy [211]. Moreover, the presence of LC3-II is a direct indication of autophagosome formation. However, the expression of these autophagy markers is significantly decreased in OA cartilage and chondrocytes [211]. Defective or reduced autophagy is apparent from the reduction of LC3-II expression. These observations are consistent in the context of ageing-related OA. Just the same, a reduction of and loss of expression of autophagy markers and, hence, a decrease of autophagy activity have also been reported in surgically induced mouse OA models, as well as OA following exposure to mechanical injury in porcine cartilage [211]. Furthermore, a reduction of these key regulators of autophagy is accompanied by increased cell death due to apoptosis [212, 213]. These observations underline the importance of autophagy in physiological and pathological (e.g. osteoarthritic) events and demonstrate that autophagy is not solely associated with ageing-related mechanisms.

Chondrocyte Senescence

Cellular senescence typically refers to the loss of the ability of mitotic cells to further divide in culture after reaching 30–40 population doublings, also known as the 'Hayflick limit' [214]. This form of replicative senescence, resulting from arrest in cell cycle progression, has been established as a protective mechanism to avoid tumour formation by preventing cells with damaged DNA from being replicated [215]. In actively dividing cells, telomeres, which are found at the ends of chromosomes are incompletely replicated during mitosis and shorten with each round of cell division [216–218]. This 'end-replication problem' is not encountered in post-mitotic or quiescent cells such as neurons or chondrocytes [219]. It is much more likely that chondrocyte senescence is a result of extrinsic factors giving rise to 'stress-induced senescence'. Stress-induced senescence can occur from various stimuli including ultraviolet radiation, oxidative damage, activated oncogenes, and chronic inflammation. Oxidative damage can, in fact, result in telomere shortening similar to that seen with replicative senescence, since chromosome ends are particularly sensitive to oxidative damage [216, 220–222].

There is increasing evidence supporting the role that chondrocyte senescence plays in the initiation and progression of OA [222–226]. The lack of cell division and cellular turnover in normal adult articular cartilage means that the chondrocytes present in the cartilage of an older individual are decades old [219]. The long lifetime of chondrocytes allows them to accumulate the detrimental changes due to both ageing and extrinsic stress, and it is an accumulation of these dysfunctional senescent cells that contributes to loss of homeostasis and tissue damage.

An altered expression of regulatory proteins that function to control growth and proliferation is exhibited in senescent cells. These include p53 and the cyclin-dependent kinase inhibitors $p21^{CIP1}$ and $p16^{INK4A}$ [215]. These regulatory proteins are involved in two pathways, p53/p21 and $p16^{INK4A}$/retinoblastoma (Rb), that are essential for induction of senescence in response to external stimuli. DNA damage or telomere shortening activates p53, which inhibits cell-cycle progression. Activated p53 also contributes to senescence by increasing p21 expression. As p21 expression declines in senescent cells, p16 is increased leading to a more stable inhibition of cell-cycle progression by inhibiting Rb [215]. Besides increased p53 and p16 expression, altered chromatin structure can be used as a marker to signify a senescent cell. Altered chromatin structure in a senescent cell is presented as foci of heterochromatin or senescence-associated heterochromatin foci (SAHFs) [227].

Not only does senescence contribute to the pathology of OA by decreasing the number of functional chondrocytes, but also senescent chondrocytes have been shown to secrete factors that favour matrix degradation. Changes in gene expression that occur once a cell becomes senescent can lead to the increased production of cytokines (e.g. IL-1, IL-6, IL-8), MMPs, and growth factors (e.g. epidermal growth factor (EGF)) by the senescent cell [228–231]. Often referred to as the senescent secretory phenotype (SASP), this form of cellular senescence has significant implications in the development and progression of OA [219, 232].

As previously alluded to, with progression of disease, chondrocytes show a decline in the proliferative and anabolic response to growth factor stimulation [233]. Chondrocytes undergoing senescence exhibit an age-related loss in their mitogenic response to growth factors, such as TGF-β [234], basic fibroblast growth factor (bFGF), platelet-derived growth factor (PDGF), and IGF-I [235, 236]. In vitro studies have shown an age-related decline in the ability of IGF-I and bone morphogenic protein-6 (BMP-6) to stimulate proteoglycan and collagen production [237, 238]. IGF-I is an important autocrine survival factor in cartilage [239]. Studies have shown that excess levels of a reactive nitrogen species, NO, reduce chondrocyte response to IGF-I [240]. Not only is there a decline in responsiveness to these growth factors, but there is also evidence for an age-related reduction in the levels of certain growth factors in cartilage [241–243]. While it is not clear why chondrocytes at this stage of disease have reduced growth factor responsiveness, it is evident that the repair capacity of senescent chondrocytes is compromised and an imbalance in anabolic and catabolic pathways favours matrix degradation.

In recent years, stress-induced senescence due to oxidative stress has been shown to play a major role in the pathogenesis and development of OA [219, 244]. A cell experiences oxidative stress when the amount of ROS exceeds the cell's antioxidant capacity. This can be a result of increased ROS production or reduced availability of antioxidants, such as glutathione and superoxide dismutase [245, 246]. An increased production of ROS may contribute to mutation in mitochondrial DNA, thus propagating mitochondrial dysfunction. Altered mitochondrial functions such as ATP production, modulation of calcium levels, and the redox state of the mitochondria increase oxidative stress in chondrocytes, which drives the cell to a senescent state [247]. ROS have been shown to be generated by chondrocytes as by-products of aerobic metabolism, as well as in response to stimulation by pro-inflammatory cytokines and growth factors, such as IL-1, TNF-α, FGF, and TGF-β [248, 249]. While in vitro studies show evidence that chondrocyte senescence is associated with oxidative stress, further studies would help to better describe the mechanism of oxidative-stress-induced chondrocyte senescence.

Conclusion

OA is a chronic degenerative joint disease that has long been considered an age-related disease of cartilage degeneration. Undeniably, age is one of the strongest predictors of OA development; however, risk factors such as genetics, gender, metabolic status, obesity, and trauma all contribute to the probability of disease development. Furthermore, it has now been established that OA is a whole joint disease. Maintenance of cartilage ECM homeostasis is the main function of chondrocytes, providing structural support and a reservoir for cytokines and growth factors – critical for cell survival and maintenance of normal joint function. A dysregulation of ECM homeostasis results in the degradation of cartilage, as well as remodelling of the subchondral bone and synovial inflammation. Due to the close interactions between cartilage, bone, and synovium, alterations in one of these tissues do not seem to occur independently from the others. As cartilage degeneration continues, loss of ECM leads to the propagation of cell death and tissue degeneration. Matrix homeostasis relies on a balance between anabolic and catabolic activities, which are dependent on the number of viable chondrocytes. Hence, the contribution of cell death is an important factor in the progression and severity of disease. With increasing age, senescent chondrocytes are less able to maintain and repair articular cartilage tissue. In addition, the chondrocytes become less responsive to anabolic stimuli and show an age-related decline in response to anabolic cytokines and growth factors. Findings in animal models support the notion of the involvement of chondrocyte senescence with the progression of cartilage degeneration and advancement of disease.

Throughout the upcoming chapters of this book, the authors have attempted to provide a comprehensive and thorough understanding of distinct joints affected by OA including hip, knee, shoulder, elbow, spine, ankle, hand and wrist. This book also covers the current imaging practice in OA, joint conservation strategies, biomarkers, present and future drugs/agents for the treatment of OA as well as safety profile of current OA therapies. Finally, this book covers recent advances in regenerative and precision OA medicine.

References

1. Zhang Y, Jordan JM. Epidemiology of osteoarthritis. Clin Geriatr Med. 2010;26(3):355–69.
2. Loeser RF. Age-related changes in the musculoskeletal system and the development of osteoarthritis. Clin Geriatr Med. 2010;26(3):371–86.
3. Lawrence RC, et al. Estimates of the prevalence of arthritis and other rheumatic conditions in the United States. Part II. Arthritis Rheum. 2008;58(1):26–35.
4. Anderson JJ, Felson DT. Factors associated with osteoarthritis of the knee in the first national Health and Nutrition Examination Survey (HANES I). Evidence for an association with overweight, race, and physical demands of work. Am J Epidemiol. 1988;128(1):179–89.
5. Felson DT, et al. Osteoarthritis: new insights. Part 1: the disease and its risk factors. Ann Intern Med. 2000;133(8):635–46.
6. Srikanth VK, et al. A meta-analysis of sex differences prevalence, incidence and severity of osteoarthritis. Osteoarthritis Cartilage. 2005;13(9):769–81.
7. Spector TD, et al. Genetic influences on osteoarthritis in women: a twin study. BMJ. 1996;312(7036):940–3.
8. Palotie A, et al. Predisposition to familial osteoarthrosis linked to type II collagen gene. Lancet. 1989;1(8644):924–7.
9. Kerkhof HJ, et al. A genome-wide association study identifies an osteoarthritis susceptibility locus on chromosome 7q22. Arthritis Rheum. 2010;62(2):499–510.
10. Felson DT, et al. Weight loss reduces the risk for symptomatic knee osteoarthritis in women. The Framingham study. Ann Intern Med. 1992;116(7):535–9.
11. Christensen R, et al. Effect of weight reduction in obese patients diagnosed with knee osteoarthritis: a systematic review and meta-analysis. Ann Rheum Dis. 2007;66(4):433–9.
12. van Saase JL, et al. Osteoarthritis and obesity in the general population. A relationship calling for an explanation. J Rheumatol. 1988;15(7):1152–8.

13. Loughlin J, et al. Association of the interleukin-1 gene cluster on chromosome 2q13 with knee osteoarthritis. Arthritis Rheum. 2002;46(6):1519–27.
14. Buckwalter JA, Mankin HJ, Grodzinsky AJ. Articular cartilage and osteoarthritis. Instr Course Lect. 2005;54:465–80.
15. Brandt KD, et al. Yet more evidence that osteoarthritis is not a cartilage disease. Ann Rheum Dis. 2006;65(10):1261–4.
16. Buckwalter JA, Mankin HJ. Articular cartilage: tissue design and chondrocyte-matrix interactions. Instr Course Lect. 1998;47:477–86.
17. Poole AR, et al. Composition and structure of articular cartilage: a template for tissue repair. Clin Orthop Relat Res. 2001;391:S26–33.
18. Eyre D. Collagen of articular cartilage. Arthritis Res. 2002;4(1):30–5.
19. Sophia Fox AJ, Bedi A, Rodeo SA. The basic science of articular cartilage: structure, composition, and function. Sports Health Multidiscip Approach. 2009;1(6):461–8.
20. Roughley PJ, Lee ER. Cartilage proteoglycans: structure and potential functions. Microsc Res Tech. 1994;28(5):385–97.
21. Watanabe H, Yamada Y, Kimata K. Roles of aggrecan, a large chondroitin sulfate proteoglycan, in cartilage structure and function. J Biochem. 1998;124(4):687–93.
22. Hardingham TE, Fosang AJ, Dudhia J. The structure, function and turnover of aggrecan, the large aggregating proteoglycan from cartilage. Eur J Clin Chem Clin Biochem J Forum Eur Clin Chem Soc. 1994;32(4):249–57.
23. Knudson CB, Knudson W. Cartilage proteoglycans. Semin Cell Dev Biol. 2001;12(2): 69–78.
24. Poole AR, et al. Contents and distributions of the proteoglycans decorin and biglycan in normal and osteoarthritic human articular cartilage. J Orthop Res. 1996;14(5):681–9.
25. Hedlund H, et al. Fibromodulin distribution and association with collagen. Matrix Biol. 1994;14(3):227–32.
26. Clark JM. The organisation of collagen fibrils in the superficial zones of articular cartilage. J Anat. 1990;171:117–30.
27. REDLER I, et al. The ultrastructure and biomechanical significance of the tidemark of articular cartilage. Clin Orthop Relat Res. 1975;112:357–62.
28. Arkill KP, Winlove CP. Solute transport in the deep and calcified zones of articular cartilage. Osteoarthritis Cartilage. 2008;16(6):708–14.
29. Green Jr WT, et al. Microradiographic study of the calcified layer of articular cartilage. Arch Pathol. 1970;90(2):151–8.
30. Samuels J, Krasnokutsky S, Abramson SB. Osteoarthritis: a tale of three tissues. Bull NYU Hosp Jt Dis. 2008;66(3):244–50.
31. Hui AY, et al. A systems biology approach to synovial joint lubrication in health, injury, and disease. Wiley Interdiscip Rev Syst Biol Med. 2012;4(1):15–37.
32. Ateshian G, Mow V, Huiskes R. Friction, lubrication, and wear of articular cartilage and diarthrodial joints. Basic Orthop Biomech Mechanobiol. 2005;3:447–94.
33. Blewis M, et al. A model of synovial fluid lubricant composition in normal and injured joints. European Cells and Materials. 2007;13:26-39.
34. Jay GD, et al. The role of lubricin in the mechanical behavior of synovial fluid. Proc Natl Acad Sci U S A. 2007;104(15):6194–9.
35. Ogston A, Stanier J. The physiological function of hyaluronic acid in synovial fluid; viscous, elastic and lubricant properties. J Physiol. 1953;119(2–3):244–52.
36. Hascall VC, Kuettner KE (eds.). Publisher: Birkhäuser Basel. Schmid TM, et al. Superficial zone protein (SZP) is an abundant glycoprotein in human synovial fluid with lubricating properties. In: The many faces of osteoarthritis. 2002. p. 159–61.
37. Kapoor M, et al. Role of proinflammatory cytokines in the pathophysiology of osteoarthritis. Nat Rev Rheumatol. 2011;7(1):33–42.
38. Goldring MB. Osteoarthritis and cartilage: the role of cytokines. Curr Rheumatol Rep. 2000;2(6):459–65.

39. Blewis ME, et al. Interactive cytokine regulation of synoviocyte lubricant secretion. Tissue Eng Part A. 2010;16(4):1329–37.
40. Futani H, et al. Relation between interleukin-18 and PGE2 in synovial fluid of osteoarthritis: a potential therapeutic target of cartilage degradation. J Immunother. 2002;25 Suppl 1:S61–4.
41. Denko CW, Boja B, Moskowitz RW. Growth factors, insulin-like growth factor-1 and growth hormone, in synovial fluid and serum of patients with rheumatic disorders. Osteoarthritis Cartilage. 1996;4(4):245–9.
42. Goldring MB, Otero M. Inflammation in osteoarthritis. Curr Opin Rheumatol. 2011;23(5):471–8.
43. Poole AR. Cartilage in health and disease. In: Koopman W, editor. Arthritis and allied conditions. A textbook of rheumatology. Philadelphia: Lippincott Williams and Wilkins; 2001.
44. Nagase H, Woessner Jr JF. Matrix metalloproteinases. J Biol Chem. 1999;274(31):21491–4.
45. Konttinen YT, et al. Analysis of 16 different matrix metalloproteinases (MMP-1 to MMP-20) in the synovial membrane: different profiles in trauma and rheumatoid arthritis. Ann Rheum Dis. 1999;58(11):691–7.
46. Tchetverikov I, et al. MMP protein and activity levels in synovial fluid from patients with joint injury, inflammatory arthritis, and osteoarthritis. Ann Rheum Dis. 2005;64(5):694–8.
47. Ishiguro N, et al. Relationship of matrix metalloproteinases and their inhibitors to cartilage proteoglycan and collagen turnover: analyses of synovial fluid from patients with osteoarthritis. Arthritis Rheum. 1999;42(1):129–36.
48. Roos H, et al. Markers of cartilage matrix metabolism in human joint fluid and serum: the effect of exercise. Osteoarthritis Cartilage. 1995;3(1):7–14.
49. Knauper V, et al. Cellular activation of proMMP-13 by MT1-MMP depends on the C-terminal domain of MMP-13. FEBS Lett. 2002;532(1–2):127–30.
50. Zhang E, et al. Aggrecanases in the human synovial fluid at different stages of osteoarthritis. Clin Rheumatol. 2013;32(6):797–803.
51. Porter S, et al. The ADAMTS metalloproteinases. Biochem J. 2005;386(Pt 1):15–27.
52. Caterson B, et al. Mechanisms involved in cartilage proteoglycan catabolism. Matrix Biol. 2000;19(4):333–44.
53. Stanton H, et al. ADAMTS5 is the major aggrecanase in mouse cartilage in vivo and in vitro. Nature. 2005;434(7033):648–52.
54. Jones GC, Riley GP. ADAMTS proteinases: a multi-domain, multi-functional family with roles in extracellular matrix turnover and arthritis. Arthritis Res Ther. 2005;7(4):160–9.
55. Yoshihara Y, et al. Matrix metalloproteinases and tissue inhibitors of metalloproteinases in synovial fluids from patients with rheumatoid arthritis or osteoarthritis. Ann Rheum Dis. 2000;59(6):455–61.
56. Martel-Pelletier J, et al. Excess of metalloproteases over tissue inhibitor of metalloprotease may contribute to cartilage degradation in osteoarthritis and rheumatoid arthritis. Lab Invest. 1994;70(6):807–15.
57. Yehia SR, Duncan H. Synovial fluid analysis. Clin Orthop Relat Res. 1975;107:11–24.
58. Kratz A, et al. Appendix: laboratory values of clinical importance. In: Longo DL et al., editors. Harrison's principles of internal medicine. 18th ed. New York: The McGraw-Hill Companies; 2012.
59. Castor CW. The microscopic structure of normal human synovial tissue. Arthritis Rheum. 1960;3(2):140–51.
60. Barland P, Novikoff AB, Hamerman D. Electron microscopy of the human synovial membrane. J Cell Biol. 1962;14(2):207–20.
61. Ropes MW, Rossmeisl EC, Bauer W. The origin and nature of normal human synovial fluid. J Clin Invest. 1940;19(6):795.
62. Sabaratnam S, et al. Size selectivity of hyaluronan molecular sieving by extracellular matrix in rabbit synovial joints. J Physiol. 2005;567(Pt 2):569–81.
63. Kushner I, Somerville JA. Permeability of human synovial membrane to plasma proteins. Relationship to molecular size and inflammation. Arthritis Rheum. 1971;14(5):560–70.

64. Pejovic M, Stankovic A, Mitrovic DR. Determination of the apparent synovial permeability in the knee joint of patients suffering from osteoarthritis and rheumatoid arthritis. Br J Rheumatol. 1995;34(6):520–4.
65. Burr DB, Gallant MA. Bone remodelling in osteoarthritis. Nat Rev Rheumatol. 2012;8(11):665–73.
66. Henrotin Y, Pesesse L, Sanchez C. Subchondral bone and osteoarthritis: biological and cellular aspects. Osteoporos Int. 2012;23 Suppl 8:S847–51.
67. Madry H, van Dijk CN, Mueller-Gerbl M. The basic science of the subchondral bone. Knee Surg Sports Traumatol Arthrosc. 2010;18(4):419–33.
68. Li G, et al. Subchondral bone in osteoarthritis: insight into risk factors and microstructural changes. Arthritis Res Ther. 2013;15(6):223.
69. Goldring MB, Goldring SR. Articular cartilage and subchondral bone in the pathogenesis of osteoarthritis. Ann N Y Acad Sci. 2010;1192:230–7.
70. Clark J, Huber J. The structure of the human subchondral plate. J Bone Joint Surg,Br. 1990;72-B(5):866–73.
71. Holmdahl DE, Ingelmark BE. The contact between the articular cartilage and the medullary cavities of the bone. Acta Orthop Scand. 1950;20(2):156–65.
72. Inoue H. Alterations in the collagen framework of osteoarthritic cartilage and subchondral bone. Int Orthop. 1981;5(1):47–52.
73. Goldring SR. Alterations in periarticular bone and cross talk between subchondral bone and articular cartilage in osteoarthritis. Ther Adv Musculoskelet Dis. 2012;4(4):249–58.
74. Lanyon LE. Osteocytes, strain detection, bone modeling and remodeling. Calcif Tissue Int. 1993;53 Suppl 1:S102–6; discussion S106–7.
75. Martin RB. Targeted bone remodeling involves BMU steering as well as activation. Bone. 2007;40(6):1574–80.
76. Imhof H, et al. Importance of subchondral bone to articular cartilage in health and disease. Top Magn Reson Imaging. 1999;10(3):180–92.
77. Suri S, Walsh DA. Osteochondral alterations in osteoarthritis. Bone. 2012;51(2):204–11.
78. Issa S, Sharma L. Epidemiology of osteoarthritis: an update. Curr Rheumatol Rep. 2006;8(1):7–15.
79. Felson DT, et al. The incidence and natural history of knee osteoarthritis in the elderly. The Framingham Osteoarthritis study. Arthritis Rheum. 1995;38(10):1500–5.
80. Saddik D, McNally EG, Richardson M. MRI of Hoffa's fat pad. Skeletal Radiol. 2004;33(8):433–44.
81. Jacobson JA, et al. MR imaging of the infrapatellar fat pad of Hoffa. Radiographics. 1997;17(3):675–91.
82. Gallagher J, et al. The infrapatellar fat pad: anatomy and clinical correlations. Knee Surg Sports Traumatol Arthrosc. 2005;13(4):268–72.
83. Vahlensieck M, et al. Hoffa's recess: incidence, morphology and differential diagnosis of the globular-shaped cleft in the infrapatellar fat pad of the knee on MRI and cadaver dissections. Eur Radiol. 2002;12(1):90–3.
84. Clockaerts S, et al. The infrapatellar fat pad should be considered as an active osteoarthritic joint tissue: a narrative review. Osteoarthritis Cartilage. 2010;18(7):876–82.
85. Ioan-Facsinay A, Kloppenburg M. An emerging player in knee osteoarthritis: the infrapatellar fat pad. Arthritis Res Ther. 2013;15(6):225.
86. Smillie IS. Diseases of the knee joint. 2nd ed. Edinburgh/New York: Churchill Livingstone; 1980.
87. Fain JN. Release of interleukins and other inflammatory cytokines by human adipose tissue is enhanced in obesity and primarily due to the nonfat cells. Vitam Horm. 2006;74:443–77.
88. Ushiyama T, et al. Cytokine production in the infrapatellar fat pad: another source of cytokines in knee synovial fluids. Ann Rheum Dis. 2003;62(2):108–12.

89. Bohnsack M, et al. Distribution of substance-P nerves inside the infrapatellar fat pad and the adjacent synovial tissue: a neurohistological approach to anterior knee pain syndrome. Arch Orthop Trauma Surg. 2005;125(9):592–7.
90. Lehner B, et al. Preponderance of sensory versus sympathetic nerve fibers and increased cellularity in the infrapatellar fat pad in anterior knee pain patients after primary arthroplasty. J Orthop Res. 2008;26(3):342–50.
91. Klein-Wieringa IR, et al. The infrapatellar fat pad of patients with osteoarthritis has an inflammatory phenotype. Ann Rheum Dis. 2011;70(5):851–7.
92. Witonski D, et al. Increased interleukin 6 and tumour necrosis factor alpha expression in the infrapatellar fat pad of the knee joint with the anterior knee pain syndrome: a preliminary report. Pol J Pathol. 2010;61(4):213–8.
93. Clements KM, et al. Cellular and histopathological changes in the infrapatellar fat pad in the monoiodoacetate model of osteoarthritis pain. Osteoarthritis Cartilage. 2009;17(6):805–12.
94. Abbink JJ, et al. Predominant role of neutrophils in the inactivation of alpha 2-macroglobulin in arthritic joints. Arthritis Rheum. 1991;34(9):1139–50.
95. Tetlow LC, Woolley DE. Effect of histamine on the production of matrix metalloproteinases-1, −3, −8 and −13, and TNFalpha and PGE(2) by human articular chondrocytes and synovial fibroblasts in vitro: a comparative study. Virchows Arch. 2004;445(5):485–90.
96. Jedrzejczyk T, et al. The infrapatellar adipose body in humans of various age groups. Folia Morphol (Warsz). 1996;55(1):51–5.
97. Sakkas LI, Platsoucas CD. The role of T cells in the pathogenesis of osteoarthritis. Arthritis Rheum. 2007;56(2):409–24.
98. Dumond H, et al. Evidence for a key role of leptin in osteoarthritis. Arthritis Rheum. 2003;48(11):3118–29.
99. Lago R, et al. A new player in cartilage homeostasis: adiponectin induces nitric oxide synthase type II and pro-inflammatory cytokines in chondrocytes. Osteoarthritis Cartilage. 2008;16(9):1101–9.
100. Toussirot E, Streit G, Wendling D. The contribution of adipose tissue and adipokines to inflammation in joint diseases. Curr Med Chem. 2007;14(10):1095–100.
101. Iliopoulos D, Malizos KN, Tsezou A. Epigenetic regulation of leptin affects MMP-13 expression in osteoarthritic chondrocytes: possible molecular target for osteoarthritis therapeutic intervention. Ann Rheum Dis. 2007;66(12):1616–21.
102. Presle N, et al. Differential distribution of adipokines between serum and synovial fluid in patients with osteoarthritis. Contribution of joint tissues to their articular production. Osteoarthritis Cartilage. 2006;14(7):690–5.
103. Koskinen A, et al. Leptin enhances MMP-1, MMP-3 and MMP-13 production in human osteoarthritic cartilage and correlates with MMP-1 and MMP-3 in synovial fluid from OA patients. Clin Exp Rheumatol. 2011;29(1):57–64.
104. Matarese G, Leiter EH, La Cava A. Leptin in autoimmunity: many questions, some answers. Tissue Antigens. 2007;70(2):87–95.
105. Fasshauer M, Paschke R, Stumvoll M. Adiponectin, obesity, and cardiovascular disease. Biochimie. 2004;86(11):779–84.
106. Gomez R, et al. Adipokines in the skeleton: influence on cartilage function and joint degenerative diseases. J Mol Endocrinol. 2009;43(1):11–8.
107. Ehling A, et al. The potential of adiponectin in driving arthritis. J Immunol. 2006;176(7):4468–78.
108. Tang CH, et al. Adiponectin enhances IL-6 production in human synovial fibroblast via an AdipoR1 receptor, AMPK, p38, and NF-kappa B pathway. J Immunol. 2007;179(8):5483–92.
109. Lotz M, Loeser RF. Effects of aging on articular cartilage homeostasis. Bone. 2012;51(2):241–8.
110. Guilak F. Biomechanical factors in osteoarthritis. Best Pract Res Clin Rheumatol. 2011;25(6):815–23.
111. Sharma AR, et al. Interplay between cartilage and subchondral bone contributing to pathogenesis of osteoarthritis. Int J Mol Sci. 2013;14(10):19805–30.

112. Scanzello CR, Goldring SR. The role of synovitis in osteoarthritis pathogenesis. Bone. 2012;51(2):249–57.
113. Berenbaum F. Osteoarthritis as an inflammatory disease (osteoarthritis is not osteoarthrosis!). Osteoarthritis Cartilage. 2013;21(1):16–21.
114. Kean WF, Kean R, Buchanan WW. Osteoarthritis: symptoms, signs and source of pain. Inflammopharmacology. 2004;12(1):3–31.
115. Bertrand J, et al. Molecular mechanisms of cartilage remodelling in osteoarthritis. Int J Biochem Cell Biol. 2010;42(10):1594–601.
116. García-Carvajal ZY, et al. Cartilage tissue engineering: the role of extracellular matrix (ECM) and novel strategies. 2013. Regenerative Medicine and Tissue Engineering, Prof. Jose A. Andrades (Ed.), ISBN: 978-953-51-1108-5, InTech, DOI: 10.5772/55917.
117. Bank RA, et al. A simplified measurement of degraded collagen in tissues: application in healthy, fibrillated and osteoarthritic cartilage. Matrix Biol. 1997;16(5):233–43.
118. Dodge GR, Poole AR. Immunohistochemical detection and immunochemical analysis of type II collagen degradation in human normal, rheumatoid, and osteoarthritic articular cartilages and in explants of bovine articular cartilage cultured with interleukin 1. J Clin Invest. 1989;83(2):647–61.
119. Aigner T, McKenna L. Molecular pathology and pathobiology of osteoarthritic cartilage. Cell Mol Life Sci. 2002;59(1):5–18.
120. Pearle AD, Warren RF, Rodeo SA. Basic science of articular cartilage and osteoarthritis. Clin Sports Med. 2005;24(1):1–12.
121. Ehrlich MG, et al. The role of proteases in the pathogenesis of osteoarthritis. J Rheumatol. 1987;14 Spec No:30–2.
122. Sellam J, Berenbaum F. The role of synovitis in pathophysiology and clinical symptoms of osteoarthritis. Nat Rev Rheumatol. 2010;6(11):625–35.
123. Pearle AD, et al. Elevated high-sensitivity C-reactive protein levels are associated with local inflammatory findings in patients with osteoarthritis. Osteoarthritis Cartilage. 2007;15(5): 516–23.
124. Sharif M, et al. Increased serum C reactive protein may reflect events that precede radiographic progression in osteoarthritis of the knee. Ann Rheum Dis. 2000;59(1):71–4.
125. Spector TD, et al. Low-level increases in serum C-reactive protein are present in early osteoarthritis of the knee and predict progressive disease. Arthritis Rheum. 1997;40(4):723–7.
126. Sturmer T, et al. Severity and extent of osteoarthritis and low grade systemic inflammation as assessed by high sensitivity C reactive protein. Ann Rheum Dis. 2004;63(2):200–5.
127. Jordan JM. Cartilage oligomeric matrix protein as a marker of osteoarthritis. J Rheumatol Suppl. 2004;70:45–9.
128. Lohmander LS, Saxne T, Heinegard DK. Release of cartilage oligomeric matrix protein (COMP) into joint fluid after knee injury and in osteoarthritis. Ann Rheum Dis. 1994;53(1):8–13.
129. Haleem-Smith H, et al. Cartilage oligomeric matrix protein enhances matrix assembly during chondrogenesis of human mesenchymal stem cells. J Cell Biochem. 2012;113(4):1245–52.
130. Halász K, et al. COMP acts as a catalyst in collagen fibrillogenesis. J Biol Chem. 2007;282(43):31166–73.
131. Zivanovic S, et al. Cartilage oligomeric matrix protein – inflammation biomarker in knee osteoarthritis. Bosn J Basic Med Sci. 2011;11(1):27–32.
132. Stolz M, et al. Early detection of aging cartilage and osteoarthritis in mice and patient samples using atomic force microscopy. Nat Nanotechnol. 2009;4(3):186–92.
133. Cohen-Solal M, Funck-Brentano T, Hay E. Animal models of osteoarthritis for the understanding of the bone contribution. Bonekey Rep. 2013;2:422.
134. Bendele AM. Animal models of osteoarthritis. J Musculoskelet Neuronal Interact. 2001;1(4):363–76.
135. Piccinini AM, Midwood KS. DAMPening inflammation by modulating TLR signalling. Mediators Inflamm. 2010;2010:672395.
136. Janeway CA, Medzhitov R. Innate immune recognition. Annu Rev Immunol. 2002;20:197.

137. Scanzello CR, Plaas A, Crow MK. Innate immune system activation in osteoarthritis: is osteoarthritis a chronic wound? Curr Opin Rheumatol. 2008;20(5):565.
138. Kim HA, et al. The catabolic pathway mediated by Toll-like receptors in human osteoarthritic chondrocytes. Arthritis Rheum. 2006;54(7):2152–63.
139. Belcher C, et al. Synovial fluid chondroitin and keratan sulphate epitopes, glycosaminoglycans, and hyaluronan in arthritic and normal knees. Ann Rheum Dis. 1997;56(5):299.
140. Scheibner KA, et al. Hyaluronan fragments act as an endogenous danger signal by engaging TLR2. J Immunol. 2006;177(2):1272.
141. Taylor KR, et al. Hyaluronan fragments stimulate endothelial recognition of injury through TLR4. J Biol Chem. 2004;279(17):17079.
142. Chevalier X, et al. Presence of ED-A containing fibronectin in human articular cartilage from patients with osteoarthritis and rheumatoid arthritis. J Rheumatol. 1996;23(6):1022–30.
143. Chevalier X, et al. Tenascin distribution in articular cartilage from normal subjects and from patients with osteoarthritis and rheumatoid arthritis. Arthritis Rheum. 1994;37(7):1013–22.
144. Midwood K, et al. Tenascin-C is an endogenous activator of Toll-like receptor 4 that is essential for maintaining inflammation in arthritic joint disease. Nat Med. 2009;15(7):774–80.
145. Cs-Szabo G, et al. Large and small proteoglycans of osteoarthritic and rheumatoid articular cartilage. Arthritis Rheum. 1995;38(5):660–8.
146. Schaefer L, et al. The matrix component biglycan is proinflammatory and signals through Toll-like receptors 4 and 2 in macrophages. J Clin Invest. 2005;115(8):2223–33.
147. Liu-Bryan R, Terkeltaub R. Chondrocyte innate immune myeloid differentiation factor 88-dependent signaling drives procatabolic effects of the endogenous Toll-like receptor 2/Toll-like receptor 4 ligands low molecular weight hyaluronan and high mobility group box chromosomal protein 1 in mice. Arthritis Rheum. 2010;62(7):2004–12.
148. Akira S. Toll-like receptor signaling. J Biol Chem. 2003;278(40):38105.
149. Buckwalter JA, Mankin HJ. Articular cartilage: degeneration and osteoarthritis, repair, regeneration, and transplantation. Instr Course Lect. 1998;47:487–504.
150. Mankin HJ, Thrasher AZ. Water content and binding in normal and osteoarthritic human cartilage. J Bone Joint Surg Am. 1975;57(1):76–80.
151. Stockwell RA. Cartilage failure in osteoarthritis: relevance of normal structure and function. A review. Clin Anat. 1991;4:161–91.
152. Radin EL, Rose RM. Role of subchondral bone in the initiation and progression of cartilage damage. Clin Orthop Relat Res. 1986;213:34.
153. Neogi T, et al. Cartilage loss occurs in the same subregions as subchondral bone attrition: a within-knee subregion-matched approach from the Multicenter Osteoarthritis study. Arthritis Rheum. 2009;61(11):1539–44.
154. Intema F, et al. In early OA, thinning of the subchondral plate is directly related to cartilage damage: results from a canine ACLT-meniscectomy model. Osteoarthritis Cartilage. 2010;18(5):691–8.
155. Burr DB, Radin EL. Microfractures and microcracks in subchondral bone: are they relevant to osteoarthrosis? Rheum Dis Clin North Am. 2003;29(4):675–85.
156. McErlain DD, et al. An in vivo investigation of the initiation and progression of subchondral cysts in a rodent model of secondary osteoarthritis. Arthritis Res Ther. 2012;14(1):R26.
157. Pfander D, Rahmanzadeh R, Scheller EE. Presence and distribution of collagen II, collagen I, fibronectin, and tenascin in rabbit normal and osteoarthritic cartilage. J Rheumatol. 1999;26(2):386–94.
158. Lee DA, Bentley G, Archer CW. The control of cell division in articular chondrocytes. Osteoarthritis Cartilage. 1993;1(2):137–46.
159. Goldring MB. The role of cytokines as inflammatory mediators in osteoarthritis: lessons from animal models. Connect Tissue Res. 1999;40(1):1–11.
160. Sandell LJ, Aigner T. Articular cartilage and changes in arthritis. An introduction: cell biology of osteoarthritis. Arthritis Res. 2001;3(2):107–13.
161. Fortier L, et al. The role of growth factors in cartilage repair. Clin Orthop Relat Res. 2011;469(10):2706–15.

162. Rothwell AG, Bentley G. Chondrocyte multiplication in osteoarthritic articular cartilage. J Bone Joint Surg Br. 1973;55(3):588–94.
163. Kirsch T, Swoboda B, Nah HD. Activation of annexin II and V expression, terminal differentiation, mineralization and apoptosis in human osteoarthritic cartilage. Osteoarthritis Cartilage. 2000;8(4):294–302.
164. Mahjoub M, Berenbaum F, Houard X. Why subchondral bone in osteoarthritis? The importance of the cartilage bone interface in osteoarthritis. Osteoporos Int. 2012;23 Suppl 8:S841–6.
165. Fuerst M, et al. Calcification of articular cartilage in human osteoarthritis. Arthritis Rheum. 2009;60(9):2694–703.
166. Hattori T, et al. SOX9 is a major negative regulator of cartilage vascularization, bone marrow formation and endochondral ossification. Development. 2010;137(6):901–11.
167. Lefebvre V, Behringer RR, de Crombrugghe B. L-Sox5, Sox6 and Sox9 control essential steps of the chondrocyte differentiation pathway. Osteoarthritis Cartilage. 2001;9 Suppl 1:S69–75.
168. Goldring MB, Tsuchimochi K, Ijiri K. The control of chondrogenesis. J Cell Biochem. 2006;97(1):33–44.
169. Kamekura S, et al. Contribution of runt-related transcription factor 2 to the pathogenesis of osteoarthritis in mice after induction of knee joint instability. Arthritis Rheum. 2006;54(8):2462–70.
170. Goldring SR. Role of bone in osteoarthritis pathogenesis. Med Clin North Am. 2009;93(1):25–35, xv.
171. von der Mark K, et al. Type X collagen synthesis in human osteoarthritic cartilage. Indication of chondrocyte hypertrophy. Arthritis Rheum. 1992;35(7):806–11.
172. Hoyland JA, et al. Distribution of type X collagen mRNA in normal and osteoarthritic human cartilage. Bone Miner. 1991;15(2):151–63.
173. Oegema Jr TR, et al. The interaction of the zone of calcified cartilage and subchondral bone in osteoarthritis. Microsc Res Tech. 1997;37(4):324–32.
174. Lane LB, Bullough PG. Age-related changes in the thickness of the calcified zone and the number of tidemarks in adult human articular cartilage. J Bone Joint Surg Br. 1980;62(3):372–5.
175. Walsh DA, et al. Angiogenesis in the synovium and at the osteochondral junction in osteoarthritis. Osteoarthritis Cartilage. 2007;15(7):743–51.
176. Cox LG, et al. Alterations to the subchondral bone architecture during osteoarthritis: bone adaptation vs endochondral bone formation. Osteoarthritis Cartilage. 2013;21(2):331–8.
177. Pfander D, et al. Vascular endothelial growth factor in articular cartilage of healthy and osteoarthritic human knee joints. Ann Rheum Dis. 2001;60(11):1070–3.
178. Walsh DA, et al. Angiogenesis and nerve growth factor at the osteochondral junction in rheumatoid arthritis and osteoarthritis. Rheumatology (Oxford). 2010;49(10):1852–61.
179. Karsdal MA, et al. Should subchondral bone turnover be targeted when treating osteoarthritis? Osteoarthritis Cartilage. 2008;16(6):638–46.
180. Lorenz H, Richter W. Osteoarthritis: cellular and molecular changes in degenerating cartilage. Prog Histochem Cytochem. 2006;40(3):135–63.
181. Grogan SP, D'Lima DD. Joint aging and chondrocyte cell death. Int J Clin Rheumtol. 2010;5(2):199–214.
182. Kuhn K, et al. Cell death in cartilage. Osteoarthritis Cartilage. 2004;12(1):1–16.
183. Kim HA, Blanco FJ. Cell death and apoptosis in osteoarthritic cartilage. Curr Drug Targets. 2007;8(2):333–45.
184. Temple MM, et al. Age- and site-associated biomechanical weakening of human articular cartilage of the femoral condyle. Osteoarthritis Cartilage. 2007;15(9):1042–52.
185. Blanco FJ, et al. Osteoarthritis chondrocytes die by apoptosis. A possible pathway for osteoarthritis pathology. Arthritis Rheum. 1998;41(2):284–9.
186. Taylor RC, Cullen SP, Martin SJ. Apoptosis: controlled demolition at the cellular level. Nat Rev Mol Cell Biol. 2008;9(3):231–41.

187. Wajant H. The Fas signaling pathway: more than a paradigm. Science. 2002;296(5573): 1635–6.
188. Kim J, et al. Mitochondrial DNA damage is involved in apoptosis caused by pro-inflammatory cytokines in human OA chondrocytes. Osteoarthritis Cartilage. 2010;18(3):424–32.
189. Thornberry NA, Lazebnik Y. Caspases: enemies within. Science. 1998;281(5381):1312–6.
190. Krysko DV, et al. Apoptosis and necrosis: detection, discrimination and phagocytosis. Methods. 2008;44(3):205–21.
191. Hashimoto S, et al. Fas/Fas ligand expression and induction of apoptosis in chondrocytes. Arthritis Rheum. 1997;40(10):1749–55.
192. Shakibaei M, Csaki C, Mobasheri A. Diverse roles of integrin receptors in articular cartilage. Adv Anat Embryol Cell Biol. 2008;197:1–60.
193. Thomas CM, et al. Chondrocyte death by apoptosis is associated with the initiation and severity of articular cartilage degradation. Int J Rheum Dis. 2011;14(2):191–8.
194. Hashimoto S, et al. Chondrocyte-derived apoptotic bodies and calcification of articular cartilage. Proc Natl Acad Sci U S A. 1998;95(6):3094–9.
195. Mobasheri A. Role of chondrocyte death and hypocellularity in ageing human articular cartilage and the pathogenesis of osteoarthritis. Med Hypotheses. 2002;58(3):193–7.
196. Wu GJ, et al. Nitric oxide from both exogenous and endogenous sources activates mitochondria-dependent events and induces insults to human chondrocytes. J Cell Biochem. 2007;101(6):1520–31.
197. Min BH, et al. Effects of ageing and arthritic disease on nitric oxide production by human articular chondrocytes. Exp Mol Med. 2001;33(4):299–302.
198. Lopez-Armada MJ, et al. Cytokines, tumor necrosis factor-alpha and interleukin-1beta, differentially regulate apoptosis in osteoarthritis cultured human chondrocytes. Osteoarthritis Cartilage. 2006;14(7):660–9.
199. Carames B, et al. Differential effects of tumor necrosis factor-alpha and interleukin-1beta on cell death in human articular chondrocytes. Osteoarthritis Cartilage. 2008;16(6):715–22.
200. Holmstrom KM, Finkel T. Cellular mechanisms and physiological consequences of redox-dependent signalling. Nat Rev Mol Cell Biol. 2014;15(6):411–21.
201. Aigner T, et al. Apoptotic cell death is not a widespread phenomenon in normal aging and osteoarthritis human articular knee cartilage: a study of proliferation, programmed cell death (apoptosis), and viability of chondrocytes in normal and osteoarthritic human knee cartilage. Arthritis Rheum. 2001;44(6):1304–12.
202. Meachim G, Collins DH. Cell counts of normal and osteo-arthritic articular cartilage in relation to the uptake of sulphate ((35)SO(4)) in vitro. Ann Rheum Dis. 1962;21(1):45–50.
203. Terman A, et al. Mitochondrial turnover and aging of long-lived postmitotic cells: the mitochondrial–lysosomal axis theory of aging. Antioxid Redox Signal. 2010;12(4):503–35.
204. Lotz MK, Carames B. Autophagy and cartilage homeostasis mechanisms in joint health, aging and OA. Nat Rev Rheumatol. 2011;7(10):579–87.
205. Mizushima N. Physiological functions of autophagy. Curr Top Microbiol Immunol. 2009;335:71–84.
206. He C, Klionsky DJ. Regulation mechanisms and signaling pathways of autophagy. Annu Rev Genet. 2009;43:67–93.
207. Hara T, et al. FIP200, a ULK-interacting protein, is required for autophagosome formation in mammalian cells. J Cell Biol. 2008;181(3):497–510.
208. Kang R, et al. The Beclin 1 network regulates autophagy and apoptosis. Cell Death Differ. 2011;18(4):571–80.
209. Tanida I, Ueno T, Kominami E. LC3 conjugation system in mammalian autophagy. Int J Biochem Cell Biol. 2004;36(12):2503–18.
210. Cuervo AM, Dice JF. Age-related decline in chaperone-mediated autophagy. J Biol Chem. 2000;275(40):31505–13.
211. Carames B, et al. Autophagy is a protective mechanism in normal cartilage, and its aging-related loss is linked with cell death and osteoarthritis. Arthritis Rheum. 2010;62(3): 791–801.

212. Marino G, et al. Self-consumption: the interplay of autophagy and apoptosis. Nat Rev Mol Cell Biol. 2014;15(2):81–94.
213. Almonte-Becerril M, et al. Cell death of chondrocytes is a combination between apoptosis and autophagy during the pathogenesis of Osteoarthritis within an experimental model. Apoptosis. 2010;15(5):631–8.
214. Hayflick L. Intracellular determinants of cell aging. Mech Ageing Dev. 1984;28(2–3):177–85.
215. Muller M. Cellular senescence: molecular mechanisms, in vivo significance, and redox considerations. Antioxid Redox Signal. 2009;11(1):59–98.
216. Goyns MH. Genes, telomeres and mammalian ageing. Mech Ageing Dev. 2002;123(7):791–9.
217. Lundblad V. Telomere end processing: unexpected complexity at the end game. Genes Dev. 2012;26(11):1123–7.
218. Watson JD. Origin of concatemeric T7 DNA. Nat New Biol. 1972;239(94):197–201.
219. Loeser RF. Aging and osteoarthritis: the role of chondrocyte senescence and aging changes in the cartilage matrix. Osteoarthritis Cartilage. 2009;17(8):971–9.
220. Itahana K, Campisi J, Dimri GP. Mechanisms of cellular senescence in human and mouse cells. Biogerontology. 2004;5(1):1–10.
221. Campisi J. Senescent cells, tumor suppression, and organismal aging: good citizens, bad neighbors. Cell. 2005;120(4):513–22.
222. Yudoh K, et al. Potential involvement of oxidative stress in cartilage senescence and development of osteoarthritis: oxidative stress induces chondrocyte telomere instability and downregulation of chondrocyte function. Arthritis Res Ther. 2005;7(2):R380–91.
223. Martin JA, Buckwalter JA. Telomere erosion and senescence in human articular cartilage chondrocytes. J Gerontol A Biol Sci Med Sci. 2001;56(4):B172–9.
224. Martin JA, Buckwalter JA. The role of chondrocyte senescence in the pathogenesis of osteoarthritis and in limiting cartilage repair. J Bone Joint Surg Am. 2003;85-A Suppl 2:106–10.
225. Price JS, et al. The role of chondrocyte senescence in osteoarthritis. Aging Cell. 2002;1(1):57–65.
226. Dai SM, et al. Catabolic stress induces features of chondrocyte senescence through overexpression of caveolin 1: possible involvement of caveolin 1-induced down-regulation of articular chondrocytes in the pathogenesis of osteoarthritis. Arthritis Rheum. 2006;54(3):818–31.
227. Zhang R, Adams PD. Heterochromatin and its relationship to cell senescence and cancer therapy. Cell Cycle. 2007;6(7):784–9.
228. Freund A, et al. Inflammatory networks during cellular senescence: causes and consequences. Trends Mol Med. 2010;16(5):238–46.
229. Campisi J, d'Adda di Fagagna F. Cellular senescence: when bad things happen to good cells. Nat Rev Mol Cell Biol. 2007;8(9):729–40.
230. Acosta JC, et al. A complex secretory program orchestrated by the inflammasome controls paracrine senescence. Nat Cell Biol. 2013;15(8):978–90.
231. Tchkonia T, et al. Cellular senescence and the senescent secretory phenotype: therapeutic opportunities. J Clin Invest. 2013;123(3):966–72.
232. Zhu Y, et al. Cellular senescence and the senescent secretory phenotype in age-related chronic diseases. Curr Opin Clin Nutr Metab Care. 2014;17(4):324–8.
233. Guerne P-A, et al. Growth factor responsiveness of human articular chondrocytes in aging and development. Arthritis Rheum. 1995;38(7):960–8.
234. Iqbal J, et al. Age-related effects of TGF-beta on proteoglycan synthesis in equine articular cartilage. Biochem Biophys Res Commun. 2000;274(2):467.
235. Martin JA, Ellerbroek SM, Buckwalter JA. Age-related decline in chondrocyte response to insulin-like growth factor-I: the role of growth factor binding proteins. J Orthop Res. 1997;15(4):491–8.
236. Loeser RF, et al. Reduction in the chondrocyte response to insulin-like growth factor 1 in aging and osteoarthritis: studies in a non-human primate model of naturally occurring disease. Arthritis Rheum. 2000;43(9):2110–20.

237. Bobacz K, et al. Expression of bone morphogenetic protein 6 in healthy and osteoarthritic human articular chondrocytes and stimulation of matrix synthesis in vitro. Arthritis Rheum. 2003;48(9):2501–8.
238. Tran-Khanh N, et al. Aged bovine chondrocytes display a diminished capacity to produce a collagen-rich, mechanically functional cartilage extracellular matrix. J Orthop Res. 2005;23(6):1354–62.
239. Loeser RF, Shanker G. Autocrine stimulation by insulin-like growth factor 1 and insulin-like growth factor 2 mediates chondrocyte survival in vitro. Arthritis Rheum. 2000;43(7):1552–9.
240. Studer RK, et al. Nitric oxide inhibits chondrocyte response to IGF-I: inhibition of IGF-IRbeta tyrosine phosphorylation. Am J Physiol Cell Physiol. 2000;279(4):C961–9.
241. Blaney Davidson EN, et al. Reduced transforming growth factor-beta signaling in cartilage of old mice: role in impaired repair capacity. Arthritis Res Ther. 2005;7(6):R1338–47.
242. Chubinskaya S, et al. Age-related changes in cartilage endogenous osteogenic protein-1 (OP-1). Biochim Biophys Acta. 2002;1588(2):126–34.
243. Loeser RF, et al. Methylation of the OP-1 promoter: potential role in the age-related decline in OP-1 expression in cartilage. Osteoarthritis Cartilage. 2009;17(4):513–7.
244. Carlo Jr MD, Loeser RF. Increased oxidative stress with aging reduces chondrocyte survival: correlation with intracellular glutathione levels. Arthritis Rheum. 2003;48(12):3419–30.
245. Finkel T, Holbrook NJ. Oxidants, oxidative stress and the biology of ageing. Nature. 2000;408(6809):239–47.
246. Jallali N, et al. Vulnerability to ROS-induced cell death in ageing articular cartilage: the role of antioxidant enzyme activity. Osteoarthritis Cartilage. 2005;13(7):614–22.
247. Grishko VI, et al. Diminished mitochondrial DNA integrity and repair capacity in OA chondrocytes. Osteoarthritis Cartilage. 2009;17(1):107–13.
248. Lo YY, Cruz TF. Involvement of reactive oxygen species in cytokine and growth factor induction of c-fos expression in chondrocytes. J Biol Chem. 1995;270(20):11727–30.
249. Jallali N, et al. Modulation of intracellular reactive oxygen species level in chondrocytes by IGF-1, FGF, and TGF-beta1. Connect Tissue Res. 2007;48(3):149–58.

Chapter 2
Hip and Knee Osteoarthritis

Ivan Dzaja and Khalid Syed

Key Points

- Osteoarthritis (OA) is the result of the loss of the ability of chondrocytes to maintain and restore articular cartilage.
- OA can be classified as primary (due to routine wear on the joint) or secondary (due to a specific etiology, i.e., posttraumatic, hemochromatosis, septic arthritis, etc.).
- Risk factors include modifiable (e.g., obesity, trauma, etc.) and nonmodifiable (e.g., age, gender, genetics, etc.) factors.
- OA leads to classic changes within the joint including loss of articular cartilage, joint space narrowing, subchondral sclerosis, formation of subchondral cysts, and osteophyte formation.
- Nonsurgical and nonpharmacologic treatment includes exercise, weight loss, and bracing.
- Pharmacologic treatment includes oral nonsteroidal anti-inflammatory medications and intra-articular injection of corticosteroids, hyaluronic acid, and plasma-rich protein.
- Surgical management includes arthroscopy, osteotomy, arthrodesis, and arthroplasty.

I. Dzaja, MD, FRCSC
Department of Surgery, University Health Network,
University of Toronto, Toronto, ON, Canada

K. Syed, MD, FRCSC (✉)
Department of Surgery, University Health Network,
University of Toronto, Toronto, ON, Canada

Toronto Western Hospital, University Health Network,
399 Bathurst St., 446, 1 East Wing, M5T 2S8 Toronto, ON, Canada
e-mail: khalid.syed@uhn.on.ca

M. Kapoor, N.N. Mahomed (eds.), *Osteoarthritis: Pathogenesis, Diagnosis, Available Treatments, Drug Safety, Regenerative and Precision Medicine*,
DOI 10.1007/978-3-319-19560-5_2

Introduction

OA is a debilitating disease that occurs most frequently in the hands, feet, knees, and spine but can develop in any synovial joint [1]. Although OA is most common in the hand, knee OA is most likely to lead to disability [1]. Incidence of symptomatic hand OA is at 100 per 100,000 compared to 240 per 100,000 for the knee [2]. About 95 % of total knee arthroplasties (TKA) and total hip arthroplasties (THA) are done for symptomatic OA. Currently, approximately 800,000 TKA and THA are performed in the USA annually, with the number expected to exceed 1.2 million by the year 2020 [3].

Clinical Evaluation

History

General symptoms associated with OA include joint pain, often worse in the morning, as well as stiffness and swelling. Advanced OA can also cause pain at rest and nighttime pain severe enough to wake the patient while sleeping. Pain is usually described as deep, aching, and poorly localized. Radiation of pain can also occur and should be considered while examining the patient.

Hip

Hip OA is usually associated with pain located in the groin; radiation of pain should be considered with hip OA. These patients may report knee pain rather than hip pain resulting from a branch of the obturator nerve. A patient may hold the hip with one hand, the so-called C-sign that is commonly seen in patients with hip pathology. Pain laterally or posteriorly over the buttock is unlikely from an intra-articular cause, and the history should be evaluated further. Differential diagnosis for articular causes of groin pain includes OA, osteonecrosis, hip dysplasia, FAI, infection, or femoral neck fractures.

Knee

The location of pain should be noted during patient history. Anterior knee pain that is exacerbated with squatting or stair climbing may indicate patellofemoral involvement. Pain at the joint line associated with mechanical symptoms may indicate meniscal pathology. Again, it is important to remember that referred pain from both the lumbar spine and ipsilateral hip may present as knee pain.

Physical Exam

A general screening musculoskeletal exam should be performed to assess for other potential pathologies. Moving on to the affected extremity, a detailed and thorough neurovascular examination should be completed and documented. Patients with OA often have altered gain secondary to both pain and deformity. Atrophy of muscles crossing the affected joint is often present in chronic disease.

Hip

Evaluation of gait is an important aspect of the hip exam. Gait can be antalgic, related to a leg-length difference or muscle weakness (Trendelenburg gait). Foot progression angle should also be noted. A detailed lumbar spine exam should be performed in addition to a distal neurovascular exam. The hip should be inspected looking for any previous scars, atrophy, or deformity. Palpation of lateral-based pain can help distinguish non-arthritic sources of pain such as greater trochanteric bursitis. Active and passive range of motion (ROM) should be assessed. It is important to stabilize the pelvis when examining the hip. ROM will usually reproduce pain in the arthritic hip, specifically flexion with internal rotation. Flexion contracture of the hip can be assessed with the Thomas test. Here, the patient lies supine on the exam table and brings one knee toward their chest while keeping the contralateral leg extended. The test is positive if the contralateral leg flexes, which is due to a tight iliopsoas.

Knee

Gait should also be examined, with specific attention to alignment and instability during gait analysis. Hip exam should be performed, as hip ROM can occasionally reproduce the knee pain. Inspection should be performed noting for any effusion, scars, deformity, and overall alignment. Ligaments should be examined assessing for any instability. Ability to correct the deformity should also be noted. The knee should then be palpated, attempting to localize areas of tenderness. ROM of the knee should be assessed, noting for flexion deformities and patellar tracking.

Imaging

Weight-bearing radiographs are effective at confirming the diagnosis of OA and also for assessment of deformity and potential operative planning. Radiographic changes associated with an arthritic joint include narrowing of the joint space, increased sclerosis or density of the subchondral bone, osteophyte formation, subchondral cyst (geode) formation, loose bodies, joint subluxation, deformity, and malalignment.

Absence of positive radiographic findings in a patient with symptoms of OA should not be interpreted as absence of disease, as the radiographs are not sensitive early in the disease process. There may also be a poor association between radiographic changes and functioning in patients with OA [4].

Hip

Standard radiographs for hip pathology should include an AP pelvis and a lateral of the affected hip joint. Hip OA is often associated with superolateral narrowing, which can then progress to global narrowing of the hip joint. Figure 2.1 demonstrates typical findings with hip OA including joint space narrowing (JSN), sclerosis, and osteophyte formation. Patients with an underlying coxa profunda may develop a more medial pattern of OA with preservation of the superior and lateral joint space. The Tönnis Classification has been established to characterize and describe radiographic findings associated with hip OA. Classification is as follows: 0, no signs of osteoarthritis; 1, mild (increased sclerosis, slight JSN, no or slight loss of head sphericity); 2, moderate (small cysts, moderate JSN, moderate loss of head sphericity); and 3, severe (large cysts, severe narrowing or obliteration of the joint space, severe deformity of the head).

Knee

Standard radiographs for knee pathology should include standing AP, lateral, merchant, and tunnel views. Figure 2.2 demonstrates some findings associated with knee OA including medial JSN. The same patient had an MRI, demonstrated in

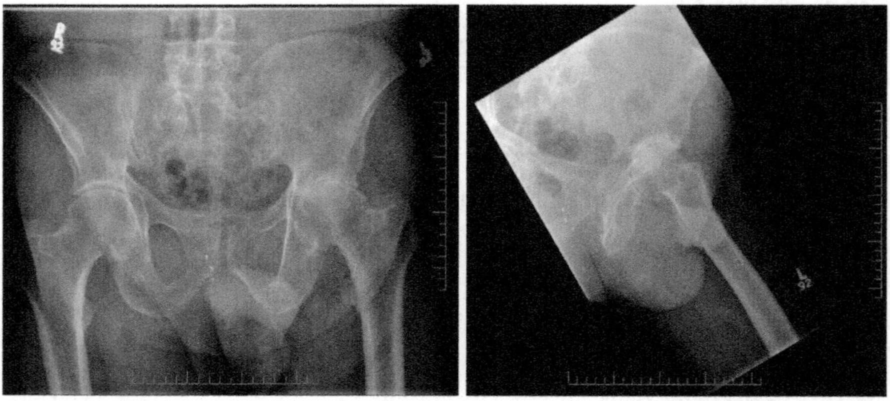

Fig. 2.1 AP pelvis and lateral radiograph of left hip showing typical findings of osteoarthritis including joint space narrowing, sclerosis, and osteophyte formation

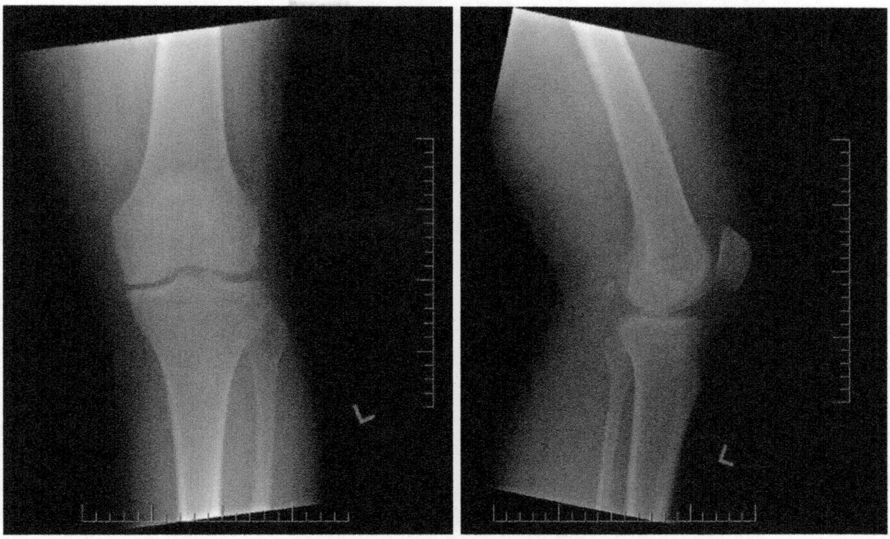

Fig. 2.2 AP and lateral radiograph of the left knee demonstrating decreased medial joint space compared to the lateral compartment

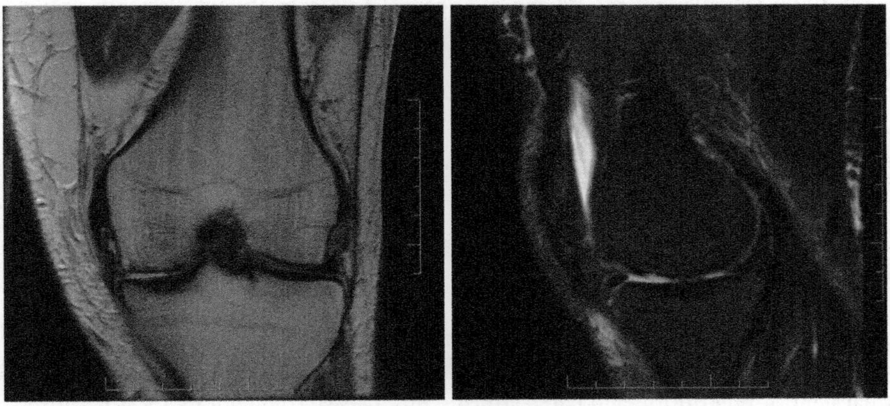

Fig. 2.3 Representative coronal and sagittal cut from a left knee MRI (same patient as in Fig. 2.2) demonstrating severe degenerative changes in the medial compartment

Fig. 2.3, which demonstrates more severe medial compartment degenerative changes than the radiographs would suggest. If the radiographs are not standing images, JSN and deformity may be minimized. Stress radiographs may be obtained to assess ligamentous instability. In patients with malalignment of the lower extremity, hip-to-ankle images can be obtained to better understand the location and cause of deformity.

Treatment

Nonsurgical and Nonpharmacologic

Nonsurgical and nonpharmacologic methods of treatment for OA do exist. An exercise program should be considered as first-line treatment for all patients with symptomatic arthritis. Strengthening the muscles surrounding the joint can help to relieve some symptoms. Weight loss in overweight patients can also help to decrease the stress the joint is forced to endure [5, 6]. Orthoses including shoe wedges and knee unloading braces can help to partially correct malalignment in the lower extremity and provide some relief.

Pharmacologic

Pharmacologic treatment can provide significant relief for patients suffering from OA. Nonsteroidal anti-inflammatory medications (NSAIDs) can help to alleviate pain due to inflammation associated with OA. These patients should be monitored by their general practitioner for adverse effects associated with use of these medications. Intra-articular injections can also be used as a treatment strategy; options include corticosteroids, hyaluronic acid (HA), as well as plasma-rich protein (PRP).

Surgical Treatment

Arthroscopy

Hip Arthroscopy

Arthroscopy can be used as a less invasive surgical procedure to treat various intra-articular hip disorders. This procedure has had an expanding role as of late in the treatment of prearthritic and early arthritic hip disease. Indications for hip arthroscopy currently include symptomatic labral tears, early articular cartilage disease (chondral flaps, chondromalacia), symptomatic hip impingement, synovitis, loose bodies, ligamentum teres ruptures, and diagnostic evaluation of the hip.

Contraindications to hip arthroscopy include advanced degenerative joint disease, disease states that limit arthroscopic access to the joint (morbid obesity, protrusio, joint ankylosis, heterotopic bone), and intra-articular hip disease (e.g., labral tears) associated with major structural abnormalities (developmental hip dysplasia) that require correction of the underlying structural problem.

Clinical results for hip arthroscopy depend on the initial indication for the procedure. Good to excellent clinical results are obtained at short-term follow-up in approximately 70–85 % of the patients treated for labral disease [7, 8]. A guarded prognosis is associated with moderate to advanced (grade IV) articular cartilage disease. The complication rate associated with hip arthroscopy is low (1–3 %). Neurovascular injury is a complication associated with this procedure.

Lateral femoral cutaneous nerve is the most at risk structure (anterior portal), while the most common neurovascular complication is a transient neuropraxia of the pudendal nerve related to traction. Other complications include deep vein thrombosis, instrumentation breakage, articular scuffing, wound hematoma, infection, and ankle strain or fracture.

Knee Arthroscopy

Knee arthroscopy is a common surgery used to treat a variety of intra-articular pathologies. With the arthritic knee, in the absence of mechanical symptoms, arthroscopic debridement is strongly recommended against [9]. At the time of arthroscopy, several strategies can be used to potentially help improve symptoms. Arthroscopic lavage and debridement of the arthritic knee is controversial but effective when properly indicated. Indications are limited to specific mechanical symptoms caused by loose bone, cartilage flaps or particles, meniscal tears, or synovial impingement. Irrigation during arthroscopy dilutes the joint fluid, which reduces the concentration of degradative enzymes. Chondroplasty, specifically removing or stabilizing diseased cartilage, can help to improve mechanical symptoms. Abrasion arthroplasty may have some benefit in this patient population. An arthroscopic shaver is used to debride cartilage defects and penetrate the subchondral bone plate to cause bleeding. The goal is to have a blood clot form, which will undergo metaplasia into fibrocartilage after several weeks. Microfracture has less of a role in more advanced diffuse OA. Here, cartilage defects are debrided to a stable rim, and the resulting exposed subchondral bone is penetrated with a small drill or awl. The goal is to create bleeding bone, which will produce a blood clot and subsequent fibrocartilage.

Osteotomy

Pelvic and Proximal Femoral Osteotomies

The goal of pelvic and proximal femoral osteotomies is to correct abnormal anatomy, thus alleviating pain, enhancing function, and preventing or delaying secondary OA. Patient selection for surgery is critical to optimize surgical outcomes. Major conditions amenable to osteotomy correction include acetabular dysplasia, post-traumatic disorders (malunion/nonunion proximal femur, including femoral neck nonunion), proximal femoral dysplasia (coxa valga), and femoral neck nonunion.

Pelvic osteotomy is a complex surgery that should be done by highly subspecialized surgeons. Indications for pelvic osteotomy include relatively young physiologic age (<55 years), symptomatic dysplasia, prearthritic or early arthritic joint disease, adequate hip motion, and correctable structural abnormality.

Relative contraindications include advanced physiologic age, morbid obesity, restricted hip motion, and moderate to advanced degenerative joint disease.

When patients are selected carefully, outcomes are favorable. Survivorship for periacetabular osteotomy with dysplasia of the hip at 20 years for Tönnis 1 and 2 is 80 % [10, 11].

High Tibial Osteotomy

High tibial osteotomy (HTO) can be considered in the younger patient with unicompartmental disease. It can be effective for treating arthritis due to a varus or valgus malalignment and can delay the need for TKA. Osteotomy of the knee is frequently combined with cartilage restoration procedures to provide a better mechanical environment for the biologic repair. HTO is ideal for the young, active patient with isolated medial or lateral compartment disease because it realigns the limb and reduces stresses on the articular cartilage of the diseased compartment.

Medial compartment arthritis in the varus malaligned limb is common and can be considered for treatment with a valgus-producing HTO. Techniques available include a lateral closing wedge osteotomy, a medial opening wedge osteotomy, or a dome osteotomy. Slight overcorrection of the varus deformity to 8–10° of valgus has produced good results [12, 13]. Lateral compartment arthritis in the valgus malaligned limb is less common. These patients can be considered for treatment with a varus-producing distal femoral osteotomy (DFO). Varus-producing osteotomy of the proximal tibia can create joint line obliquity; as such, the osteotomy should be carried out in the distal femur.

Contraindications to HTO include tricompartmental arthritic change, >15° flexion contracture, less than 90° of knee flexion, loss of lateral meniscus in a valgus-producing HTO, or loss of medial meniscus in a varus-producing DFO. Complications of HTO or DFO include recurrence of deformity, 60 % failure rate after 3 years when there is failure to overcorrect or if patient is overweight, loss of posterior slope or patella baja, and shortened patellar tendon, which decreases the distance of patellar tendon from the inferior joint line. This can be caused by:

- Raising tibiofemoral joint line in opening wedge osteotomy
- Retropatellar scarring and tendon contracture
- Bony impingement of the patella on the tibia

Other complications include compartment syndrome, peroneal nerve palsy (more common in lateral opening wedge), malunion, or nonunion.

Results associated with osteotomy of either the distal femur or proximal tibia will depend on appropriate patient selection. Valgus-producing HTO has been successful in approximately 50–85 % of patients at 10 years (96 % at 5 years, 80 % at 10 years, 57 % at 15 years) [13–15].

When considering osteotomy around the knee, it is important to realize challenges with TKA after osteotomy should the patient continue to have symptomatic arthritis. TKA is technically challenging because of previous incisions, scar tissue, retained hardware, and tibial and femoral abnormalities. Patella baja seen after HTO makes exposure more difficult and increases the need for lateral release. Survivorship of TKA after HTO does not seem to be affected, as several studies have shown excellent long-term results [16].

Arthrodesis

Hip

Hip arthrodesis is an uncommon procedure used to treat advanced hip degeneration in a very specific patient population. The position of fusion is critical for optimizing function and minimizing deterioration of neighboring joints. The preferred position of fusion is 25–30° of hip flexion, 0–5° of adduction, and 5–10° of lower extremity external rotation. Indications should be carefully considered and include young age (<30 years of age), high activity level (e.g., manual labor), severe pain and stiffness, posttraumatic arthritis or end-stage disease associated with previous infection, and normal neighboring joints (lumbar spine, contralateral hip, ipsilateral knee). Similarly, contraindications to arthrodesis include disease in neighboring joints (lumbar spine, ipsilateral knee, contralateral hip), major limb-length discrepancy (>2.0 cm), and active infection.

Patients with previous fusions may eventually want the procedure reversed. Indication for fusion takedown includes back or knee pain, leg-length discrepancy, or malposition of the fusion. Patients should be counseled on expected outcomes, as the rehabilitation is prolonged because of profound hip abductor weakness and the associated limp.

Knee

Knee arthrodesis is also an uncommon procedure and indications should be carefully selected. The most common indication is the unrevisable TKA (usually because of infection). Less common indications include septic arthritis, osteomyelitis, posttraumatic arthritis in a young manual laborer, painful ankylosis, neuropathic knee, and paralytic deformity. Contraindications to knee fusion include bilateral knee involvement or ipsilateral hip arthrodesis.

Position of fusion is important and can vary based on patient anatomy or leg-length discrepancy. If the limb-length discrepancy is <2 cm, arthrodesis should be placed in 5–7° of valgus and 15° of flexion. If the limb-length discrepancy is 2–4 cm, arthrodesis should be placed with the knee in full extension. If the limb-length discrepancy is >4 cm, consider bone grafting or a prosthetic spacer to limit gait abnormalities. Prior to fusion, the leg can be immobilized in a cast to prepare the patient for the fusion.

Complications associated with knee arthrodesis include painful nonunion, infection, deep venous thrombosis (DVT), peroneal nerve palsy, and wound dehiscence. Long-term complications include hip, spine, and ankle pain due to the altered gait pattern.

Arthroplasty

Hip

Total hip arthroplasty (THA) has proved to be an extremely successful surgery at relieving pain and improving function. Technical aspects of the surgery should be respected to improve chances of a good outcome. Achieving stability of the articulation between the ball and socket is critical. THA stability is determined by the following variables:

(a) *Component design*: The primary determinant of arc range (or the total arc of motion available between the ball and cup before dislocation) is the head-neck ratio. Other component design characteristics can affect the arc range. An example includes skirted heads, which leads to smaller head-neck ratios and excursion distance (or the distance the head must travel to dislocate after primary impingement).
(b) *Component alignment*: Ideal cup alignment to minimize chance of dislocation is 45° of cup abduction and 15° of cup anteversion. Stem alignment should be in 10–15° of anteversion.
(c) *Soft tissue tensioning*: The abductor complex helps to restore tension via head offset and neck length. Trochanteric deficiency or escape leads to deficient abductor complex contributing to hip instability.

Potential complications associated with THA include heterotopic ossification (HO) or calcification of the soft tissue around the hip. Risk factors for the formation of HO include prolonged surgical time, subtype of OA (hypertrophic), and handling of soft tissues during surgery. The Brooker classification characterizes the amount of HO visible on radiographs: I, islands; II, bone spurs leaving at least 1 cm between bony surfaces; III, spurs from pelvis and proximal femur with space less than 1 cm; and IV, radiographic ankyloses. Vascular injury during screw insertion has a low incidence (less than 1 %) [17]. Although less common than nerve injury, it can be life threatening. Wasielewski proposed the hip quadrant system as a guide for safe screw insertion [18]. Screws are safest when inserted posterior and superior to line A (a line drawn between the ASIS and the center of the acetabulum) and line B (line perpendicular to line A). Nerve injury has an incidence ranging from 0 to 3 % [19]. The peroneal branch of the sciatic nerve is most commonly injured. Risk factors for nerve injury include revision surgery, congenital hip dislocation, female gender, and lengthening the extremity by greater than 4 cm. Dislocation has an incidence of 1–3 %, with 70 % occurring within the first month after surgery [20, 21]. Risk factors for dislocation include female gender, prior hip surgery (most significant risk factor), posterior approach, and malposition of components. Initial treatment of a dislocated THA includes closed reduction. If component malposition is present soon after hip arthroplasty, immediate revision arthroplasty may be required. Venous thromboembolic events are common after THA in patients that are not on prophylaxis (incidence of DVT being 45–57 % in unprotected patients). Pulmonary embolism (PE) occurs in 0.7–2 % of patients with THA without prophylaxis [22, 23]. After THA, patients should therefore be protected with some form of anticoagulant to minimize the chance of these events.

Knee

Similar to THA, TKA has proven to be a reliable surgery at relieving symptoms and improving function. Technical goals of TKA include restoring mechanical alignment (restoring the joint line allows proper function of preserved ligaments). Elevating the joint line can lead to midflexion instability and patellofemoral tracking problems. Lowering the joint line can lead to lack of flexion and flexion instability, balancing ligaments by creating equal flexion and extension gaps, maintaining a normal Q angle (angle formed from the intersection of the extensor mechanism axis above the patella with the axis of the patellar tendon), and thus ensuring proper patellar femoral tracking. Errors that increase the Q angle include internal rotation of the femoral prosthesis, medialization of the femoral component, internal rotation of the tibial prosthesis, or placing the patellar prosthesis lateral on the patella.

Ligament balancing in TKA is crucial to obtaining a stable knee. The goal is to achieve equal symmetric flexion and extension gaps. In a varus-aligned knee, most ligament balancing occurs at the time of exposure through controlled posteromedial release. Femoral and tibial osteophytes should be removed followed by the meniscus. Deep medial collateral ligament (MCL) release can be performed. Reduction osteotomy (placing the tibial tray as far lateral as possible and recutting the tibia around it) is another technique to help with balancing. Superficial MCL release, medial epicondyle osteotomy, and lateral collateral ligament tightening are other options available to the surgeon once other methods have been exhausted. With valgus deformity, balancing follows different steps. Care should be taken to prevent overly aggressive release of the medial side during exposure. Valgus knees are often found to have hypoplastic lateral femoral condyles. As such, secondary checks should be used when determining femoral rotation, such as Whiteside's line (a vertical line extending from the deepest part of the trochlear groove and the center of the intercondylar notch) and the epicondylar axis. Osteophytes should be resected and soft tissue released as deemed appropriate can be helpful to balance a valgus knee. The iliotibial band can be released if the knee is tight in extension, and the popliteus can be released if the knee is tight in flexion. Alternatively, a laminar spreader can be inserted to open up the lateral compartment, and tight structures can be released as they are encountered.

Knee prostheses come in varying levels of constraint. Unconstrained knees are available in posterior cruciate-retaining and posterior cruciate-substituting designs. If increased constraint is required, constrained nonhinged (varus-valgus constrained) implants are available. Finally, constrained hinges are available for grossly unstable knees.

There are many potential complications associated with TKA. Some of these include:

(a) *Instability:* This complication accounts for 10–20 % of all TKA revisions [24, 25]. It can occur in the mediolateral (axial instability) and the anteroposterior (flexion instability) planes. Factors leading to instability include ligament imbalance, component malalignment or failure, bone loss from over-resection of femur, bone loss from femoral or tibial component loosening, soft tissue laxity of collateral ligaments, or connective tissue disorders.
(b) *Rotational malalignment:* Patellofemoral (PF) maltracking must be avoided when performing a TKA. The most common complications in TKA involve abnormal patellar tracking. Surgeons must avoid an increased Q angle to avoid increased lateral patellar subluxation forces. Femoral component internal rotation should be avoided because it causes lateral patellar tilt and a net increase in the Q angle. The femoral component should be placed in 3° of external rotation to the neutral axis to maintain a symmetric flexion gap. The femoral component should be biased to the lateralized position because medialization places the trochlear groove in a medial position and increases the Q angle. Midpoint of the tibial component should align over the medial third of the tibial tubercle, and care should be taken to avoid an internally rotated position and err toward external rotation. Internal rotation of the tibia results in external rotation of the tubercle and increases the Q angle. The patella should be placed medially and superiorly on the undersurface of the patella.
(c) *Vascular injury*: Incidence of these injuries is low. To minimize these events, one should avoid sharp dissection in the posterior compartment of the knee. Posterior retractor placement must also be performed carefully and should be biased medially away from the popliteal artery (artery has been shown to lie 9 mm posterior to the posterior cortex of the tibia at 90° of flexion). If arterial injury is suspected, drop tourniquet to check artery. Popliteal artery injury can lead to acute ischemia, compartment syndrome, and potential amputation.
(d) *Nerve palsy*: Incidence is reported at 0.3 %. In patients with severe valgus, rate of peroneal nerve injury increases to 3–4 % [26, 27]. If a peroneal nerve injury is suspected following TKA, the leg should be immediately flexed and all compressive dressings should be removed. Initial management should include use of ankle foot orthoses and physiotherapy to maintain a supple joint.
(e) *Wound complications:* These can be challenging for both surgeon and patient. Systemic risk factors include diabetes, vascular disease, rheumatoid arthritis, nutritional status, and obesity.
(f) *Stiffness*: Poor motion after TKA leads to suboptimal outcomes. Patient factors that affect ROM include preoperative ROM, body habitus, patient compliance,

and pain tolerance. Technical factors affecting ROM include overstuffing the patellofemoral joint, mismatched extension and flexion gaps, inaccurate balancing, component malposition, oversized components, joint line elevation, and excessive tightening of the extensor mechanism at closure.

Conclusions

OA is a common cause of pain and disability, which can develop in any synovial joint. Symptoms include activity related pain, rest pain, as well as nighttime pain. ROM of the affected joint demonstrates a painful and stiff arc of motion. Radiographs demonstrate JSN, increased sclerosis at the joint surfaces, osteophyte formation, and subchondral cysts. Nonoperative treatment includes physiotherapy, weight loss, orthoses, NSAIDs, and intra-articular injections. Surgical management includes arthroscopy, osteotomy, arthrodesis, and arthroplasty.

References

1. Pereira D, et al. The effect of osteoarthritis definition on prevalence and incidence estimates: a systematic review. Osteoarthritis Cartilage. 2011;19(11):1270–85.
2. Oliveria SA, et al. Incidence of symptomatic hand, hip, and knee osteoarthritis among patients in a health maintenance organization. Arthritis Rheum. 1995;38(8):1134–41.
3. Kurtz S, et al. Projections of primary and revision hip and knee arthroplasty in the United States from 2005 to 2030. J Bone Joint Surg Am. 2007;89(4):780–5.
4. Cicuttini FM, et al. Association of pain with radiological changes in different compartments and views of the knee joint. Osteoarthritis Cartilage. 1996;4(2):143–7.
5. Messier SP, et al. Exercise and dietary weight loss in overweight and obese older adults with knee osteoarthritis: the arthritis, diet, and activity promotion trial. Arthritis Rheum. 2004;50(5): 1501–10.
6. Christensen R, et al. Effect of weight reduction in obese patients diagnosed with knee osteoarthritis: a systematic review and meta-analysis. Ann Rheum Dis. 2007;66(4):433–9.
7. McCormick F, et al. Predictors of hip arthroscopy outcomes for labral tears at minimum 2-year follow-up: the influence of age and arthritis. Arthroscopy. 2012;28(10):1359–64.
8. Ha YC, Kim KC, Shin YE. Patient satisfaction after arthroscopic repair of acetabular labral tears. Clin Orthop Surg. 2014;6(2):159–64.
9. Kirkley A, et al. A randomized trial of arthroscopic surgery for osteoarthritis of the knee. N Engl J Med. 2008;359(11):1097–107.
10. Dahl LB, et al. Clinical and radiological outcome after periacetabular osteotomy: a cross-sectional study of 127 hips operated on from 1999–2008. Hip Int. 2014;24(4):369–80.
11. Matheney T, et al. Intermediate to long-term results following the bernese periacetabular osteotomy and predictors of clinical outcome: surgical technique. J Bone Joint Surg Am. 2010;92(Suppl 1 Pt 2):115–29.
12. El-Azab HM, et al. Limb alignment after open-wedge high tibial osteotomy and its effect on the clinical outcome. Orthopedics. 2011;34(10):e622–8.
13. Majima T, et al. Progression of joint arthrosis 10 to 15 years after high tibial osteotomy. Clin Orthop Relat Res. 2000;381:177–84.

14. Naudie D, et al. The Install Award. Survivorship of the high tibial valgus osteotomy. A 10- to –22-year followup study. Clin Orthop Relat Res. 1999;(367):18–27.
15. Floerkemeier S, et al. Outcome after high tibial open-wedge osteotomy: a retrospective evaluation of 533 patients. Knee Surg Sports Traumatol Arthrosc. 2013;21(1):170–80.
16. van Raaij TM, et al. Total knee arthroplasty after high tibial osteotomy. A systematic review. BMC Musculoskelet Disord. 2009;10:88.
17. Wilson JS, et al. Vascular injuries associated with elective orthopedic procedures. Ann Vasc Surg. 2003;17(6):641–4.
18. Wasielewski RC, et al. Acetabular anatomy and the transacetabular fixation of screws in total hip arthroplasty. J Bone Joint Surg Am. 1990;72(4):501–8.
19. Brown GD, Swanson EA, Nercessian OA. Neurologic injuries after total hip arthroplasty. Am J Orthop (Belle Mead NJ). 2008;37(4):191–7.
20. Bourne RB, Mehin R. The dislocating hip: what to do, what to do. J Arthroplasty. 2004;19(4 Suppl 1):111–4.
21. Alberton GM, High WA, Morrey BF. Dislocation after revision total hip arthroplasty: an analysis of risk factors and treatment options. J Bone Joint Surg Am. 2002;84-A(10):1788–92.
22. O'Reilly RF, Burgess IA, Zicat B. The prevalence of venous thromboembolism after hip and knee replacement surgery. Med J Aust. 2005;182(4):154–9.
23. Fender D, et al. Mortality and fatal pulmonary embolism after primary total hip replacement. Results from a regional hip register. J Bone Joint Surg Br. 1997;79(6):896–9.
24. Parratte S, Pagnano MW. Instability after total knee arthroplasty. Instr Course Lect. 2008;57:295–304.
25. Vince KG, Abdeen A, Sugimori T. The unstable total knee arthroplasty: causes and cures. J Arthroplasty. 2006;21(4 Suppl 1):44–9.
26. Schinsky MF, et al. Nerve injury after primary total knee arthroplasty. J Arthroplasty. 2001;16(8):1048–54.
27. Nercessian OA, Ugwonali OF, Park S. Peroneal nerve palsy after total knee arthroplasty. J Arthroplasty. 2005;20(8):1068–73.

Chapter 3
Shoulder and Elbow Osteoarthritis

Timothy Leroux and Christian Veillette

Key Points

Shoulder

- Shoulder osteoarthritis (OA) is common.
- Primary shoulder OA is the most common form.
- The most common type of secondary shoulder OA is rotator cuff arthropathy and is believed to be related to a decoupling of forces about the humeral head.
- Typical presentation is activity-related shoulder pain and loss of shoulder range of motion.
- Physical exam should include an assessment of the rotator cuff and axillary nerve.
- Standard radiographs are often sufficient to make diagnosis, but cross-sectional imaging may be indicated to identify bone loss (CT) or soft tissue deficiencies (MRI/ultrasound).
- Nonoperative care can include physical therapy, pharmacotherapy, and intra-articular injections (cortisone and hyaluronic acid), but evidence for or against these treatments is limited.

T. Leroux, MD, Med
Division of Orthopaedic Surgery, Department of Surgery, University of Toronto, Toronto, ON, Canada

C. Veillette, MD, MSc, FRCSC (✉)
Division of Orthopaedic Surgery, Department of Surgery,
Toronto Western Hospital – University Health Network, 399 Bathurst Street,
East Wing Rm 1-440, Toronto, ON M5T 2S8, Canada

University of Toronto, Toronto, ON, Canada
e-mail: christian.veillette@uhn.ca

M. Kapoor, N.N. Mahomed (eds.), *Osteoarthritis: Pathogenesis, Diagnosis, Available Treatments, Drug Safety, Regenerative and Precision Medicine*,
DOI 10.1007/978-3-319-19560-5_3

- Surgical management of end-stage shoulder OA includes arthroscopic debridement, interposition arthroplasty (glenoid resurfacing), humeral head resurfacing, hemiarthroplasty, anatomic total shoulder arthroplasty, and, in low demand patients with a deficient rotator cuff, reverse total shoulder arthroplasty.
- In young patients with end-stage shoulder OA, arthroplasty has high failure rates secondary to either glenoid erosion (hemiarthroplasty) or glenoid component loosening (anatomic total shoulder arthroplasty).
- For older patients with end-stage shoulder OA and an intact rotator cuff, anatomic total shoulder arthroplasty is recommended.

Elbow

- Symptomatic elbow OA is rare.
- Secondary elbow OA is the most common form.
- Following elbow trauma, radiographic changes consistent with elbow OA are common, but symptoms infrequent.
- Typical presentation of patients with symptomatic elbow OA includes complaints of motion loss and impingement.
- Physical exam should include an assessment of the collateral ligaments and ulnar nerve.
- In addition to standard elbow radiographs, cross-sectional imaging (CT) is often useful to determine osteophyte distribution and presence of loose bodies.
- Nonoperative management of elbow OA should include activity modification, while the utility of pharmacotherapy, physiotherapy, bracing, and intra-articular injections (cortisone and hyaluronic acid) has not been fully elucidated.
- The mainstay of surgical management is elbow debridement, performed either open or arthroscopically.
- Total elbow arthroplasty should be reserved for older patients with minimal physical demands.
- For patients with OA isolated to the radiocapitellar joint, an isolated radiocapitellar joint arthroplasty has demonstrated favorable early outcomes.

Introduction

OA of the shoulder or elbow can significantly impact quality of life. Despite this, our understanding of how to appropriately manage patients with symptomatic OA of the shoulder or elbow is quite limited. The use of shoulder and elbow arthroplasty appears to be rising exponentially, but these options are costly, and although outcomes tend to be favorable, they are dependent upon appropriate patient selection. In this chapter, we will discuss management options and outcomes but also explore the epidemiology, etiology, and work-up of patients with shoulder and elbow OA.

Epidemiology

Shoulder

Glenohumeral OA is a debilitating condition akin to other chronic medical conditions such as congestive heart failure, diabetes, and acute myocardial infarction [1]; moreover, it can limit shoulder function resulting in anxiety, depression, activity limitations, and poor job performance [2]. Despite this, the overall prevalence of glenohumeral OA in the general North American population has not been studied [3]. A 2011 Korean study found the prevalence of radiographic primary and secondary glenohumeral OA in the general population to be 16.1 % and 1.9 %, respectively, and that risk increased with age [3]. Of note, female sex and obesity did not influence radiographic glenohumeral OA risk [3].

Studies have sought to understand the utilization of shoulder arthroplasty – the end-stage management of OA. It has been observed that the rate of shoulder arthroplasty in the United States has increased significantly over the past decade (47,000 in 2008 compared to 19,000 in 1998) [4]. This has been attributed to a growing elderly population, public awareness, advances in implant design and availability, and increasing number of shoulder and elbow surgeons [4, 5]. Interestingly, the increase in the rate of total shoulder arthroplasty was significantly greater than shoulder hemiarthroplasty, which may reflect the Food and Drug Administration approval of the reverse total shoulder arthroplasty in November 2003 [4]. It has been estimated that the annual rate of total shoulder arthroplasty in the United States will increase between 192 and 322 % from 2007 to 2015 [6].

Elbow

OA of the elbow is rare, with a prevalence believed to be less than 2 % in the general population [7]. It is more commonly seen in males with a history of repetitive use of their dominant upper extremity, such as manual laborers, throwing athletes, weight lifters, and those who use walking aids (crutches) [7, 8].

In the United States, the utilization of elbow arthroplasty to manage end-stage OA has increased significantly over the past two decades [9]. Despite this, population data suggests that the number of total elbow arthroplasty procedures performed annually to manage OA remains quite low (of the 1,155 total elbow arthroplasty procedures undertaken in New York State over a 10-year period, 88–91 % of the associated diagnoses were inflammatory arthritis or trauma [10]).

Etiology

Shoulder

The etiology of glenohumeral OA can be divided into primary (idiopathic) and secondary causes. Primary OA is the most common cause of glenohumeral OA [11] and is the most common diagnosis among patients undergoing total shoulder arthroplasty (77 %) and shoulder hemiarthroplasty (43 %) [4]. Secondary causes of glenohumeral OA include rotator cuff deficiency, previous arthroscopic shoulder surgery, fracture, and recurrent instability.

The relationship between glenohumeral OA and rotator cuff deficiency remains a hotly debated topic. Three theories have been proposed to explain how a rotator cuff tear can result in the development of rotator cuff arthropathy – a unique pattern of changes in the glenohumeral joint characterized by anterosuperior migration and femoralization of the proximal humerus, collapse of the proximal aspect of the humeral articular surface, and acetabularization of the coracoacromial arch [12, 13]. These theories include:

1. An inflammatory-mediated destruction of the articular cartilage resulting from the accumulation of calcium phosphate crystals which trigger the release of collagenases and proteases
2. Malnutrition of the cartilage resulting from loss of nourishing factors in the subacromial space through the torn rotator cuff
3. Abnormal physical stresses on the articular cartilage secondary to a loss of force couples around the shoulder and the resulting anterosuperior migration of the humeral head [13, 14]

Basic science studies have suggested that the latter theory best accounts for the observed cartilage degeneration [14], and biomechanical studies have supported the notion that a critical tear size is necessary to sufficiently disrupt joint kinematics initiating this cascade (a full thickness supraspinatus tear with 50 % of the infraspinatus), ultimately resulting in humeral head migration and the development of rotator cuff arthropathy [15]. Despite this evidence, full thickness rotator cuff tears are common in the older, general population (the prevalence of cuff tears in persons >60 years and >70 years is 28 % and 50 %, respectively) [16, 17]; however, rotator cuff arthropathy is not common, and further study is necessary to better understand why only a percentage of patients with full thickness rotator cuff tears develop rotator cuff arthropathy [18].

Chondrolysis following arthroscopic shoulder surgery, a phenomenon termed postarthroscopic glenohumeral chondrolysis (PAGCL), has been reported [19, 20]. Although rare, it is a challenging problem that tends to arise in younger, male patients rather than the typical older patient with primary glenohumeral OA [19–21]. The underlying pathophysiology has yet to be completely elucidated; however, it does appear to be multifactorial, and case reports have linked this pathology to the use of intra-articular pain pumps, radiofrequency devices, and implants/anchors during arthroscopic surgery [19–21].

Fractures that disrupt or malalign the glenohumeral articular surface can result in glenohumeral OA, commonly referred to as posttraumatic arthropathy [22–24]. The pathogenesis of posttraumatic OA is not well understood, but it is believed that multiple factors lead to its onset, including cartilage injury at the time of the initial trauma, biological response of bleeding and inflammation, and chronic cartilage overload secondary to articular surface incongruity, joint instability, and glenohumeral malalignment [24, 25]. Unfortunately, the literature on the epidemiology of this clinical entity is quite sparse and is largely focused on management.

Glenohumeral OA can also arise in patients who have sustained a previous glenohumeral dislocation, commonly referred to as dislocation arthropathy [26, 27]. Again, the pathogenesis is not completely understood but is believed to be similar to the development of OA following fracture (discussed above) [24]. The prevalence of this disease has been investigated, including a study with 25-year follow-up that found the rate of glenohumeral OA in patients managed nonsurgically following a glenohumeral dislocation was 60 % [28]. In another study, the rate of radiographic glenohumeral OA 13 years following arthroscopic labral repair was similar (68 %); however, most radiographic changes were mild, and most patients were asymptomatic [29]. It appears that patient age at the time of first dislocation influences OA severity in the long-term, whereby older age is associated with more severe disease on follow-up radiographs [28–30]. Similarly, increased time between labral repair and the first dislocation and the number of previous dislocations have been shown to influence OA risk in the unstable shoulder [31].

Elbow

Similar to glenohumeral OA, elbow OA has typically been divided into primary (idiopathic) and secondary causes. Secondary causes include fracture, repetitive stress, valgus extension overload, osteochondritis dissecans, and synovial chondromatosis [8].

It has been acknowledged that our understanding of elbow OA, particularly its etiology, is largely unknown. For instance, many patients develop radiographic signs of OA following elbow trauma (at a median of 19.5 years following surgical fixation of an elbow fracture, the prevalence of moderate-to-severe elbow OA on radiographs to be 23 %[32]), but symptoms vary, and few seek treatment [32]. The lack of evidence likely stems from the rarity of this disease and the relative paucity of studies that have sought to delineate the factors that predispose an elbow to OA [8].

Several biomechanical studies have improved our understanding of the relationship between repetitive stress and elbow OA. First, the elbow has been shown to be a load-bearing joint, whereby normal daily activity can generate forces up to half the body weight across the ulnohumeral joint [33], and heavy lifting and overhead throwing can generate forces three and six times the body weight, respectively [8, 34, 35]. Second, forces tend to be directed toward the margins of the articular surface, decreasing load sharing across the joint [36]. Collectively, a high force over a small surface area has the potential to damage the exposed articular surface, particularly with long exposure periods such as repetitive use.

Clinical and Radiographic Assessment

Shoulder

Patients with glenohumeral OA typically present with a long history of progressive activity-related shoulder pain that is relieved with rest. It is not uncommon for patients to also complain of pain at rest and pain at night, and these complaints tend to be more frequently reported in advanced stages of the disease. The pain is often localized deep in the shoulder and described as a dull ache. In addition to pain, patients may report a loss of shoulder function, including range of motion and strength. They may also report instability, locking, or crepitus. A thorough history of past shoulder complaints, injuries, and surgeries may reveal secondary causes of glenohumeral OA, such as rotator cuff deficiency, fracture, and glenohumeral instability. Management plans are often dictated by a failure of nonsurgical management, and it is important to inquire about previous attempts to modify painful activities; past injections, including the injected substance, the number of injections, the location of the injections (subacromial vs. glenohumeral), and their success; and previous trials of physiotherapy, including the number of sessions, the quality of the sessions (manipulation- vs. modality-based physiotherapy), and their success. Lastly, glenohumeral OA can be quite disabling, and clinicians should inquire about its impact on quality of life [37].

Physical exam tends to be quite variable, and the findings often overlap with a number of other shoulder pathologies. Typically, patients with glenohumeral OA have joint line tenderness; pain with shoulder motion; loss of both active and passive range of motion, the latter being more indicative of advanced disease; global shoulder weakness; and crepitus. An exam of the rotator cuff should be attempted to exclude deficiency, and a thorough neurovascular exam with care to document the motor and sensory function of the axillary nerve.

In patients with glenohumeral OA, the mainstay of diagnosis is imaging. Standard radiographs, including anteroposterior, lateral (transscapular), and axillary views, are sufficient to visualize the characteristic features of glenohumeral OA, including narrowing of the joint space, osteophyte formation, subchondral sclerosis, and subchondral cysts (see Fig. 3.1). On the anteroposterior image, it is not uncommon to see "the goat's beard," a large inferomedial humeral head osteophyte. Radiographs can also be used to assess for secondary causes of glenohumeral OA, including the classic features of rotator cuff arthropathy (anterosuperior migration and femoralization of the proximal humerus, collapse of the proximal aspect of the humeral articular surface, and acetabularization of the coracoacromial arch [12, 13]), recurrent glenohumeral instability (humeral head defects and glenoid bone loss [38]), and previous fracture (deformity and articular incongruity [24, 25]). Advanced imaging should be considered in situations where a soft tissue defect or bone loss will impact management, such as rotator cuff deficiency (MRI or ultrasound) or glenoid bone loss (CT scan).

A thorough history, physical exam, and appropriate imaging can be useful to exclude other common pathologies that may mimic glenohumeral OA, including rotator cuff tears, labral tears, inflammatory arthritis, impingement, adhesive capsu-

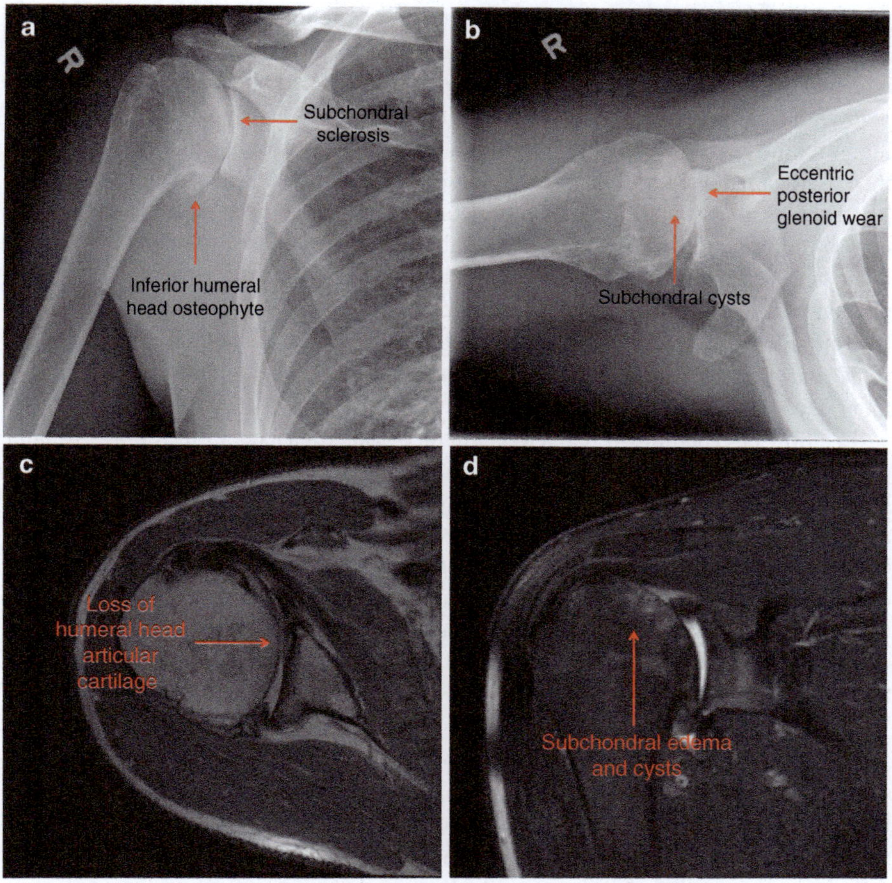

Fig. 3.1 Shoulder osteoarthritis. (**a**, **b**) Demonstration of the typical radiographic appearance of primary shoulder osteoarthritis in the anteroposterior and axillary views, respectively. Typical radiographic features include an inferior humeral head osteophyte (**a**), subchondral sclerosis (**a**), subchondral cysts (**b**), and eccentric posterior glenoid wear (**b**). (**c**, **d**) Demonstration of corresponding coronal and axial MRI views of the same patient, respectively. In these images, there is complete loss of articular cartilage on the humeral head (**c**), subchondral cysts (**d**), and subchondral bone edema (**d**)

litis, and cervical disk disease. A review of these pathologies is beyond the scope of this chapter, but the clinician should seek to exclude them during each patient assessment.

Elbow

Compared to OA of other joints in the body, elbow OA is unique in that it is characterized by hypertrophic osteophyte formation and capsular contracture alongside a relative preservation of both articular cartilage and joint space [7]. These features account for the typical patient complaints of loss of motion (capsule contraction) and pain at terminal extension or flexion (impingement from an osteophyte on the olecranon and coronoid, respectively). Similar to the clinical assessment of glenohumeral OA, it is important to determine degree of pain and disability, including pain with activity, pain at rest, pain at night, location of pain, loss of motion, locking, crepitus, and instability. As alluded to above, patients commonly report increased pain at the terminal ends of motion, which is the hallmark of impingement [8]. There is an association between repetitive stress and elbow OA, and it is important to inquire about vocation (manual labor) and recreational demands (overhead sports and weight lifting) [8]. A thorough history of past elbow complaints, injuries, and surgeries would be helpful to exclude secondary causes of elbow OA, such as fracture. Furthermore, any past attempts at nonsurgical (activity modification, injections, and physiotherapy) or surgical management would help guide future management decisions.

In elbow OA, pathology tends to begin on the lateral aspect of the elbow [8], and physical examination can reveal an effusion in the lateral soft spot (a point on the lateral elbow bordered by the tip of the olecranon, the lateral epicondyle, and the radial head) and lateral joint line tenderness. Additionally, elbow OA may result in decreased active and passive range of motion, pain at the terminal ends of motion, crepitus, and instability. It is imperative to document the integrity of the collateral ligaments, as this can guide surgical management [39]. Lastly, a detailed neurovascular exam should be performed with care to document the sensory and motor function of the ulnar nerve.

As in glenohumeral OA, the mainstay of diagnosis is imaging. Standard radiographs with anteroposterior and lateral views are usually sufficient to make the diagnosis of elbow OA. Pathology tends to begin in the radiocapitellar joint, and loss of ulnohumeral joint space signifies more advanced disease [8, 39]. Visualization of loose bodies and a more advanced perspective of osteophyte distribution can be difficult with standard radiographs, and this would be an indication for a CT scan [8, 39, 40].

Classification Systems

Shoulder

Several shoulder-specific classification systems have been developed to describe the stages of primary glenohumeral OA, including glenoid morphology and erosion (the Walch classification), the formation of an inferior humeral head osteophyte (the Samilson and Prieto classification [27] and the modified versions of this classification made by Allain et al. [41] and Gerber [42]), the loss of glenohumeral joint space (the Weinstein classification [43]), and the constellation of classic radiographic changes, including joint space narrowing, subchondral sclerosis, osteophyte formation, and subchondral cysts (the Guyette classification [44]). The Samilson and Prieto classification was originally developed for dislocation arthropathy [27] but is now commonly used in primary glenohumeral OA [45]. All of the aforementioned classification systems have demonstrated excellent intra- and inter-observer reliability and are suitable for clinical and scientific use [45].

Classification systems have also been developed to describe the stages of cuff tear arthropathy, including glenoid erosion (the Sirveaux classification [46]), and the classic collection of radiographic changes, including anterosuperior migration of the humeral head, acetabularization of the coracoacromial arch, femoralization of the humeral head, and narrowing of the glenohumeral joint space (the Favard classification [47], the Visotsky-Seebauer classification [48], and the Hamada classification [49]). Evidence suggests that the Sirveaux classification demonstrates the best overall reliability [47]; however, it does not address the changes in humeral head position and morphology [46]. The Visotsky-Seebauer and Hamada classification systems reliably characterize both humeral head and glenoid changes and have been recommended for clinical and scientific use [47].

Elbow

At present, the Rettig classification [50] is the only classification system available to stage radiographic changes in elbow OA, including radiocapitellar joint space narrowing and instability, and the development of marginal ulnohumeral osteophytes (the Rettig classification [50]). This classification system has demonstrated good correlation with clinical outcomes (pain and function) [50]; however, intra- and inter-observer reliability has not been established.

Nonoperative Management

Nonoperative interventions are the first-line management for both glenohumeral and elbow OA, including rest, anti-inflammatory medication, long-term activity modification, intra-articular injections, physiotherapy, and bracing; however, the efficacy of these interventions is quite variable. Emerging biological therapies, such as intra-articular injections of platelet-rich plasma or stem cells, should be considered experimental in the shoulder and elbow [51].

Shoulder

In 2010, the American Academy of Orthopaedic Surgeons released clinical practice guidelines for the treatment of glenohumeral OA [52]. In this publication, the authors concluded that evidence was not sufficient to recommend for or against the use of physical therapy, pharmacotherapy (nonsteroidal anti-inflammatories, acetaminophen, and opioids), and intra-articular corticosteroid injections to manage patients with glenohumeral OA [52]. At the time of the publication, one industry-funded level IV study suggested that viscosupplementation (hyaluronic acid) significantly decreased pain, increased range of motion, and improved quality of life up to 6 months postinjection [53]. The clinical practice guidelines do acknowledge the weakness of this study [52], and a recent randomized trial suggests that, as compared to placebo injections, there may be no significant clinical improvement following intra-articular hyaluronic acid injections [54].

Elbow

Given the relationship between repetitive stress and the development of elbow OA, the mainstay of nonoperative management is long-term activity modification [7], which can be challenging when activity modification impacts employment (manual labor) [8]. Intra-articular corticosteroid or hyaluronic acid injections may provide short-term (<3 months) improvement in symptoms [8, 55], but the evidence is sparse, and their benefit in the long-term has not been demonstrated. Similarly, anti-inflammatory medications, bracing, and physiotherapy are often recommended, but their benefit for patients with elbow OA has not been studied.

Operative Management

Surgical options for patients with OA include procedures that preserve the native joint and those that replace the native joint (arthroplasty). A general approach to management of these patients would be to fully exhaust all nonoperative measures, followed by an emphasis on joint preservation rather than joint replacement.

Shoulder

A number of surgical procedures have been described to manage glenohumeral OA, including those that are joint preserving (arthroscopic debridement, osteotomy, and interposition arthroplasty) and joint replacing (humeral head resurfacing, humeral head replacement with or without glenoid reaming, and total shoulder replacement) [11, 56]. Based upon the 2010 American Academy of Orthopaedic Surgeons clinical practice guidelines for the treatment of glenohumeral OA, humeral head replacement and total shoulder replacement were recommended; however, total shoulder replacement was the preferred treatment [52], as it has demonstrated superior clinical outcomes (decreased pain, improved range of motion, and increased strength) and a lower revision rate in the short term (6.5 % vs. 10.2 %) [57, 58]. Recent long-term evidence suggests that clinical improvements following total shoulder arthroplasty are sustained up to 15 years but revision rates may be as high as 30 % [59]. Additional studies are needed to substantiate these long-term findings.

Surgical management of glenohumeral OA in the young patient (<60 years of age) is challenging for a number of reasons, including higher activity levels, greater functional expectations, and limited lifespan of prosthetic joint replacement in this demographic [56]. Arthroscopic debridement is often the first-line surgical management for these patients, as it also has value in diagnosing and characterizing cartilage lesions [56]. It tends to be more efficacious in patients with mild OA [60], small cartilage defects (<2 cm^2) [61], and disease that only affects one side of the joint (humeral head or glenoid) [62]. An alternative joint-preserving procedure is glenoid interposition arthroplasty, which involves the interposition of a graft to resurface the glenoid (commonly used grafts are lateral meniscus and Achilles tendon allografts) [56]. Early results of this procedure were favorable, but more recent evidence suggests it has failure rate of over 50 % at a mean follow-up of 2.8 years [63]. Interestingly, the American Academy of Orthopaedic Surgeons clinical guidelines could not recommend for or against arthroscopic debridement or interposition arthroplasty [52].

As alluded to above, joint replacement in the young patient can be challenging given the high failure rates [56]. Of the options available, humeral head resurfacing has the theoretical advantage of preserving bone stock, but the evidence is quite sparse and no high-level comparative trials have been undertaken to determine survivorship. The ultimate challenge of shoulder replacement in young patients is management of the glenoid. For instance, it has been shown that humeral head replacement decreases pain and improves motion, but its survival in patients under the age of 50 is only 83 % and 73 % at 10 and 15 years, respectively [64]. Most concerning, however, was the degree and progression of glenoid erosion, which can complicate future revision procedures [56]. Similar improvements in pain and function have been observed for young patients undergoing total shoulder replacement, but the concern in this population is glenoid component loosening [56]. In fact, studies have demonstrated a high rate of radiolucency about the glenoid component [56], which may translate into a higher risk for failure and need for revision in these young patients. Given its functional limitations, reverse total shoulder replacement has generally not been considered an option for young patients; furthermore, recent evidence suggests a lower satisfaction rate [65] and higher complication rate [66] in this patient demographic, and the long-term survivability has yet to be determined.

Surgical management of rotator cuff arthropathy is also challenging, but the advent of the reverse total shoulder arthroplasty has improved this. The biomechanical concept of this implant is to increase the efficiency of the deltoid for abduction – an activity that a rotator-deficient shoulder would otherwise have difficulty doing [18]. A second advantage of this implant is that it is semi-constrained, preventing superior migration and instability often seen following total shoulder replacement performed in rotator-deficient shoulders [18]. Although reverse total shoulder replacement improves patient function, its use is limited by high failure rates in patients who do not have low functional demands (generally used in patients over the age of 70) [18]. In higher-demand patients with rotator cuff arthropathy and an intact coracoacromial arch and anterior deltoid, humeral head replacement has been the mainstay of treatment [18]. Again, glenoid erosion and failure are a concern, but less so with increasing age. A difficult situation is the high-demand patient with rotator cuff arthropathy who does not have an intact coracoacromial arch or anterior deltoid. In these cases, superior escape is a dreaded complication of humeral head replacement, and arthrodesis may be a consideration if the patient cannot tolerate the functional demands of a reverse total shoulder arthroplasty [13]. Lastly, anatomic total shoulder replacement is not advisable in rotator-deficient shoulders due to high failure rates [52].

Elbow

Similar to glenohumeral OA, surgical management of elbow OA can be categorized into joint preserving (open or arthroscopic debridement, otherwise known as ulnohumeral arthroplasty) and joint replacement (radiocapitellar replacement and total elbow replacement). The mainstay of elbow OA is joint debridement, which can be done either open or arthroscopically. The goals of either approach are to remove loose bodies and osteophytes, debride frayed articular cartilage, and perform a capsule release [67]. The advantages of an arthroscopic debridement would be less complications (open has been associated with instability, heterotopic bone formation, ulnar neuropathy) [68], pain, and bleeding [69]; however, it may be difficult to perform a complete debridement (as can be performed in an open debridement) and requires expertise and equipment that may not be readily available [68]. Short-term results suggest an improvement in pain and functional outcome scores following either procedure, but the evidence supporting an improvement in range of motion is mixed [68]. Despite short-term improvements, long-term studies following open joint debridement suggest that the rate of recurrence is high (loss of motion [70, 71], progression in radiographic OA changes [68], and there is recurrence of osteophytes [70]), but similar studies do not exist for arthroscopic joint debridement. Lastly, it is advised to decompress the ulnar nerve following ulnohumeral arthroplasty, as postoperative ulnar neuropathy can be as high as 28 % [72].

Beyond joint debridement, few surgical options are available. Although the results of total elbow arthroplasty in elbow OA are good (improvement in pain, range of motion, and functional outcome scores [73]), the indications for its use are limited to elderly patients with minimal physical demands. Furthermore, much of the evidence on elbow arthroplasty pertains to patients with inflammatory arthritis – a vastly different population with lower expectations as compared to the patient with primary or posttraumatic elbow OA. In the young patient with elbow OA (commonly posttraumatic), elbow arthroplasty has a high failure rate (among young patients with posttraumatic elbow OA, the rate of revision was 37 % at a mean follow-up of 91 months [74]; at 9 years follow-up for elbow arthroplasty performed in patients with posttraumatic elbow OA, there was a 19 % failure rate; and 75 % of these failures were in patients under 60 years of age at the time of the replacement [75]). In the older population, revision and complication rates are improved, albeit still higher than commonly performed joint replacements such as hip, knee, and shoulder [76]. For instance, a systematic review found the overall complication rate to be approximately 25 %, with a higher loosening rate among patients with a preoperative diagnosis of posttraumatic OA [76]. Given the technical demands of the procedure, it is not surprising that provider volume has an impact on outcome following total elbow arthroplasty, whereby surgeons who perform more than ten per year have lower revision rates [77]. An alternative to the total elbow arthroplasty is radiocapitellar replacement, and although early outcomes following radiocapitellar replacement have been encouraging [78–80], long-term outcomes and survivability remain unknown [73].

Outcome Assessment

The primary purpose of an outcome scoring system is to establish the severity of impairment, track the response to treatment, compare treatments, and report outcomes in a meaningful way [8]. There are two primary types of outcome scoring systems: physician-completed or patient-completed questionnaires. There is a recent emphasis on the latter, which have become the gold standard in the orthopedic literature [81, 82]. To deem a scoring system valid, it must demonstrate reliability, consistency, and reproducibility [82].

Shoulder

There are a number of shoulder scoring systems [82]; however, the Western Ontario Osteoarthritis of the Shoulder Index (WOOS) [83] is the only scoring system to be specifically developed, validated, and recommended for use in patients with primary glenohumeral OA [84]. Initially developed to be used as the primary outcome measure in clinical trials involving patients with symptomatic primary glenohumeral OA [85], the WOOS is a 19-item, patient-completed scoring system that assesses four domains: pain and physical symptoms; sport, recreation, and work; lifestyle function; and emotion function. A minimal clinically important difference (change in score that is clinically relevant) has not been determined for the WOOS [84]. For general assessment of the shoulder, the American Shoulder and Elbow Surgeons Shoulder Score [86], the University of California Los Angeles Shoulder Score [87], the Disabilities of the Arm, Shoulder, and Hand Score [88], and the Single Assessment Numeric Evaluation [89] have all been recommended [84], whereas the American Shoulder and Elbow Surgeons Shoulder Score [86] and the Shoulder Pain and Disability Index [90] were found to be the most responsive instruments for assessment of patient improvement following total shoulder arthroplasty [91] – a treatment for end-stage glenohumeral OA.

Elbow

At present, no scoring system has been created specifically for patients with elbow OA; however, a recent review of the literature identified 12 commonly used elbow-specific scoring systems [81], including the Liverpool Elbow Score [92], the Elbow Functional Assessment [93], the Mayo Elbow Performance Score [94], the American Shoulder and Elbow Surgeons Elbow Score [95], the Hospital for Special Surgery Elbow Assessment Scale [96], the shortened version of the Hospital for Special Surgery Elbow Assessment Scale [97], the Ewald Scoring System [98], the Broberg and Morrey rating system [99], the Pritchard Score [94], the Oxford Elbow Score [100], the Patient-Rated Elbow Evaluation [95], and the Patient-Rated Tennis Elbow Evaluation [101]. Despite the plethora of elbow-specific scoring systems, the authors concluded that only the Oxford Elbow Score was validated using high-quality methodology on heterogeneous patient populations, including elbow OA [81]. Briefly, the Oxford Elbow Score is a patient-completed outcome measure that comprises three scales, including elbow function, pain, and social-psychological domains, and is scored on a 100-point scale (0–100) [100]. The minimal clinically important difference for the elbow function, pain, and social-psychological domains was approximately 10, 18, and 18 points, respectively [102].

Conclusions

Management of patients with shoulder or elbow OA is complex. Although favorable outcomes have been reported following arthroplasty of the shoulder or elbow, success appears to be highly dependent upon appropriate patient selection, and evidence pertaining to outcomes is quite limited. As explored in this chapter, clinicians who manage patients with shoulder or elbow OA should not only be familiar with the various treatment options but also the outcomes and limitations of each. Perhaps most importantly, patients should be appropriately counseled and realistic expectations established.

References

1. Gartsman GM, et al. Self-assessment of general health status in patients with five common shoulder conditions. J Shoulder Elbow Surg. 1998;7(3):228–37.
2. Memel DS, et al. General practitioners miss disability and anxiety as well as depression in their patients with osteoarthritis. Br J Gen Pract. 2000;50(457):645–8.
3. Oh JH, et al. The prevalence of shoulder osteoarthritis in the elderly Korean population: association with risk factors and function. J Shoulder Elbow Surg. 2011;20(5):756–63.
4. Kim SH, et al. Increasing incidence of shoulder arthroplasty in the United States. J Bone Joint Surg Am. 2011;93(24):2249–54.
5. Adams JE, et al. Shoulder arthroplasty in Olmsted County, Minnesota, 1976–2000: a population-based study. J Shoulder Elbow Surg. 2006;15(1):50–5.

6. Day JS, et al. Prevalence and projections of total shoulder and elbow arthroplasty in the United States to 2015. J Shoulder Elbow Surg. 2010;19(8):1115–20.
7. Cheung EV, Adams R, Morrey BF. Primary osteoarthritis of the elbow: current treatment options. J Am Acad Orthop Surg. 2008;16(2):77–87.
8. Gramstad GD, Galatz LM. Management of elbow osteoarthritis. J Bone Joint Surg Am. 2006;88(2):421–30.
9. Kamineni S. Observations on the epidemiology of total elbow arthroplasties in a statewide database: is it time for a national U.S. joint registry? Commentary on an article by David M. Gay, MD, et al.: "Indications and reoperation rates for total elbow arthroplasty: an analysis of trends in New York State". J Bone Joint Surg Am. 2012;94(2), e12.
10. Gay DM, et al. Indications and reoperation rates for total elbow arthroplasty: an analysis of trends in New York State. J Bone Joint Surg Am. 2012;94(2):110–7.
11. Millett PJ, Gobezie R, Boykin RE. Shoulder osteoarthritis: diagnosis and management. Am Fam Physician. 2008;78(5):605–11.
12. Neer CS, Craig EV, Fukuda H. Cuff-tear arthropathy. J Bone Joint Surg Am. 1983;65(9):1232–44.
13. Feeley BT, Gallo RA, Craig EV. Cuff tear arthropathy: current trends in diagnosis and surgical management. J Shoulder Elbow Surg. 2009;18(3):484–94.
14. Kramer EJ, et al. Evaluation of cartilage degeneration in a rat model of rotator cuff tear arthropathy. J Shoulder Elbow Surg. 2013;22(12):1702–9.
15. Oh JH, et al. Does a critical rotator cuff tear stage exist?: a biomechanical study of rotator cuff tear progression in human cadaver shoulders. J Bone Joint Surg Am. 2011;93(22):2100–9.
16. Sher JS, et al. Abnormal findings on magnetic resonance images of asymptomatic shoulders. J Bone Joint Surg Am. 1995;77(1):10–5.
17. Milgrom C, et al. Rotator-cuff changes in asymptomatic adults. The effect of age, hand dominance and gender. J Bone Joint Surg Br. 1995;77(2):296–8.
18. Ecklund KJ, et al. Rotator cuff tear arthropathy. J Am Acad Orthop Surg. 2007;15(6):340–9.
19. McNickle AG, et al. Postsurgical glenohumeral arthritis in young adults. Am J Sports Med. 2009;37(9):1784–91.
20. Solomon DJ, et al. Glenohumeral chondrolysis after arthroscopy: a systematic review of potential contributors and causal pathways. Arthroscopy. 2009;25(11):1329–42.
21. Yeh PC, Kharrazi FD. Postarthroscopic glenohumeral chondrolysis. J Am Acad Orthop Surg. 2012;20(2):102–12.
22. Boileau P, et al. Shoulder arthroplasty for the treatment of the sequelae of fractures of the proximal humerus. J Shoulder Elbow Surg. 2001;10(4):299–308.
23. Boileau P, et al. Proximal humerus fracture sequelae: impact of a new radiographic classification on arthroplasty. Clin Orthop Relat Res. 2006;442:121–30.
24. Schenker ML, et al. Pathogenesis and prevention of posttraumatic osteoarthritis after intraarticular fracture. J Am Acad Orthop Surg. 2014;22(1):20–8.
25. Anderson DD, et al. Post-traumatic osteoarthritis: improved understanding and opportunities for early intervention. J Orthop Res. 2011;29(6):802–9.
26. Marx RG, et al. Development of arthrosis following dislocation of the shoulder: a case–control study. J Shoulder Elbow Surg. 2002;11(1):1–5.
27. Samilson RL, Prieto V. Dislocation arthropathy of the shoulder. J Bone Joint Surg Am. 1983;65(4):456–60.
28. Hovelius L, Saeboe M. Neer Award 2008: arthropathy after primary anterior shoulder dislocation – 223 shoulders prospectively followed up for twenty-five years. J Shoulder Elbow Surg. 2009;18(3):339–47.
29. Kavaja L, et al. Arthrosis of glenohumeral joint after arthroscopic Bankart repair: a long-term follow-up of 13 years. J Shoulder Elbow Surg. 2012;21(3):350–5.
30. Buscayret F, et al. Glenohumeral arthrosis in anterior instability before and after surgical treatment: incidence and contributing factors. Am J Sports Med. 2004;32(5):1165–72.
31. Cameron ML, et al. The prevalence of glenohumeral osteoarthrosis in unstable shoulders. Am J Sports Med. 2003;31(1):53–5.

32. Guitton TG, et al. Incidence and risk factors for the development of radiographic arthrosis after traumatic elbow injuries. J Hand Surg Am. 2010;35(12):1976–80.
33. An KN, et al. Determination of muscle and joint forces: a new technique to solve the indeterminate problem. J Biomech Eng. 1984;106(4):364–7.
34. Amis AA, et al. The derivation of elbow joint forces, and their relation to prosthesis design. J Med Eng Technol. 1979;3(5):229–34.
35. Goldberg VM, et al. Total elbow arthroplasty. J Bone Joint Surg Am. 1988;70(5):778–83.
36. An KN, et al. Pressure distribution on articular surfaces: application to joint stability evaluation. J Biomech. 1990;23(10):1013–20.
37. Matsen FA, Ziegler DW, DeBartolo SE. Patient self-assessment of health status and function in glenohumeral degenerative joint disease. J Shoulder Elbow Surg. 1995;4(5):345–51.
38. Chen AL, et al. Management of bone loss associated with recurrent anterior glenohumeral instability. Am J Sports Med. 2005;33(6):912–25.
39. Sears BW, et al. Posttraumatic elbow arthritis in the young adult: evaluation and management. J Am Acad Orthop Surg. 2012;20(11):704–14.
40. Ward WG, Belhobek GH, Anderson TE. Arthroscopic elbow findings: correlation with preoperative radiographic studies. Arthroscopy. 1992;8(4):498–502.
41. Allain J, Goutallier D, Glorion C. Long-term results of the Latarjet procedure for the treatment of anterior instability of the shoulder. J Bone Joint Surg Am. 1998;80(6):841–52.
42. Gerber C. Latissimus dorsi transfer for the treatment of irreparable tears of the rotator cuff. Clin Orthop Relat Res. 1992;275:152–60.
43. Weinstein DM, et al. Arthroscopic debridement of the shoulder for osteoarthritis. Arthroscopy. 2000;16(5):471–6.
44. Guyette TM, et al. Results of arthroscopic subacromial decompression in patients with subacromial impingement and glenohumeral degenerative joint disease. J Shoulder Elbow Surg. 2002;11(4):299–304.
45. Elsharkawi M, et al. Reliability of radiologic glenohumeral osteoarthritis classifications. J Shoulder Elbow Surg. 2013;22(8):1063–7.
46. Sirveaux F, et al. Grammont inverted total shoulder arthroplasty in the treatment of glenohumeral osteoarthritis with massive rupture of the cuff. Results of a multicentre study of 80 shoulders. J Bone Joint Surg Br. 2004;86(3):388–95.
47. Kappe T, et al. Reliability of radiologic classification for cuff tear arthropathy. J Shoulder Elbow Surg. 2011;20(4):543–7.
48. Visotsky JL, et al. Cuff tear arthropathy: pathogenesis, classification, and algorithm for treatment. J Bone Joint Surg Am. 2004;86-A Suppl 2:35–40.
49. Hamada K, et al. Roentgenographic findings in massive rotator cuff tears. A long-term observation. Clin Orthop Relat Res. 1990;254:92–6.
50. Rettig LA, Hastings H, Feinberg JR. Primary osteoarthritis of the elbow: lack of radiographic evidence for morphologic predisposition, results of operative debridement at intermediate follow-up, and basis for a new radiographic classification system. J Shoulder Elbow Surg. 2008;17(1):97–105.
51. Anz AW, et al. Application of biologics in the treatment of the rotator cuff, meniscus, cartilage, and osteoarthritis. J Am Acad Orthop Surg. 2014;22(2):68–79.
52. Izquierdo R, et al. Treatment of glenohumeral osteoarthritis. J Am Acad Orthop Surg. 2010;18(6):375–82.
53. Silverstein E, Leger R, Shea KP. The use of intra-articular hylan G-F 20 in the treatment of symptomatic osteoarthritis of the shoulder: a preliminary study. Am J Sports Med. 2007;35(6):979–85.
54. Kwon YW, Eisenberg G, Zuckerman JD. Sodium hyaluronate for the treatment of chronic shoulder pain associated with glenohumeral osteoarthritis: a multicenter, randomized, double-blind, placebo-controlled trial. J Shoulder Elbow Surg. 2013;22(5):584–94.
55. van Brakel RW, Eygendaal D. Intra-articular injection of hyaluronic acid is not effective for the treatment of post-traumatic osteoarthritis of the elbow. Arthroscopy. 2006;22(11):1199–203.

56. Denard PJ, Wirth MA, Orfaly RM. Management of glenohumeral arthritis in the young adult. J Bone Joint Surg Am. 2011;93(9):885–92.
57. Bryant D, et al. A comparison of pain, strength, range of motion, and functional outcomes after hemiarthroplasty and total shoulder arthroplasty in patients with osteoarthritis of the shoulder. A systematic review and meta-analysis. J Bone Joint Surg Am. 2005;87(9):1947–56.
58. Radnay CS, et al. Total shoulder replacement compared with humeral head replacement for the treatment of primary glenohumeral osteoarthritis: a systematic review. J Shoulder Elbow Surg. 2007;16(4):396–402.
59. Raiss P, et al. Longitudinal observational study of total shoulder replacements with cement: fifteen to twenty-year follow-up. J Bone Joint Surg Am. 2014;96(3):198–205.
60. Ogilvie-Harris DJ, Wiley AM. Arthroscopic surgery of the shoulder. A general appraisal. J Bone Joint Surg Br. 1986;68(2):201–7.
61. Saltzman MD, et al. Comparison of patients undergoing primary shoulder arthroplasty before and after the age of fifty. J Bone Joint Surg Am. 2010;92(1):42–7.
62. Kerr BJ, McCarty EC. Outcome of arthroscopic débridement is worse for patients with glenohumeral arthritis of both sides of the joint. Clin Orthop Relat Res. 2008;466(3):634–8.
63. Strauss EJ, et al. The high failure rate of biologic resurfacing of the glenoid in young patients with glenohumeral arthritis. J Shoulder Elbow Surg. 2014;23(3):409–19.
64. Sperling JW, Cofield RH, Rowland CM. Neer hemiarthroplasty and Neer total shoulder arthroplasty in patients fifty years old or less. Long-term results. J Bone Joint Surg Am. 1998;80(4):464–73.
65. Muh SJ, et al. Early follow-up of reverse total shoulder arthroplasty in patients sixty years of age or younger. J Bone Joint Surg Am. 2013;95(20):1877–83.
66. Ek ET, et al. Reverse total shoulder arthroplasty for massive irreparable rotator cuff tears in patients younger than 65 years old: results after five to fifteen years. J Shoulder Elbow Surg. 2013;22(9):1199–208.
67. Morrey BF. Primary degenerative arthritis of the elbow. Treatment by ulnohumeral arthroplasty. J Bone Joint Surg Br. 1992;74(3):409–13.
68. Vincent JI, Vandervoort AA, Macdermid JC. A literature synthesis indicates very low quality, but consistent evidence of improvements in function after surgical interventions for primary osteoarthritis of the elbow. Arthritis. 2013;2013:487615.
69. O'Driscoll SW. Arthroscopic treatment for osteoarthritis of the elbow. Orthop Clin North Am. 1995;26(4):691–706.
70. Oka Y, Ohta K, Saitoh I. Debridement arthroplasty for osteoarthritis of the elbow. Clin Orthop Relat Res. 1998;351:127–34.
71. Wada T, et al. Débridement arthroplasty for primary osteoarthritis of the elbow. J Bone Joint Surg Am. 2004;86-A(2):233–41.
72. Antuña SA, et al. Ulnohumeral arthroplasty for primary degenerative arthritis of the elbow: long-term outcome and complications. J Bone Joint Surg Am. 2002;84-A(12):2168–73.
73. Giannicola G, et al. Radial head, radiocapitellar and total elbow arthroplasties: a review of recent literature. Injury. 2014;45(2):428–36.
74. Celli A, Morrey BF. Total elbow arthroplasty in patients forty years of age or less. J Bone Joint Surg Am. 2009;91(6):1414–8.
75. Throckmorton T, et al. Failure patterns after linked semiconstrained total elbow arthroplasty for posttraumatic arthritis. J Bone Joint Surg Am. 2010;92(6):1432–41.
76. Voloshin I, et al. Complications of total elbow replacement: a systematic review. J Shoulder Elbow Surg. 2011;20(1):158–68.
77. Jenkins PJ, et al. Total elbow replacement: outcome of 1,146 arthroplasties from the Scottish Arthroplasty Project. Acta Orthop. 2013;84(2):119–23.
78. Heijink A, Morrey BF, Cooney WP. Radiocapitellar hemiarthroplasty for radiocapitellar arthritis: a report of three cases. J Shoulder Elbow Surg. 2008;17(2):e12–5.
79. Giannicola G, et al. Hemilateral resurfacing arthroplasty in posttraumatic degenerative elbow resulting from humeral capitellum malunion. J Shoulder Elbow Surg. 2010;19(1):e12–7.

80. Kepler CK, et al. Radiocapitellar prosthetic arthroplasty for capitellar nonunion. J Shoulder Elbow Surg. 2010;19(2):e13–7.
81. The B, et al. Elbow-specific clinical rating systems: extent of established validity, reliability, and responsiveness. J Shoulder Elbow Surg. 2013;22(10):1380–94.
82. Roller AS, et al. Outcome instruments for the shoulder. Arthroscopy. 2013;29(5):955–64.
83. Lo IK, Griffin S, Kirkley A. The development of a disease-specific quality of life measurement tool for osteoarthritis of the shoulder: The Western Ontario Osteoarthritis of the Shoulder (WOOS) index. Osteoarthritis Cartilage. 2001;9(8):771–8.
84. Wright RW, Baumgarten KM. Shoulder outcomes measures. J Am Acad Orthop Surg. 2010;18(7):436–44.
85. Kirkley A, Griffin S, Dainty K. Scoring systems for the functional assessment of the shoulder. Arthroscopy. 2003;19(10):1109–20.
86. Richards RR, et al. A standardized method for the assessment of shoulder function. J Shoulder Elbow Surg. 1994;3(6):347–52.
87. Amstutz HC, Sew Hoy AL, Clarke IC. UCLA anatomic total shoulder arthroplasty. Clin Orthop Relat Res. 1981;155:7–20.
88. Hudak PL, Amadio PC, Bombardier C. Development of an upper extremity outcome measure: the DASH (disabilities of the arm, shoulder and hand) [corrected]. The Upper Extremity Collaborative Group (UECG). Am J Ind Med. 1996;29(6):602–8.
89. Williams GN, et al. Comparison of the Single Assessment Numeric Evaluation method and two shoulder rating scales. Outcomes measures after shoulder surgery. Am J Sports Med. 1999;27(2):214–21.
90. Roach KE, et al. Development of a shoulder pain and disability index. Arthritis Care Res. 1991;4(4):143–9.
91. Angst F, et al. Responsiveness of six outcome assessment instruments in total shoulder arthroplasty. Arthritis Rheum. 2008;59(3):391–8.
92. Sathyamoorthy P, et al. Development and validation of an elbow score. Rheumatology (Oxford). 2004;43(11):1434–40.
93. de Boer YA, et al. Clinical reliability and validity of elbow functional assessment in rheumatoid arthritis. J Rheumatol. 1999;26(9):1909–17.
94. Turchin DC, Beaton DE, Richards RR. Validity of observer-based aggregate scoring systems as descriptors of elbow pain, function, and disability. J Bone Joint Surg Am. 1998;80(2):154–62.
95. MacDermid JC. Outcome evaluation in patients with elbow pathology: issues in instrument development and evaluation. J Hand Ther. 2001;14(2):105–14.
96. Inglis AE, Pellicci PM. Total elbow replacement. J Bone Joint Surg Am. 1980;62(8):1252–8.
97. Figgie MP, et al. Results of reconstruction for failed total elbow arthroplasty. Clin Orthop Relat Res. 1990;253:123–32.
98. Ewald FC. Total elbow replacement. Orthop Clin North Am. 1975;6(3):685–96.
99. Broberg MA, Morrey BF. Results of delayed excision of the radial head after fracture. J Bone Joint Surg Am. 1986;68(5):669–74.
100. Dawson J, et al. The development and validation of a patient-reported questionnaire to assess outcomes of elbow surgery. J Bone Joint Surg Br. 2008;90(4):466–73.
101. Rompe JD, Overend TJ, MacDermid JC. Validation of the Patient-rated Tennis Elbow Evaluation Questionnaire. J Hand Ther. 2007;20(1):3–10; quiz 11.
102. Dawson J, et al. Comparative responsiveness and minimal change for the Oxford Elbow Score following surgery. Qual Life Res. 2008;17(10):1257–67.

Chapter 4
Lumbar Spine Osteoarthritis

Y. Raja Rampersaud, Akihiro Nakamura, and Stephen J. Lewis

Key Points

- Spinal degeneration is often not considered in the same context as osteoarthritis (OA); however, the degenerative changes in the disc and, in particular, the synovial facet joints are consistent with those of OA elsewhere.

Y.R. Rampersaud, MD, FRCSC (✉)
Division of Orthopaedic Surgery, Department of Surgery, Toronto Western Hospital, University Health Network, University of Toronto, Toronto, ON, Canada

Arthritis Program, Toronto Western Hospital, University Health Network, University of Toronto, Toronto, ON, Canada

Spinal Program, Krembil Neuroscience Center, Toronto Western Hospital, University Health Network, University of Toronto, Toronto, ON, Canada

Division of Orthopaedic Surgery, Department of Surgery, University of Toronto, Toronto Western Hospital, University Health Network, 399 Bathurst St. East Wing, 1-441, Toronto, ON M5T-2S8, Canada
e-mail: raja.rampersaud@uhn.ca

A. Nakamura, MD
Division of Genetics and Development, Toronto Western Research Institute, University Health Network, Toronto, ON Canada

S.J. Lewis, MD, MSc, FRCSC
Division of Orthopaedic Surgery, Department of Surgery, Toronto Western Hospital, University Health Network, University of Toronto, Toronto, ON, Canada

Arthritis Program, Toronto Western Hospital, University Health Network, University of Toronto, Toronto, ON, Canada

Spinal Program, Krembil Neuroscience Center, Toronto Western Hospital, University Health Network, University of Toronto, Toronto, ON, Canada

M. Kapoor, N.N. Mahomed (eds.), *Osteoarthritis: Pathogenesis, Diagnosis, Available Treatments, Drug Safety, Regenerative and Precision Medicine*,
DOI 10.1007/978-3-319-19560-5_4

- The main clinical symptoms of lumbar spine OA (i.e., facet joint OA) are low back pain and associated leg symptoms (pain, numbness, and weakness).
- Various factors contribute to the degenerative changes, including age, biomechanical factors, systemic factors, genetics, and lifestyle.
- Although there is no universal nonsurgical or surgical treatment for spine OA, exercise and activity modification is typically accepted as an effective form of initial management.
- For end-stage disease, nonsurgical treatment has limited efficacy and surgical intervention in appropriately selected patients is associated with good patient-reported outcomes that are comparable to those associated with total knee replacement for OA.
- This chapter focuses on the latest knowledge on lumbar spine OA and associated clinical presentations to enable further understanding from both a clinical and a research perspective.

Introduction

Each spinal segment, except one cervical spine level (C1–C2), consists of an anterior situated intervertebral disc and smaller paired posterior facet joints (also termed the zygapophyseal joint), thereby comprising a "three-joint complex." Intervertebral disc degeneration and vertebral osteophyte formation do not share the exact same pathophysiological process of degeneration associated with osteoarthritis, in part due to a lack of synovial structures, and thus do not meet the definition of OA. However, the facet joint is a synovial joint (hyaline cartilage overlying subchondral bone, a synovial membrane, and a joint capsule) that shares the same pathophysiologic attributes of appendicular OA [1, 2]. Due to the wide variety of confounding factors, the interplay between disc degeneration and spine OA as they relate to clinical sequelae and OA as a whole remains unclear [3]. Given the increasing prevalence and tremendous disease burden of low back pain (LBP) and the overlap with that of OA [4–7], spine OA represents an important area of clinical and research focus.

OA is a major cause of disability and is one of the most frequent musculoskeletal disorders [8, 9]. LBP, including that caused by spine OA, is ranked as the single leading cause of disability worldwide [8, 9]. From a societal perspective, the annual economic burden of spine OA, including health-care costs and lost work hours, has been estimated in billions of dollars [10]. Clinically, OA is characterized by cartilage deterioration, persistent inflammation, synovial fibrosis, sclerosis of the subchondral bone, and osteophyte formation at the joint margin [11]. OA is observed throughout the appendicular and axial skeleton, affecting both weight-bearing and non-weight-bearing joints. There exists a tremendous amount of clinical and basic science research in OA. However, in the spine due to a historical focus on disc degeneration and the association of spine degeneration with neurologically induced symptoms and sequelae, the epidemiologic, clinical, and basic research focus of appendicular OA and spine degeneration typically occurs in isolation from each other. Furthermore, the study of facet joint OA is grossly deficient.

A variety of both mechanical and nonmechanical factors can contribute to the pathogenesis of spine OA [3]. Aging is the most common risk factor; however, others such as genetic and systemic factors similar to what have been demonstrated for knee OA [1] may also play significant roles for the pathogenesis and warrant exploration and discussion. In particular, the identification of spine OA specific microRNAs (miRNAs) may have potential of being biomarkers that both enable early disease detection and enable targeted treatment(s). At present, we still rely on clinical diagnosis of facetogenic-based symptoms (i.e., extension-based LBP and/or neurogenic claudication relieved by forward flexion) and correlation with imaging such as computed tomography (CT) and magnetic resonance imaging (MRI) [12, 13]. However, imaging does not always correlate with clinical symptoms, with many asymptomatic individuals demonstrating significant structural abnormalities on spine imaging [14]. Consequently, in the absence of red flags (e.g., suspicion of cancer, infection, fracture, or neurological deficits), imaging is not required, nor recommended, for LBP that is manageable and nonprogressive. The treatment options for spine OA ranges from self-management to complex surgery. Although generally associated with a favorable natural history and manageable by conservative means [13], approximately 20 % of patients with spine OA have progressive or persistent severe symptoms that undergo surgical management [15]. Surgery is typically aimed at addressing the structural changes that have led to increasing nerve compression due to facet joint and ligamentous hypertrophy (i.e., lumbar spinal stenosis (LSS) causing neurogenic claudication) and/or failure of both facet joint and the disc, leading to spinal instability with resultant degenerative spondylolisthesis (slippage of one vertebrae over the next in the anterior-posterior plane) and/or degenerative scoliosis (coronal/rotational plane deformity that develops in late adulthood).

In this chapter, we focus on the latest knowledge on lumbar spine OA, including the epidemiology, pathogenesis, clinical characteristics, and treatments options. In addition, we will touch on areas requiring further research to improve our understanding of spine OA and its role in the overall bigger picture of OA.

Anatomy and Kinematics of the Spine

Basic knowledge of spine structure is necessary to understand spine OA. The human spine consists of 33 bony vertebrae: 7 cervical, 12 thoracic, 5 lumbar, 5 sacral (fused), and 4 coccygeal (usually fused). At every spine level below the second cervical vertebra, the term "three-joint complex" is often used in describing the spinal structure, which is formed by the three articulations between two vertebral levels: one disc and two facet joints (Fig. 4.1). Together, with the ligamentous

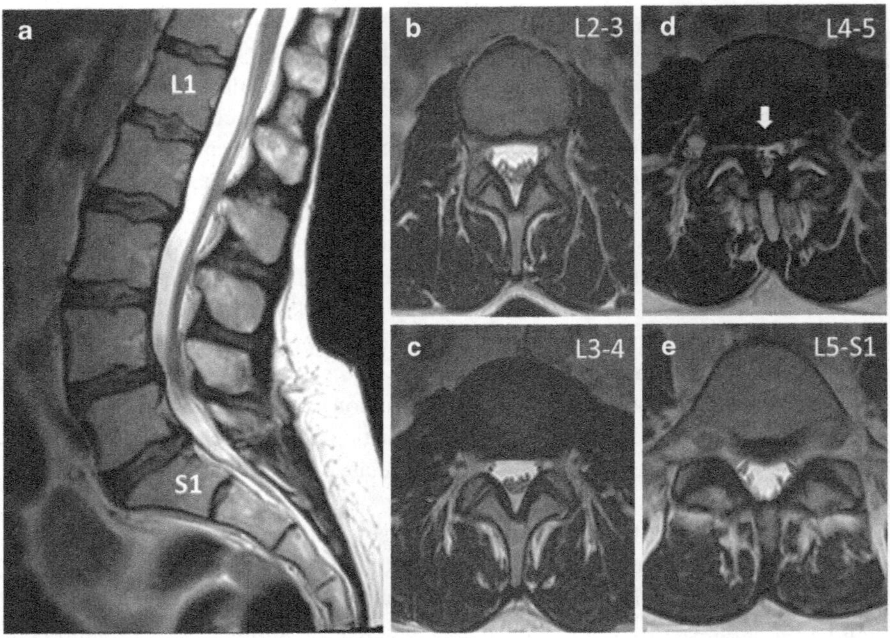

Fig. 4.1 (**a**) Midsagittal MRI demonstrating the L1–S1 vertebrae in a 47-year-old female. (**b–d**) Axial views of the facet joint from L2–L3 to L5–S1 vertebrae. Each vertebra connects to an adjacent vertebra with two facet joints (**b–e**) and intervertebral disc to form the three-joint complex that makes up the spine functional unit. As can be seen, the orientation of the facet joints progressively changes from a more horizontal orientation at L5–S1 to a more oblique or vertical orientation at L2–L3. This enables complex kinematics of the lumbar spine. Also demonstrated in (**d**) is the evidence of facet joint OA, with hypertrophy of the bony articulations and the ligament that is resulting in stenosis of the spinal canal (*white arrow*) compared to other levels where the facets are essentially normal in appearance. In addition, there is minimal disc degeneration in this particular patient

structures, the pairing of two vertebrae is termed the functional spinal unit. Although these three joints are closely related to each other functionally, the facet joints are anatomically distinct from the disc because they are true synovial joints, containing hyaline cartilage, synovial membrane, and a fibrous joint capsule [16]. The facet joints form an articulation between the inferior articular process of the vertebrae above and the superior articular process of the vertebrae below and enable the significant multiplanar motion of the spine. In the lumbar region, the facet joints are inclined to a nearly vertical and oblique orientation and are curvilinear, such that they limit rotation as well as forward displacement, but allow significant flexion [17, 18]. Clinically, the range of motion for the lumbar spine varies significantly and depends on age (reduces with increasing age), sex (greater in women than men), the presence or absence of LBP (reduced with LBP), and most significantly the method of measurement [19]. In healthy individuals, flexion has been reported to range between 23° and 92°, extension 17–56°, lateral flexion 28–44°, and rotation 5–15° (in either direction). The spinal musculature is also critical to spinal kinematic and dynamic stability. The musculature controls the movement of the spine and dynamically stabilizes the spinal functional units throughout physiologic spinal movement [20].

Joint alignment, load distribution, and wide range of movement are thought to be major anatomical factors in the development and progression of spinal OA (see below) [21].

Prevalence

The exact incidence of spine OA is impossible to pinpoint due to the fact that the degenerative process is initiated years before the clinical symptoms and morphologic abnormalities are detected. In addition, many patients with mild and/or episodic symptoms do not seek health care. Nevertheless, cross-sectional population-based studies in adults give a reasonable estimate of the prevalence of spine OA. The lumbar region is the most common sight of spine OA. However, it must be clear that one has to consider the gross difference between symptomatic prevalence and radiographic or cadaveric prevalence of facet joint OA. For example, a recent population-based clinical study showed that the prevalence of symptomatic lumbar facet joint OA was 7.4 % [22]. Comparatively, cadaveric studies of the lumbar spine reported that at least 50 % of the population demonstrates lumbar facet joint OA [23]. It is well established that the radiographic prevalence of spine OA increases with age similar to other synovial joints. Kalichman et al., from the Framingham Heart Study, reported OA of the facet joints was present in 24.0 % of <40-year-olds, 44.7 % of 40–49-year-olds, 74.2 % of 50–59-year-olds, 89.2 % of 60–69-year-olds, and 69.2 % of >70-year-olds [24]. Surprisingly, even for individuals who are less than 40 years old, the presence of facet joint OA ranges from 3.4 to 36 % [1, 22, 25]. In terms of gender, data is limited and thus it is not clear which gender is more radiographically or clinically affected by spinal OA [25]. However, Kalichman et al. [26] have demonstrated a greater ratio of degenerative spondylolisthesis in women. Recent work by Goode et al. from the Johnston County Osteoarthritis Project has also shown facet joint OA is radiographically greater in women (61.6 %) than men (51.6 %); however, facet joint OA was not correlated to self-reported LBP.

Joint Areas Affected

Almost all studies showed that the level of L4–L5 is the most affected region among lumbar spines, followed by L3–L4 or L5–S1 [23, 24, 27, 28]. Kalichman et al. reported the prevalence at the spinal level and noted that the prevalence of facet joint OA was 15.1 % at L2–L3, 30.6 % at L3–L4, 45.1 % at L4–L5, and 38.2 % at L5–S1 [24].

Disc degeneration is considered as another important factor for progressing spine OA. Recent studies revealed that disc degeneration precedes the changes of OA in other joints such as the knee and hip and is more common [29–31]. Bajwa et al.

reported in the 340 specimens of a cadaveric human study that 35 % of specimens of age younger than 29 years had evidence of degenerative disc and 17 % of them had hip OA changes. At 70 years, 100 % of specimens had evidence of disc degeneration and 50 % of hip OA changes. They found that there was a significant association between lumber disc degeneration and hip OA changes and lumbar degeneration precedes hip degeneration [31]. Fujiwara and his colleague reported the relationship between facet joint OA and disc degeneration on the lumbar study assessing 84 lumbar facet joints by MRI [29]. They found all patients with facet joint OA had some degrees of disc degeneration, even the population under 40 years old. In addition, they noted that disc degeneration was the primary event leading to facet joint OA, due to increased loading of facets that occurs as a result of disc degeneration. A similar study reported by Vernon-Rogerts and Pirie showed that disc degeneration occurred in advance of facet joint OA and the formation of osteophytes [30]. In a community-based population study, Suri et al. demonstrated similar findings for the majority of individuals [32]. However, 22 % of the individuals studied demonstrate patterns of degeneration, beginning in the posterior joints. The authors found that increased age and BMI and female sex may be related to the occurrence of isolated posterior degeneration in these individuals. In a preliminary work for our center, we have found that this occurrence may also be associated with spino-pelvic parameters, in particular a higher pelvic incidence, which is a fixed anatomical relationship between the pelvis and sacrum that imparts greater lumbar lordosis and, hence, increased facet loading (Fig. 4.2) particularly at the lower lumbar levels [33]. The pelvic incidence in women is typically greater than men.

Symptoms of Spine OA

Activity-limiting LBP, in particular, has a worldwide lifetime prevalence of approximately 39 % and a similar annual prevalence of 38 % [9]. LBP is second only to the common cold in frequency [34], is the most common reason for time-off work, and has a total social cost of more than $100 billion annually [35]. Up to 85 % of patients never receive a definitive diagnosis and are classified as having nonspecific pain [36]. The source of LBP remains a very controversial topic, and a detailed discussion is not within the scope of this chapter, but suffice it to say that LBP, as is OA pain, is multifactorial involving both peripheral and central mechanisms [3].

As noted above, the prevalence of radiographic spine OA compared with symptomatic spine OA is grossly different. Previous studies assessing the association between LBP and imaging characteristics of spinal degeneration are listed in Table 4.1. The majority of studies have found that disc space narrowing (DSN) is the most significant radiographic factor associated with LBP. In a recent study of community-based US older adults, Suri et al. are the first to demonstrate that severe facet joint OA was more common in participants with back pain than those without (63.2 % vs. 46.7 %; $p=0.03$) [37]. In the study of 252 patients who were participants in the Framingham Heart Study multivariable analysis, adjusting for sociode-

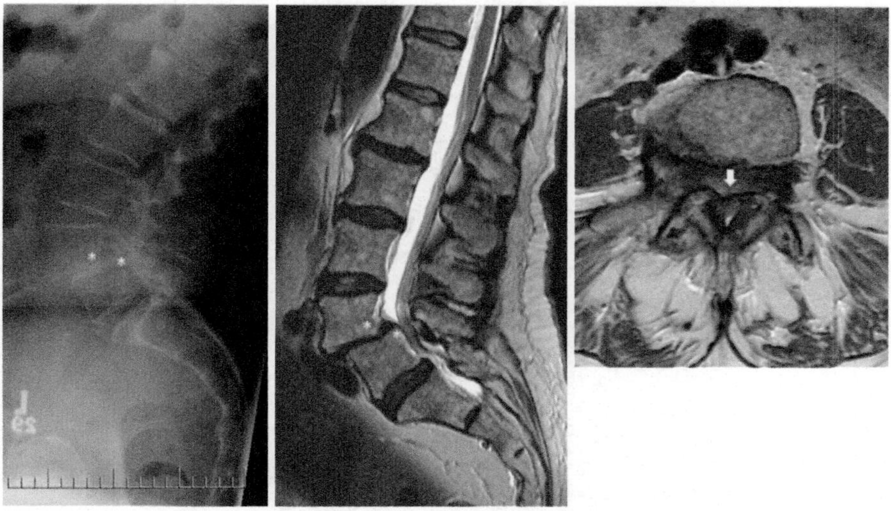

Fig. 4.2 Lateral standing radiograph, midsagittal MRI, and axial MRI at L4–L5 in a 71-year-old female with a degenerative spondylolisthesis at L4–L5 and associated back pain and neurogenic claudication with less than one-block walking tolerance. As marked by the *white asterisks*, the L4 vertebra has slipped forward on the L5 vertebra. In combination with the facet joint OA, this causes severe spinal stenosis to the point where the spinal fluid is no longer seen (*white arrow*) compared to the degree of stenosis demonstrated in Fig. 4.1. This particular patient has a high pelvic incidence (74°; normal is approximately 50 ± 10°) which gives her higher than normal lordosis, which increases the loading of the facet joints and decreases the load on the disc. Complete disc collapse is seen at the L4–L5 level, with relative normal discs above and below

mographics, health factors, and disc height narrowing, the association of severe facet joint OA remained significant (odds ratio of 2.15 (95 % confidence interval, 1.13–4.08)), with a greater number of joints with severe facet joint OA also conferring a greater odds of having frequent back pain. Interestingly, disc height narrowing was independently associated with back pain in younger adults < age 60 years, but not in older adults. These findings conflict with prior studies [4, 24, 38] showing no association or only minimal association between facet joint OA and LBP. In these studies, patients were relatively younger and the severity of OA was not considered. Interestingly, studies that have investigated edema of the lumbar facet joint have showed significant correlation with LBP [39, 40]. Bone marrow edema is considered a possible cause of pain in the musculoskeletal system [41]; however, its diagnostic or prognostic capacity function remains unclear in the spine.

Osteophytes resulting from facet joint OA and/or ligamentous hypertrophy that is associated with facet joint OA (i.e., spinal stenosis) may directly impinge on the spinal nerve roots or the spinal cord which may cause severe pain and/or neurologically based back and leg symptoms, commonly termed neurogenic claudication [13, 42]. It is estimated that LSS causing neurogenic claudication affects about 20 % of people older than 65 years and about half of that group suffer serious restrictions in their daily routines [13, 43]. In a recent study by Battie et al., the authors demon-

Table 4.1 Previous studies shown the association between low back pain and clinical images of the spine

	Imaging modality	Mean age (years)	Sample size	Country	FOA OR (95 % CI)	DSN OR (95 % CI)	OST OR (95 % CI)
Savage et al. [143]	MRI	36	149	The UK	4.4 (0.9–21)	N/A	N/A
Pye et al. [144]	Radiograph	65	585	The UK	N/A	1.7 (1.1–2.4)	0.7 (0.4–1.4)
Kjaer et al. [38]	MRI	40	412	Denmark	1.1 (0.7–1.6)	1.8 (1.2–2.7)	N/A
Kalichman et al. [24]	CT	53	188	The USA	1.0 (0.5–2.1)	[a]K–L ≥ 2	[b]K–L ≥ 3
Muraki et al. [145]	Radiograph	74	2,288	Japan	N/A	[a]Men = 1.4 (0.9–2.4) Women = 1.8 (1.4–2.4)	[b]Men = 1.2 (0.7–1.9) Women = 1.0 (0.7–1.4)
de Schepper et al. [146]	Radiograph	65	2,819	The Netherlands	N/A	1.4 (1.1–1.7)	1.2 (1.0–1.5)
Kalichman et al. [147]	CT	53	187	The USA	0.8 (0.3–1.9)	1.4 (0.6–3.3)	N/A
Goode et al. [4]	Radiograph	60	840	The USA	0.8 (0.6–1.2)	1.4 (1.0–1.8)	1.1 (0.8–1.5)
Suri et al. [37]	CT	67	252	The USA	2.2 (1.1–4.0)	0.7 (0.4–1.3)	N/A

FOA facet joint osteoarthritis, *DSN* disc space narrowing, *OST* osteophyte

[a,b] Used Kellgren-Lawrence grading

strated that the associated health burden of LSS on health-related quality of life was significant and is about the same or greater than diabetes, heart disease, arthritis, or stroke. The hallmark of neurogenic claudication is spinal symptoms that are relieved by forward flexion (e.g., sitting or walking in a flexed posture using a "shopping cart") [12]. The physical exam is often normal; however, in more severe cases of LSS, static objective neurological deficits may occur.

Diagnosis

The diagnosis of spinal OA is ultimately based on medical history and physical examination and confirmed by imaging. The most common presentation is LBP with or without radicular or claudicant leg symptoms that are typically brought on by standing or walking (i.e., erect posture) and relieved by forward flexion of the spine [12, 13, 44]. Due to multiple potential sources, the presentation of symptomatic spine OA must be differentiated from other common causes of LBP [44, 45].

Differential Diagnosis

In clinical practice, patients with LBP regardless of presentation must be screened for red flags (e.g., fevers, unexplained weight loss, progressive neurological deficit) that are associated with more serious but less common causes of back pain (such as infection, cancer, or fracture) and represent an indication for urgent or emergent investigation in patients who present with LBP [46, 47]. With respect to facet joint OA, it is important that the typical clinical presentation of other mechanical LBP disorders be excluded as they all can increase progressively with age (often coexisting) (Table 4.2) [44].

Imaging

It is important to note that the severity of symptoms, treatment decisions, outcomes of treatment, and even the existence of symptoms do not strongly correlate with spinal imaging [14, 48, 49]. For example, 22–51 % of asymptomatic individuals have been shown to demonstrate MRI irregularities in their lumbar spine, with this number increasing to between 57 and 80 % for those over the age of 60 [50, 51].

Multiple modalities exist that can assess spine OA including radiography, CT, MRI, and hybrid single-photon emission computed tomography/CT (SPECT/CT). Plain radiograph, CT, and MRI are most commonly used in clinical practice (Table 4.3, Fig. 4.2).

Table 4.2 Common clinical presentation of mechanical low back pain

Clinical observation	Spine osteoarthritis causing LBP	Herniated disc causing radiculopathy	Spinal stenosis (end-stage spine OA causing claudication)	Degenerative disc causing LBP
Age (in years)	>40	30–50	>60	30–50
Straight leg raising (SLR) test	No	Yes	Yes (after standing and walking; SLR is typically negative)	No
Leg pain, numbness, or tingling	No	Yes	Yes	No
Dominant location	Back	Back/leg (unilateral)	Leg (unilateral or bilateral)	Back
Onset	Insidious	Acute	Insidious	Insidious
Increased with standing erect	Yes	No	Yes	Variable
Increased with sitting	No	Yes	No	Yes
Increased with forward bending	No	Yes	No	Yes

Modified from Hall et al. [45]

Table 4.3 Utility of clinical images to detect OA changes in the spine

	Disc		Facet joint						
	Degeneration	Intervertebral narrowing	Joint space narrowing	Osteophyte of articular process	Hypertrophy of articular process	Sclerosis	Subchondral erosion	Subchondral cysts	Subchondral edema
Radiography	x	√	√	√	x	√	x	x	x
CT	x	√√	√√	√√	√√	√√	√√	√	x
MRI	√√	√√	√√	√√	√√	x	√√	√√	√√

Modified from Gellhorn et al. [1]
x no utility, √ moderate utility, √√ good utility

Radiographs

Due to their inexpensive cost and universal availability, radiographs remain the most common initial imaging choice of many bone and joint disorders [52]. They are typically limited to picking up gross abnormalities of the bone and to a lesser degree the soft tissue; however, due to the ability to easily image in an upright/loaded or dynamic posture(s), they are superior for the assessment of malalignment or instability of the spine. For spine OA, radiographs are limited to detecting disc degeneration by narrowed intervertebral spaces and the appearance of osteophytes (Table 4.3). Similarly, it is relatively easy to identify gross facet osteophytes (i.e., hypertrophy) and severe joint-space narrowing of facet joints (on oblique views) but very limited with respect to detecting lower grades of hypertrophy of articular process, subchondral erosion, and subchondral cysts. Pathria et al. divided the radiographic features of facet joints into four groups [52]. Normal facets were classified as grade 0, facets with joint-space narrowing as grade 1, facets with narrowing plus sclerosis or hypertrophy as grade 2, and facets with severe degenerative disease encompassing narrowing, sclerosis, and osteophytes as grade 3. They demonstrated that the sensitivity and specificity for oblique radiographs to distinguish between the presence and absence of degenerative disease in the lumbar facet joints in patients with LBP were 55 and 69 %, respectively. Since the specificity was high but the sensitivity was not as good for early or middle stage, they concluded that the utility of radiographs should be limited only when patients with LBP are being screened. Currently, unless there exist significant clinical concerns of serious underlying pathology, radiographic screening or other forms of imaging are strongly discouraged for the aforementioned reasons [14].

CT

The axial nature of CT provides much more detailed bony information for spine OA, especially with respect to facet joint changes compared with standard radiographs [53]. As shown in Table 4.3, CT can detect almost all changes seen in the spine OA, although it is not as useful as MRI in depicting the disc degeneration and subchondral cysts. Specifically, Leone et al. reported that CT clearly delineates most degenerative changes including articular process hypertrophy, osteophytes, subchondral sclerosis, and capsular and ligamentous calcification [54]. However, exposure to the radiation dose associated with CT should always be considered particularly when serial imaging is required.

MRI

MRI depicts internal structures of joint based on their chemical composition [55]. A major advantage of MRI in the evaluation of OA is its ability to evaluate non-calcified tissues. The periarticular soft tissues such as the ligaments, tendons, muscles, synovium, and cartilage are directly visualized and are readily evaluated with MRI. However, with the exception of edema, MRI is less sensitive to detect bony OA changes of spinal structures [56]. More recent imaging techniques utilizing fat-suppressed MRI sequences, which are more fluid sensitive than conventional MRI such as fat-suppressed T2-weighted images (e.g., short T1 inversion-recovery [STIR] sequences). MRI has no radiation exposure, although there are several contraindications including orbital metallic foreign bodies, cardiac pacemakers or implanted defibrillators, and cochlear implants [57] and other metallic implanted devices.

Comparison of CT and MRI

Weishaupt et al. investigated the coefficient between MRI and CT in the assessment of facet joint OA [58]. They were using a four-point scale similar to that of Pathria, and images of both CT and MRI were assessed by two musculoskeletal radiologists independently. As a result, the weighted kappa coefficients for MRI versus CT were 0.61 and 0.49, for readers 1 and 2, respectively (0.41–0.60 = moderate, 0.61–0.80 = substantial). Looking at the agreement between CT and MRI imaging within one grade, it was at 95 % and 97 %, respectively. In addition, the majority of disagreements were in mild grades. From a clinical perspective, the authors suggested that the agreement between CT and MRI was adequate and, thus, a CT in the situation of existing MRI is not required for grading the severity of facet joint OA.

Fujiwara et al. reported that CT is better able to demonstrate the degenerative bony changes of facet joints; however, the detection of joint effusions and juxtafacet synovial cysts is less sensitive than MRI [29].

Leone et al. examined nine human autopsy specimens with CT and MRI and compared them with histopathologic findings. CT delineated the most degenerative changes including articular process hypertrophy, osteophytes, subchondral sclerosis, and capsular and ligamentous calcification. On the other hand, MRI was better able to depict cartilage surface tears in specimens demonstrating mild and advanced stages of degeneration [54].

SPECT/CT

Recently, hybrid SPECT/CT imaging has been introduced for spine OA. SPECT/CT provides functional imaging and is used to detect microcalcification due to increased osteoblastic activity [59]. Hosam et al. reported identification of potential pain generators in 92 % of cervical spine scans and 86 % of lumbar spine scans with SPECT/CT supported by a good response to the intra-articular steroid injections. The most common method for diagnosing a facetogenic source of LBP is with low-volume intra-articular and medial branch blocks, both of which are associated with high false-positive rates. SPECT/CT may represent a noninvasive alternative. Dolan et al. noted that there are 95 and 79 % response rates at 1 month and 3 months, respectively, after injection therapy in patients with SPECT-positive facets [60].

Pneumaticos et al. also reported that significant improvement in LBP was shown only when SPECT-positive facet joints were subjected to injection therapy [61]. Hariankar et al. investigated the correlation of SPECT/CT findings with clinical features and MRI findings. They concluded SPECT/CT had less sensitivity for detecting facet arthropathy but is likely to be more specific as compared to MRI [62]. Furthermore, because of its significantly higher accuracy, SPECT/CT could be the conventional nuclear medical procedure of choice for patients with lower back pain after lumbar fusion surgery to clarify the pathogenesis of persistent pain [63].

Diagnostic Blocks

Facet pain often overlaps disc pain and may coexist with disc disease. In 1976, Mooney and Robertson introduced a technique of injecting steroid preparations and local anesthetic into the facet joint [64]. It is generally accepted in clinical practice that diagnostic blocks are the most reliable and minimally invasive procedures for diagnosing facet joints as pain generators [65]. Intra-articular injections and medial branch block (MBB) are readily available and are equally effective [66]. Due to their location, size, and orientation, facet blocks are performed under radiographic guidance such as CT or fluoroscopy. Ultrasound-guided blocks have been proposed, although they may be less likely to detect low-volume intravascular uptake and are less accurate in obese woman [67]. It is well known that single diagnostic blocks have been shown to be associated with a high false-positive rate [68] and repeated blocks are recommended. The use of local anesthetics enables the determination of pain relief and is used for diagnostic purposes, whereas the use of corticosteroids may provide short-term therapeutic relief (see section "Treatment" below).

Pathogenesis/Risk Factors

Degenerative spine OA is a multifactorial process, with contributions from both systemic and local factors. Genetic predisposition and mechanical factors can contribute to both disc degeneration and facet joint OA with disc degeneration typically proceeding that of facet joint [69]. Spine OA can lead to associated subconditions, such as spinal instability and deformity (see section "Treatment" below).

Aging

Aging is a normal process in all structures. Similar to other sites, advanced age is one of the strongest risk factors associated with spine OA [70]. The prevalence of disc degeneration clearly increases with age, in both the cervical and the lumbar spine. Aging leads to degenerative changes starting with subtle biochemical alterations followed by microstructural and finally gross structural changes of the spinal unit. The human intervertebral disc is one of the tissues most vulnerable to degeneration in the human body with degeneration beginning as early as the second decade of life [71]. The disc itself has great variation in the matrix organization, composition, cell morphology, and activities in different regions of the disc. The annulus is a collagen-rich, concentrically organized tissue. Its outer cells are thin and elongated, while the cells of the inner annulus are rounded. The annulus protects the nucleus pulposus. The nucleus pulposus consists of chondrocytes that produce and maintain a well-hydrated proteoglycan-rich matrix. These cells have a notochordal origin and are replaced in the first decade of life by rounded chondrocyte-like cells. The disc does not have a uniform cell density. The cell density is greatest in the regions closest to the blood supply, which is generally near the end plate and at the periphery of the annulus. Aggrecan is the most prevalent proteoglycan in the disc, making up approximately 70 % of the nucleus and 25 % of the annulus. Studies have demonstrated that aging leads to the decrease of nutrient supply to the intradiscal chondrocytes [72], which in turn lead to loss of proteoglycans. As a result, a loss of glycosaminoglycans leads to the decrease in hydration of the disc, as well as the loss of mechanical competence and ability of the disc to withstand and distribute load in a normal manner [73]. These changes lead to the migration of inflammatory cells and the production of various cytokines and proteases [74], which contribute to further cellular and matrix degradation. As noted above, degeneration of the facet joints can occur secondary to disc degeneration. The altered mechanics caused by disc degeneration, including loss of disc height and segmental instability (increased micro- or macro-motion), leads to increased and unbalanced loading on the facet joints and results in cartilage alteration [71]. In addition to those two main aging processes, the aging of the ligaments, muscles, and bones is reported as a contributing factor to spinal aging [75, 76].

Genetics

For disc degeneration, the contribution of various factors including vitamin D receptor, genes encoding the collagen IX molecule, aggrecan, collagen I, and matrix metalloproteinase 3 have been reported [3, 77]. Recent studies related to miRNAs are beginning to shed light on the mechanisms of disc degeneration, as well as OA of other joints [78–81]. We are not aware of any study that has specifically looked at or identified definitive factors or pathways for facet joint OA; however, we would postulate that they would be similar to OA in other joints.

Although there are many hurdles for the translocation of current research into clinical practice at this time, several pathways related to miRNAs are expected to be targets for disease modification of OA or disc degeneration. In addition, miRNAs may also prove to be reliable biomarkers for the severity of OA and determination of treatment response. At present, miRNA expression from facet joints has not been reported. We feel that specific assessment of the facet joint concurrently with changes in the disc is required for further understanding of the pathogenesis for spine OA.

Systemic Factors

Recently, metabolic syndrome (MetS) has been reported as an independent risk factor for OA [82]. MetS is a combination disorder including dyslipidemia, hypertension, diabetes or insulin resistance, and obesity [83] and increases the risk of cardiovascular diseases. Longitudinal hyperglycemia may disrupt chondrocyte homeostasis via multiple direct and indirect mechanisms [84, 85], hypertension may decrease the blood flow in the subchondral microvessels and impair subchondral bone remodeling [86], and hyperlipidemia may also affect chondrogenesis, osteogenesis, and mesenchymatous cell differentiation [87]. Our group investigated the association between MetS and spine OA [88] and found that patients with severe spine OA had more composition of factors of MetS than those with early spine OA statistically [88], although significant further investigation is required.

Obesity has been well established as a risk factor for OA in weight-bearing joints such as the hip and knee, with mechanical overload being the causative link [89–91]. However, studies have also identified obesity as a predictor of OA in non-weight-bearing joints such as the hands, which supports the influence of an independent systemic metabolic effect. It has been demonstrated that white adipose tissue (WAT) secretes inflammatory mediators into the systemic circulation and negatively impacts cartilage degeneration [90, 92, 93]. Although a comprehensive understanding of the association between obesity and OA in both weight-bearing and non-weight-bearing joints is lacking, adipokines such as adiponectin, leptin, and visfatin seem to play important roles [94]. It has been shown that adipokines stimulate similar chondrocyte activation as that seen with mechanical stress and proinflammatory cytokines [95, 96].

Mechanical Factors

The lumbar spine transmits loads between intervertebral levels through the "three-joint complex." The percentage of load transferred through the anterior or posterior spine depends on the spinal posture and the degree of disc degeneration [97]. The lumbar facet joints may normally carry up to 33 % of the total compressive load [98, 99], which increases to 47 % in the presence of facet joint spondylosis and up to 70 % in the presence of intervertebral disc degeneration [100]. Disc degeneration, including loss of disc height and segmental instability, leads to the asymmetrical stress distribution. Increased degree of degeneration may be influenced by the variation of pelvic incidence and associated lordosis from one individual to the next.

Inflammation

Although OA is not classified as an inflammatory disorder, inflammation is a major factor associated with the risk of both progression of cartilage loss and symptoms of the disease, including joint pain, swelling, and stiffness [101]. The cytokine mediators detected in the synovial fluid of OA can come from the three-joint sources: the cartilage, the subchondral bone, and the synovium. Synovitis, involving infiltration of mononuclear cells into the synovial membrane and production of proinflammatory mediators, including interleukin-1β (IL-1β), tumor necrosis factor-α (TNF-α), and chemokines, is common in early-stage and late-stage disease [101]. In spine OA, only a few studies related to inflammation are available. Igarashi et al. reported IL-1β positivity in a third of cases with facet joint OA. In addition, the presence of IL-1β in facet joint cartilage was associated with leg pain and poorer quality of life [102]. Similarly, Xu et al. revealed that overexpression of MMP-1 induced by IL-1β plays an important role in the inflammatory process of lumbar facet joint degeneration [103]. As more attention has been focused on the association of inflammation in peripheral OA, the role of inflammation in the pathogenesis of spine OA requires further investigation.

Treatments

The treatment of spinal OA consists of various approaches comprising self-management, supervised exercise therapy, medical management, interventional procedures, and surgery. The goals of therapy for patients with spinal OA are to control pain, minimize disability, improve the quality of life, and educate the patient about their role in chronic disease management.

Nonsurgical Treatment

Exercise

Spine OA pain is exacerbated by activities that involve lumbar extension such as standing and walking; thus, treatments are directed at avoiding those positions and promoting exercises that involve flexion of the lumbar spine. Flexion exercises will increase the relative space of the posterior spinal elements (i.e., unloads the facet joints), which opens up the spinal canal and the foramina to help alleviate the symptoms of neural compression and/or facet overload. Simply stretching in the flexed position will provide temporary relief for these patients. An exercise program can be formulated under the guidance of a physiotherapist, chiropractor, kinesiologist, or personal trainer. The desire and encouragement of others to have a good (i.e., "erect") posture generally aggravates the spine OA back and/or leg pain. Significant education is required to undo this counterintuitive reasoning and to promote "bad posture" to help alleviate the symptoms. While the use of a walker will greatly improve walking tolerance by allowing ambulation with the spine in a flexed position, many patients are resistant to using these devices for reasons of practicality and vanity.

Pharmacotherapy

Oral medications for spine OA are the same as those commonly used in patients with peripheral OA. Nonsteroidal anti-inflammatory drugs (NSAIDs) and acetaminophen are widely used as first-line drugs for the treatment of LBP or neck pain. NSAIDs might be considered for younger patients without significant renal, gastric, or cardiovascular comorbidity. Acetaminophen should be considered for patients without hepatic compromise who cannot tolerate NSAIDs, although it is not typically useful for LBP [104]. Although there is no evidence to support chronic use of muscle relaxants [105], they have been understood as more effective agents than placebo for short-term relief of acute LBP (RR 0.80, 95 % CI 0.71–0.89), regardless of etiology [106]. Opioid therapy is occasionally indicated for severe pain and should be prescribed for short-term use on a fixed schedule [107] with monitoring of side effects such as sedation, confusion, nausea, and constipation. Several other medications, including anticonvulsants and tricyclic antidepressants, have been also used clinically. Tricyclic antidepressants have been found to be beneficial in the setting of chronic back pain but have not been studied for acute back pain or spine OA [108].

Interventional Procedures

The use of glucocorticoid injections into the epidural space or facet joint to treat neurogenic claudication or facet joint pain, respectively, is still a controversial subject. Despite significant increase in the utilization of these interventions, evidence-based reviews have concluded that there is not sufficient evidence to support their ubiquitous use [109, 110]. The overall risk of these intervention is actually quite low; however, they are not without the potential for very rare but severe neurological complications (e.g., paraplegia) [111]. Globally, epidural steroid injections are the most commonly performed pain procedure; however, multiple reviews suggest they offer little if any benefit for low back pain and only short-term benefit for leg symptoms [112–114]. Facet joint intervention typically involves image-guided steroid injection, medical branch nerve block, or facet joint radiofrequency denervation (FJRD). There is no strong consensus regarding the treatment efficacy of FJRD and how it compares with nerve blockades and joint infiltration with anesthetics and/or corticosteroids [115]. A recent review by Falco et al. [116] suggests there is good evidence for the use of FJRD and fair to good evidence for lumbar facet joint nerve blocks for the treatment of chronic lumbar facet joint pain resulting in 6–12-month pain relief and functional improvement. They noted that there was limited evidence for intra-articular facet joint injections.

In a recent systematic review of nonoperative treatment of spine OA (i.e., stenosis) causing neurogenic claudication, Ammendolia et al.[117] noted that most current nonoperative treatment had no or limited (effect size and/or duration) impact in patients with neurogenic claudication.

Surgical Treatment

The rate of spine surgery has steadily increased in recent decades, even after adjustment for the aging of the population [118]. The only absolute indication for surgery in spine OA is in the uncommon scenario of a progressive neurological deficit or cauda equina syndrome. Otherwise, surgical treatment is a preference-based decision for patients that have significant symptoms that have not been well controlled with appropriate nonsurgical treatment methods. In the current surgical practice, LSS patients without instability or deformity most commonly undergo direct spinal decompression (removal of bony and ligamentous structures causing neural compression) [119]. Those with significant back pain, instability, or deformity typically undergo decompression along with instrumented fusion (placement of bone screws into the spine to stabilize the movement and facilitate bony bridging of one vertebra to the other (i.e., fusion)) [119]. The majority of surgery for spine OA is in patients with stenosis-related back and leg symptoms. In select cases, surgery for isolated axial low back pain may also be indicated, particularly in those with associated instability or deformity (see below).

Overall, the best evidence regarding patient-reported outcomes has been from the Spine Patient Outcomes Research Trial (SPORT). In general, better outcomes are reported for patients choosing to proceed with surgery compared to continued nonoperative treatment for patients with lumbar stenosis or degenerative spondylolisthesis (see below) [120]. In addition, surgical intervention appears to be cost-effective in this scenario. Furthermore, patients with leg dominant symptoms tend to have the best overall outcomes [121]. Compared to the generally accepted excellent outcomes of primary hip and knee replacement for OA, work from our center has demonstrated comparable improvement in patient-reported health-related quality of life (HRQoL) and cost per quality-adjusted life year following spine surgery for level 1–2 spine OA compared to total knee replacement at a minimum of 5 years' follow-up [122, 123]. Total hip replacement was associated with superior outcomes compared to both spine surgery and total knee replacement. Spine surgery, however, was associated with a significantly higher long-term reoperation rate compared to either hip or knee replacement surgery.

Morbidity of Surgical Care

The best available adverse event (AE) data stem from the multicenter SPORT studies for LSS and degenerative spondylolisthesis [119]. In general, the intraoperative complication rate was 12 %, with dural tears (10 %), which typically did not affect outcome, representing the most common AE. The majority of postoperative events are medical adverse events (AEs) (7 %), with urinary tract infections being the most common. Major medical AEs such as myocardial infarction or pulmonary embolism are uncommon (<1 %). The wound infection rate was 2 %. While the majority of infections are curable with appropriate treatment, there may be permanent negative effects regarding pain and function. Permanent neurological injury was less than 1 % with varying impact on postoperative outcome. The reoperation rate (same or adjacent level) at 2 and 4 years for decompression and fusion was 12 and 15 %, respectively [124]. The reoperation rate for decompression alone is similar (8 and 13 % at 2 and 4 years, respectively) [125].

Distinct Spine OA Subpopulations

Spine OA has two distinct radiographic subgroups that demonstrate secondary instability (termed degenerative lumbar spondylolisthesis) and/or deformity (termed degenerative scoliosis). Although, clinically similar to other spine OA patients, these patients often require different decision-making regarding management, particularly from a surgical perspective.

Degenerative Lumbar Spondylolisthesis (DLS)

In this subgroup, the arthritic changes result in the forward movement of one spinal vertebra over the other, often referred to as a "slip" [126]. DLS creates increased narrowing of the spinal canal and instability (hypermobility) of the spine. The prevalence of LSS with DLS in the general population is estimated at 6 % [127] and progressively increases from the fifth to the eighth decade of life [128]. DLS typically occurs in patients over the age of 50 and is five times more common in women than men [127]. The majority of DLS patients have a grade 1 listhesis (i.e., <25 % slip), and nearly 60 % of patients with DLS will have recurrent/persistent symptoms [127]. Limited studies looking at demographic and radiographic predictors of progression of degenerative spondylolisthesis have found contradictory results regarding the significance of facet angles, facet fluid volumes, or pelvic incidence at the relevant vertebral levels [129–131].

Nonoperative treatment of DLS is as noted in section "Treatment" for spine OA. In current surgical practice, LSS patients without DLS typically undergo decompression (removal of bony and ligamentous structures causing neural compression). On the other hand, decompression along with instrumented fusion (placement of bone screws into the spine to stabilize the movement and facilitate bony bridging of one vertebra to the other (i.e., fusion)) is recommended for those with DLS [126] (Fig. 4.3). Current decompression techniques that preserve the stabilizing midline spinal anatomy have been proposed as an effective and less morbid alternative to fusion for patients with stable DLS (i.e., <3–5 mm of motion on flexion/extension radiographs or supine to standing (i.e., unloaded to loaded films)) [132–134]. Overall, the surgical outcomes for DLS, which is typically limited to level 1–2 surgery, seem to more durable and provide greater cost-effectiveness compared to surgery for LSS [120].

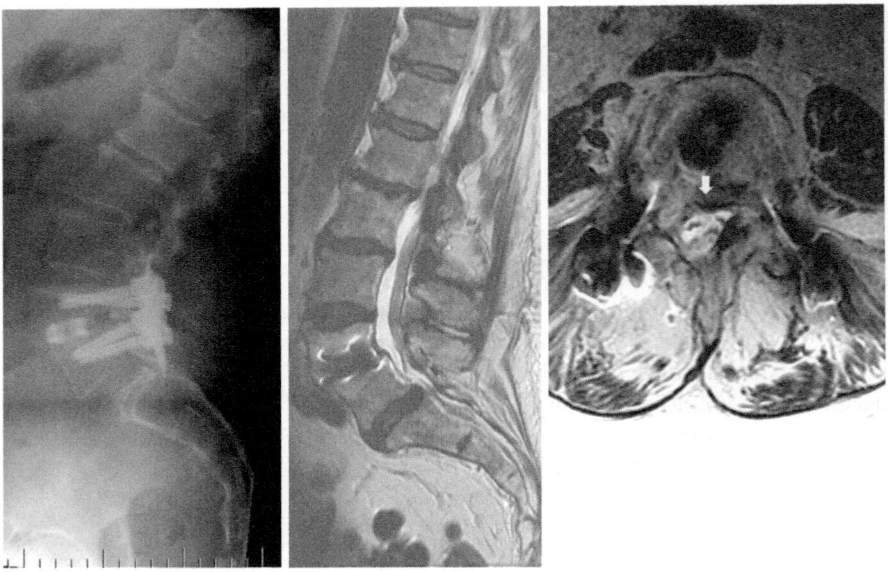

Fig. 4.3 Five-year postsurgical lateral standing radiograph, midsagittal MRI, and axial MRI at L4–L5 in the same patient as in Fig. 4.2. Due to the instability, the patient required a decompression of the spinal canal (*white arrow*) and spinal fusion with instrumentation that is seen on the lateral radiograph. This resulted in dramatic reduction of her pain and improvement of her functional ability

Degenerative Scoliosis

Degenerative scoliosis is defined as an abnormal coronal curvature of the spine greater than 10° that develops in adulthood in the absence of a preexisting childhood deformity [135]. It is considered to be "de novo," another term used to describe the deformity, as it is felt to arise through asymmetrical degeneration of the discs or facets [136]. It occurs almost exclusively in the lumbar spine and is often associated with the progression of the coronal plane deformity over time. Secondary listhesis, generally in the coronal or rotational plane, may occur as well. The associated spine OA generally occurs on the concave part of the curve (increased loading). This can be on the concavity of the main curve, the concavity of the fractional lumbosacral curve, or concavity at both sites [137] (Fig. 4.4). The etiology, epidemiology, clinical course, and treatment of degenerative scoliosis remain unclear.

Etiology

Spinal deformities are associated with asymmetrical disc wear. Whether this is a result of asymmetrical wear of the disc resulting in the deformity or the deformity leading to the asymmetrical disc wear is not known [138]. These deformed discs

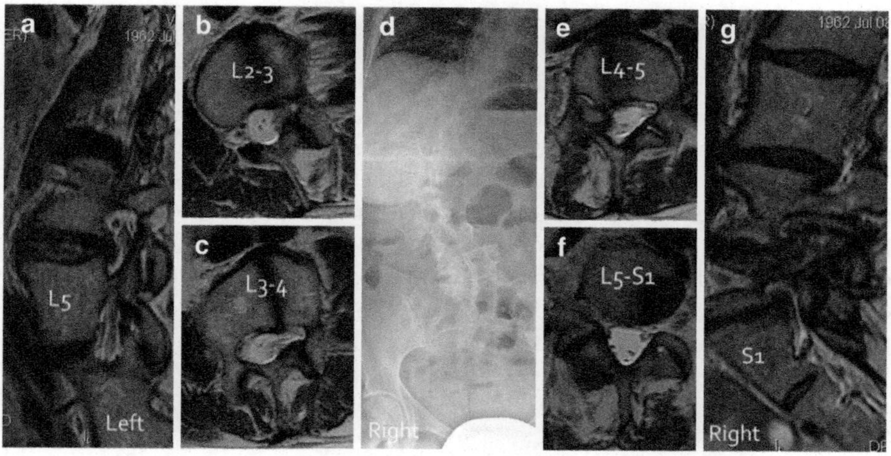

Fig. 4.4 Spinal stenosis in the setting of a coronal plane deformity will develop on the concave side of the curve. For example, a lumbar curve with a right convex apex at L1–L2 (**d**). Stenosis will develop on the left concave aspect at the curve apex (**b**, **c**). Because of the main curve, a secondary fractional curve develops in the lumbosacral region with an opposite configuration to the main curve. This results in lumbosacral stenosis on the right side (**e**–**g**), which is the concave side for the lumbosacral fractional curve. Because the distal lumbar levels are more prone to stenosis secondary to smaller foramens and underlying degeneration, nerve compression most often occurs in the fractional curve. Note the wide open foramens in the lower lumbar region on the convex left (**a**) compared with the tight distal foramens (**g**) on the concave side of the fractional lumbosacral curve. For these reasons, a right lumbar degenerative scoliosis with an upper lumbar apex will most often lead to right-sided neurological symptoms of the distal lumbar roots

often have calcifications and osteophytes on the concave side of the disc with noted changes in cell number and collagen types and composition of the disc matrix.

Demographics

Adult scoliosis has a prevalence rate of up to 10 % in some series. The adult de novo degenerative type is generally seen in patients older than 40 years without a previous history of scoliosis [138]. The most common site for the curves is in the lumbar spine without a thoracic component. The Cobb angle measurement of these curves is often less than 10°; however, the majority of curves that require treatment are greater than 20°. Males and females are equally affected. Characteristic radiographic features can include a coronal plane deformity, a rotational deformity to the apex vertebra, and a lateral or rotational listhesis of one or more vertebrae with varying degrees of sagittal plane (i.e., leaning forward) deformity. The curves can progress over time, usually at about a mean rate of 3° per year [139]. Unlike idiopathic curves, which tend to be left-sided lumbar curves (the convexity of the curve points to the left), the curves in adult degenerative scoliosis have similar distributions of right- and left-sided curves.

Clinical Presentation

Patients with adult-onset scoliosis present essentially the same as other spine OA patients with back and/or leg pain [140]; however, leg pain is frequently unilateral, secondary to the asymmetrical degeneration of the disc and facet joints [141, 142]. As the curves are usually less than 30°, few patients complain of spinal deformity as a primary complaint. For mild curves, a small prominence may be apparent in the lumbar region on the convexity of the curve. For patients with larger deformities, evidence of global sagittal and/or coronal imbalance (i.e., head/trunk is not centered over the pelvis) may be evident. Patients with progressive curves and symptoms can be profoundly limited in function and quality of life.

Treatment

Conservative treatment is as outlined above for spine OA. Specific to degenerative scoliosis, brace treatment has no role in the treatment of spinal stenosis in association with degenerative scoliosis [138]. While radiographic parameters are not considered surgical indications per se, patients requiring surgery generally have significant spinal stenosis in association with progression of the curve, lateral listhesis, and increasing symptomatology. There is a large gamut of surgical treatments that can range from a limited decompression to a large multilevel instrumentation with osteotomies.

Decompression Alone

Similar to patients with spondylolisthesis, decompression alone for degenerative scoliosis is generally reserved for patients with normal sagittal and coronal balance, presenting with leg dominant pain secondary to spinal stenosis [132]. Back pain should be minimal or absent, and radiographically, there should be no sagittal or coronal plane listhesis. Care during surgery must be taken in these cases to preserve as much of the anatomy as possible, as progression of the curve and worsening of the symptoms can be associated with these limited procedures.

Decompression and Limited Fusion

In patients with well-balanced spines in the coronal and sagittal planes with focal levels of degeneration and listhesis, a decompression and fusion of only the affected level is a reasonable option [140]. This allows for a more complete decompression at the affected level without the concern of focal progression of the deformity. This can help alleviate the symptoms without subjecting the patient to a large procedure. This can be an excellent compromise in older patients or those with serious medical comorbidities.

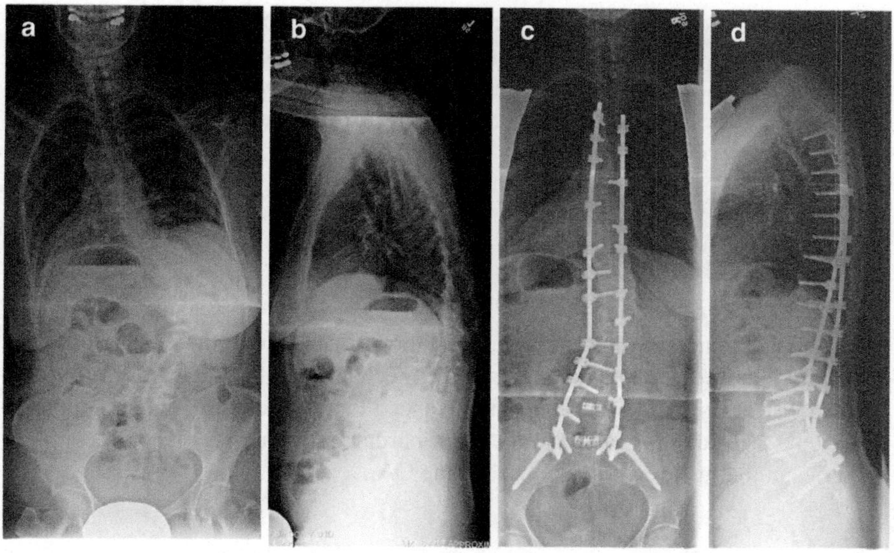

Fig. 4.5 Preoperative standing posteroanterior (**a**) and lateral (**b**) views of the patient depicted in Fig. 4.4. A pedicle screw-based construct extending from T4 to the pelvis was performed restoring her coronal (**c**) and sagittal balance (**d**). Interbody devices placed posteriorly were placed at L4–L5 and L5–S1 to help promote fusion at these levels. A decompression was performed from L2 to S1 to relieve the spinal stenosis

Decompression and Fusion of the Entire Lumbar Curve

Patients with reasonable sagittal and coronal balance with large symptomatic curves are candidates for fusion of the entire curve with partial correction of the deformity and decompression of the affected levels. These patients often have larger curves (Cobb angles greater than 30°) with levels of sagittal or lateral listhesis. The fusions extend along the entire curve and generally require fusion to the sacrum and pelvis. The choice of the proximal level of the fusion can be somewhat controversial but often either extends to L2, when there is no deformity or rotation in the upper lumbar levels, or crosses the thoracolumbar junction to T10 or T11. For patients with structural deformities in the thoracic spine, kyphosis or scoliosis, the constructs can extend proximally up to T4 (Fig. 4.5). Patients with sagittal or coronal imbalance will require spinal osteotomies in conjunction with the fusion to rebalance the spine [138]. A variety of techniques exist regarding fusion and correction of alignment [138].

Morbidity of Surgical Care

Despite the highest degree of planning and attention to perioperative care, spinal deformity surgeries are associated with a relatively high complication rate. Short-term complications include deep wound infection, dural tears, the need for blood transfusions, and others. Relatively common later complications include failure to fuse at one or more levels and junctional failures, most frequently at the proximal end of the construct. Despite the high complication rates, outcomes from these procedures are quite successful, with the majority of patients enjoying improved function and quality of life [138].

Future Directions

Increased genomic and proteomic investigations that include the facet joints will hopefully increase our understanding of the mechanisms of spine degeneration and ultimately lead to the development of advanced diagnostics (i.e., biomarkers) and treatments that can mitigate the tremendous burden of disease and need for complex surgeries in the treatment of advanced spine OA.

Conclusion

Spinal degeneration is often not considered in the same context as OA; however, the degenerative changes in the disc and particular the synovial facet joints are consistent with those of OA elsewhere. The main clinical symptoms of lumbar spine OA (i.e., facet joint OA) are low back pain and/or associated leg symptoms (pain, numbness, and weakness). Various factors contribute to the degenerative changes, including age, biomechanical factors, systemic factors, genetics, and lifestyle. Although there is no universal nonsurgical or surgical treatment for spine OA, exercise and activity modification is typically accepted as an effective form of initial management. For end-stage disease, nonsurgical treatment has limited efficacy and surgical intervention in appropriately selected patients is associated with good patient-reported outcomes that are comparable to those associated with total knee replacement for OA. Further research in spine OA pathophysiology, biomarkers, and early disease management is critically required to mitigate the increasing socioeconomic burden of spine OA.

References

1. Gellhorn AC, Katz JN, Suri P. Osteoarthritis of the spine: the facet joints. Nat Rev Rheumatol. 2013;9(4):216–24.
2. Borenstein D. Does osteoarthritis of the lumbar spine cause chronic low back pain? Curr Rheumatol Rep. 2004;6(1):14–9.
3. Goode AP, Carey TS, Jordan JM. Low back pain and lumbar spine osteoarthritis: how are they related? Curr Rheumatol Rep. 2013;15(2):305.

4. Goode AP, Marshall SW, Renner JB, Carey TS, Kraus VB, Irwin DE, Sturmer T, Jordan JM. Lumbar spine radiographic features and demographic, clinical, and radiographic knee, hip, and hand osteoarthritis. Arthritis Care Res. 2012;64(10):1536–44.
5. March L, Smith EU, Hoy DG, Cross MJ, Sanchez-Riera L, Blyth F, Buchbinder R, Vos T, Woolf AD. Burden of disability due to musculoskeletal (MSK) disorders. Best Pract Res Clin Rheumatol. 2014;28(3):353–66.
6. Hoy DG, Smith E, Cross M, Sanchez-Riera L, Buchbinder R, Blyth FM, Brooks P, Woolf AD, Osborne RH, Fransen M, et al. The global burden of musculoskeletal conditions for 2010: an overview of methods. Ann Rheum Dis. 2014;73(6):982–9.
7. Perruccio AV, Power JD, Badley EM. Revisiting arthritis prevalence projections – it's more than just the aging of the population. J Rheumatol. 2006;33(9):1856–62.
8. Vos T, Flaxman AD, Naghavi M, Lozano R, Michaud C, Ezzati M, Shibuya K, Salomon JA, Abdalla S, Aboyans V, et al. Years lived with disability (YLDs) for 1160 sequelae of 289 diseases and injuries 1990–2010: a systematic analysis for the Global Burden of Disease Study 2010. Lancet. 2012;380(9859):2163–96.
9. Hoy D, Bain C, Williams G, March L, Brooks P, Blyth F, Woolf A, Vos T, Buchbinder R. A systematic review of the global prevalence of low back pain. Arthritis Rheum. 2012;64(6):2028–37.
10. Dartmouth Medical School, Center for the Evaluative Clinical Sciences, Maine Medical Center & Center for Outcomes Research and Evaluation. The Dartmouth atlas of musculoskeletal health care (2000).
11. Spector TD, Hart DJ, Byrne J, Harris PA, Dacre JE, Doyle DV. Definition of osteoarthritis of the knee for epidemiological studies. Ann Rheum Dis. 1993;52(11):790–4.
12. Suri P, Rainville J, Kalichman L, Katz JN. Does this older adult with lower extremity pain have the clinical syndrome of lumbar spinal stenosis? JAMA. 2010;304(23):2628–36.
13. Genevay S, Atlas SJ. Lumbar spinal stenosis. Best Pract Res Clin Rheumatol. 2010;24(2):253–65.
14. Chou R, Qaseem A, Owens DK, Shekelle P. Diagnostic imaging for low back pain: advice for high-value health care from the American College of Physicians. Ann Intern Med. 2011;154(3):181–9.
15. Chen E, Tong KB, Laouri M. Surgical treatment patterns among Medicare beneficiaries newly diagnosed with lumbar spinal stenosis. Spine J. 2010;10(7):588–94.
16. Tischer T, Aktas T, Milz S, Putz RV. Detailed pathological changes of human lumbar facet joints L1-L5 in elderly individuals. Eur Spine J. 2006;15(3):308–15.
17. Farfan HF, Cossette JW, Robertson GH, Wells RV, Kraus H. The effects of torsion on the lumbar intervertebral joints: the role of torsion in the production of disc degeneration. J Bone Joint Surg Am. 1970;52(3):468–97.
18. Asano S, Kaneda K, Umehara S, Tadano S. The mechanical properties of the human L4-5 functional spinal unit during cyclic loading. The structural effects of the posterior elements. Spine. 1992;17(11):1343–52.
19. Laird RA, Gilbert J, Kent P, Keating JL. Comparing lumbo-pelvic kinematics in people with and without back pain: a systematic review and meta-analysis. BMC Musculoskelet Disord. 2014;15:229.
20. Crisco 3rd JJ, Panjabi MM. The intersegmental and multisegmental muscles of the lumbar spine. A biomechanical model comparing lateral stabilizing potential. Spine. 1991;16(7):793–9.
21. Kettler A, Wilke HJ. Review of existing grading systems for cervical or lumbar disc and facet joint degeneration. Eur Spine J. 2006;15(6):705–18.
22. Tian W, Lv Y, Liu Y, Xiao B, Han X. The high prevalence of symptomatic degenerative lumbar osteoarthritis in Chinese adults: a population-based study. Spine. 2014;39(16):1301–10.
23. Eubanks JD, Lee MJ, Cassinelli E, Ahn NU. Prevalence of lumbar facet arthrosis and its relationship to age, sex, and race: an anatomic study of cadaveric specimens. Spine. 2007;32(19):2058–62.

24. Kalichman L, Li L, Kim DH, Guermazi A, Berkin V, O'Donnell CJ, Hoffmann U, Cole R, Hunter DJ. Facet joint osteoarthritis and low back pain in the community-based population. Spine. 2008;33(23):2560–5.
25. Jentzsch T, Geiger J, Zimmermann SM, Slankamenac K, Nguyen-Kim TD, Werner CM. Lumbar facet joint arthritis is associated with more coronal orientation of the facet joints at the upper lumbar spine. Radiol Res Pract. 2013;2013:693971.
26. Kalichman L, Guermazi A, Li L, Hunter DJ. Association between age, sex, BMI and CT-evaluated spinal degeneration features. J Back Musculoskelet Rehabil. 2009;22(4):189–95.
27. Miller JA, Schmatz C, Schultz AB. Lumbar disc degeneration: correlation with age, sex, and spine level in 600 autopsy specimens. Spine. 1988;13(2):173–8.
28. Kelsey JL, White 3rd AA. Epidemiology and impact of low-back pain. Spine. 1980;5(2):133–42.
29. Fujiwara A, Tamai K, Yamato M, An HS, Yoshida H, Saotome K, Kurihashi A. The relationship between facet joint osteoarthritis and disc degeneration of the lumbar spine: an MRI study. Eur Spine J. 1999;8(5):396–401.
30. Vernon-Roberts B, Pirie CJ. Degenerative changes in the intervertebral discs of the lumbar spine and their sequelae. Rheumatol Rehabil. 1977;16(1):13–21.
31. Bajwa NS, Toy JO, Young EY, Cooperman DR, Ahn NU. Disk degeneration in lumbar spine precedes osteoarthritic changes in hip. Am J Orthop (Belle Mead, NJ). 2013;42(7):309–12.
32. Suri P, Miyakoshi A, Hunter DJ, Jarvik JG, Rainville J, Guermazi A, Li L, Katz JN. Does lumbar spinal degeneration begin with the anterior structures? A study of the observed epidemiology in a community-based population. BMC Musculoskel Disord. 2011;12:202.
33. Labelle H, Roussouly P, Berthonnaud E, Dimnet J, O'Brien M. The importance of spino-pelvic balance in L5-s1 developmental spondylolisthesis: a review of pertinent radiologic measurements. Spine. 2005;30(6 Suppl):S27–34.
34. Walker BF. The prevalence of low back pain: a systematic review of the literature from 1966 to 1998. J Spinal Disord. 2000;13(3):205–17.
35. Katz JN. Lumbar disc disorders and low-back pain: socioeconomic factors and consequences. J Bone Joint Surg Am. 2006;88 Suppl 2:21–4.
36. Cassidy JD, Carroll LJ, Cote P. The Saskatchewan health and back pain survey. The prevalence of low back pain and related disability in Saskatchewan adults. Spine. 1998;23(17):1860–6; discussion 1867.
37. Suri P, Hunter DJ, Rainville J, Guermazi A, Katz JN. Presence and extent of severe facet joint osteoarthritis are associated with back pain in older adults. Osteoarthritis Cartilage. 2013;21(9):1199–206.
38. Kjaer P, Leboeuf-Yde C, Korsholm L, Sorensen JS, Bendix T. Magnetic resonance imaging and low back pain in adults: a diagnostic imaging study of 40-year-old men and women. Spine. 2005;30(10):1173–80.
39. Friedrich KM, Nemec S, Peloschek P, Pinker K, Weber M, Trattnig S. The prevalence of lumbar facet joint edema in patients with low back pain. Skeletal Radiol. 2007;36(8):755–60.
40. Mainka T, Lemburg SP, Heyer CM, Altenscheidt J, Nicolas V, Maier C. Association between clinical signs assessed by manual segmental examination and findings of the lumbar facet joints on magnetic resonance scans in subjects with and without current low back pain: a prospective, single-blind study. Pain. 2013;154(9):1886–95.
41. Meizer R, Radda C, Stolz G, Kotsaris S, Petje G, Krasny C, Wlk M, Mayerhofer M, Landsiedl F, Aigner N. MRI-controlled analysis of 104 patients with painful bone marrow edema in different joint localizations treated with the prostacyclin analogue iloprost. Wien Klin Wochenschr. 2005;117(7–8):278–86.
42. Issack PS, Cunningham ME, Pumberger M, Hughes AP, Cammisa Jr FP. Degenerative lumbar spinal stenosis: evaluation and management. J Am Acad Orthop Surg. 2012;20(8):527–35.
43. Battie MC, Jones CA, Schopflocher DP, Hu RW. Health-related quality of life and comorbidities associated with lumbar spinal stenosis. Spine J. 2012;12(3):189–95.
44. Borenstein D. Mechanical low back pain – a rheumatologist's view. Nat Rev Rheumatol. 2013;9(11):643–53.

45. Hall H, McIntosh G, Boyle C. Effectiveness of a low back pain classification system. Spine J. 2009;9(8):648–57.
46. Henschke N, Maher CG, Refshauge KM, Herbert RD, Cumming RG, Bleasel J, York J, Das A, McAuley JH. Prevalence of and screening for serious spinal pathology in patients presenting to primary care settings with acute low back pain. Arthritis Rheum. 2009;60(10):3072–80.
47. Deyo RA, Weinstein JN. Low back pain. N Engl J Med. 2001;344(5):363–70.
48. Cheng F, You J, Rampersaud YR. Relationship between spinal magnetic resonance imaging findings and candidacy for spinal surgery. Can Fam Physician Medecin de famille canadien. 2010;56(9):e323–30.
49. Beattie PF, Meyers SP, Stratford P, Millard RW, Hollenberg GM. Associations between patient report of symptoms and anatomic impairment visible on lumbar magnetic resonance imaging. Spine. 2000;25(7):819–28.
50. Jensen MC, Brant-Zawadzki MN, Obuchowski N, Modic MT, Malkasian D, Ross JS. Magnetic resonance imaging of the lumbar spine in people without back pain. N Engl J Med. 1994;331(2):69–73.
51. Boden SD, Davis DO, Dina TS, Patronas NJ, Wiesel SW. Abnormal magnetic-resonance scans of the lumbar spine in asymptomatic subjects. A prospective investigation. J Bone Joint Surg Am. 1990;72(3):403–8.
52. Pathria M, Sartoris DJ, Resnick D. Osteoarthritis of the facet joints: accuracy of oblique radiographic assessment. Radiology. 1987;164(1):227–30.
53. Carrera GF, Haughton VM, Syvertsen A, Williams AL. Computed tomography of the lumbar facet joints. Radiology. 1980;134(1):145–8.
54. Leone A, Aulisa L, Tamburrelli F, Lupparelli S, Tartaglione T. The role of computed tomography and magnetic resonance in assessing degenerative arthropathy of the lumbar articular facets. Radiol Med. 1994;88(5):547–52.
55. Prost R, Czervionke LF. How does an MR scanner operate? AJNR Am J Neuroradiol. 1994;15(7):1383–6.
56. Grenier N, Kressel HY, Schiebler ML, Grossman RI, Dalinka MK. Normal and degenerative posterior spinal structures: MR imaging. Radiology. 1987;165(2):517–25.
57. Shellock FG, Morisoli S, Kanal E. MR procedures and biomedical implants, materials, and devices: 1993 update. Radiology. 1993;189(2):587–99.
58. Weishaupt D, Zanetti M, Boos N, Hodler J. MR imaging and CT in osteoarthritis of the lumbar facet joints. Skeletal Radiol. 1999;28(4):215–9.
59. Matar HE, Navalkissoor S, Berovic M, Shetty R, Garlick N, Casey AT, Quigley AM. Is hybrid imaging (SPECT/CT) a useful adjunct in the management of suspected facet joints arthropathy? Int Orthop. 2013;37(5):865–70.
60. Dolan AL, Ryan PJ, Arden NK, Stratton R, Wedley JR, Hamann W, Fogelman I, Gibson T. The value of SPECT scans in identifying back pain likely to benefit from facet joint injection. Br J Rheumatol. 1996;35(12):1269–73.
61. Pneumaticos SG, Chatziioannou SN, Hipp JA, Moore WH, Esses SI. Low back pain: prediction of short-term outcome of facet joint injection with bone scintigraphy. Radiology. 2006;238(2):693–8.
62. Harisankar CN, Mittal BR, Bhattacharya A, Singh P, Sen R. Utility of single photon emission computed tomography/computed tomography imaging in evaluation of chronic low back pain. Indian J Nucl Med. 2012;27(3):156–63.
63. Sumer J, Schmidt D, Ritt P, Lell M, Forst R, Kuwert T, Richter R. SPECT/CT in patients with lower back pain after lumbar fusion surgery. Nucl Med Commun. 2013;34(10):964–70.
64. Mooney V, Robertson J. The facet syndrome. Clin Orthop Relat Res. 1976;115:149–56.
65. Bani A, Spetzger U, Gilsbach JM. Indications for and benefits of lumbar facet joint block: analysis of 230 consecutive patients. Neurosurg Focus. 2002;13(2), E11.
66. Marks RC, Houston T, Thulbourne T. Facet joint injection and facet nerve block: a randomised comparison in 86 patients with chronic low back pain. Pain. 1992;49(3):325–8.
67. Santiago AE, Leal PC, Bezerra EH, Giraldes AL, Ferraro LC, Rezende AH, Sakata RK. Ultrasound-guided facet block to low back pain: a case report. Rev Bras Anestesiol. 2014;64(4):278–80.

68. Dreyfuss P, Schwarzer AC, Lau P, Bogduk N. Specificity of lumbar medial branch and L5 dorsal ramus blocks. A computed tomography study. Spine. 1997;22(8):895–902.
69. Dunlop RB, Adams MA, Hutton WC. Disc space narrowing and the lumbar facet joints. J Bone Joint Surg. 1984;66(5):706–10.
70. Lewin T. Osteoarthritis in lumbar synovial joints. A morphologic study. Acta Orthop Scand Suppl. 1964;73(Suppl):71–112.
71. Benoist M. Natural history of the aging spine. Eur Spine J. 2003;12 Suppl 2:S86–9.
72. Boos N, Weissbach S, Rohrbach H, Weiler C, Spratt KF, Nerlich AG. Classification of age-related changes in lumbar intervertebral discs: 2002 Volvo Award in basic science. Spine. 2002;27(23):2631–44.
73. Wilder DG, Pope MH, Frymoyer JW. The biomechanics of lumbar disc herniation and the effect of overload and instability. J Spinal Disord. 1988;1(1):16–32.
74. Rannou F, Corvol MT, Hudry C, Anract P, Dumontier MF, Tsagris L, Revel M, Poiraudeau S. Sensitivity of anulus fibrosus cells to interleukin 1 beta. Comparison with articular chondrocytes. Spine. 2000;25(1):17–23.
75. Panjabi MM, Goel VK, Takata K. Physiologic strains in the lumbar spinal ligaments. An in vitro biomechanical study 1981 Volvo Award in Biomechanics. Spine. 1982;7(3):192–203.
76. Kalichman L, Klindukhov A, Li L, Linov L. Indices of paraspinal muscles degeneration: reliability and association with facet joint osteoarthritis: feasibility study. J Spinal Disord Tech. 2013 [Epub ahead of print] Doi: 10.1097/BSD.0b013e31828be943.
77. Chan D, Song Y, Sham P, Cheung KM. Genetics of disc degeneration. Eur Spine J. 2006;15 Suppl 3:S317–25.
78. Yamasaki K, Nakasa T, Miyaki S, Ishikawa M, Deie M, Adachi N, Yasunaga Y, Asahara H, Ochi M. Expression of MicroRNA-146a in osteoarthritis cartilage. Arthritis Rheum. 2009;60(4):1035–41.
79. Swingler TE, Wheeler G, Carmont V, Elliott HR, Barter MJ, Abu-Elmagd M, Donell ST, Boot-Handford RP, Hajihosseini MK, Munsterberg A, et al. The expression and function of microRNAs in chondrogenesis and osteoarthritis. Arthritis Rheum. 2012;64(6):1909–19.
80. Miyaki S, Asahara H. Macro view of microRNA function in osteoarthritis. Nat Rev Rheumatol. 2012;8(9):543–52.
81. Song YQ, Karasugi T, Cheung KM, Chiba K, Ho DW, Miyake A, Kao PY, Sze KL, Yee A, Takahashi A, et al. Lumbar disc degeneration is linked to a carbohydrate sulfotransferase 3 variant. J Clin Invest. 2013;123(11):4909–17.
82. Sellam J, Berenbaum F. Is osteoarthritis a metabolic disease? Joint Bone Spine. 2013;80(6):568–73.
83. Grundy SM, Cleeman JI, Daniels SR, Donato KA, Eckel RH, Franklin BA, Gordon DJ, Krauss RM, Savage PJ, Smith Jr SC, et al. Diagnosis and management of the metabolic syndrome: an American Heart Association/National Heart, Lung, and Blood Institute Scientific Statement. Circulation. 2005;112(17):2735–52.
84. Rosa SC, Rufino AT, Judas FM, Tenreiro CM, Lopes MC, Mendes AF. Role of glucose as a modulator of anabolic and catabolic gene expression in normal and osteoarthritic human chondrocytes. J Cell Biochem. 2011;112(10):2813–24.
85. Uchida K, Urabe K, Naruse K, Ogawa Z, Mabuchi K, Itoman M. Hyperlipidemia and hyperinsulinemia in the spontaneous osteoarthritis mouse model, STR/Ort. Exp Anim. 2009;58(2):181–7.
86. Imhof H, Sulzbacher I, Grampp S, Czerny C, Youssefzadeh S, Kainberger F. Subchondral bone and cartilage disease: a rediscovered functional unit. Invest Radiol. 2000;35(10):581–8.
87. Aspden RM, Scheven BA, Hutchison JD. Osteoarthritis as a systemic disorder including stromal cell differentiation and lipid metabolism. Lancet. 2001;357(9262):1118–20.
88. Gandhi R, Woo KM, Zywiel MG, Rampersaud YR. Metabolic syndrome increases the prevalence of spine osteoarthritis. Orthop Surg. 2014;6(1):23–7.
89. Bourne R, Mukhi S, Zhu N, Keresteci M, Marin M. Role of obesity on the risk for total hip or knee arthroplasty. Clin Orthop Relat Res. 2007;465:185–8.
90. Grotle M, Hagen KB, Natvig B, Dahl FA, Kvien TK. Obesity and osteoarthritis in knee, hip and/or hand: an epidemiological study in the general population with 10 years follow-up. BMC Musculoskelet Disord. 2008;9:132.

91. Sowers MF, Yosef M, Jamadar D, Jacobson J, Karvonen-Gutierrez C, Jaffe M. BMI vs. body composition and radiographically defined osteoarthritis of the knee in women: a 4-year follow-up study. Osteoarthritis Cartilage. 2008;16(3):367–72.
92. Hart DJ, Spector TD. The relationship of obesity, fat distribution and osteoarthritis in women in the general population: the Chingford Study. J Rheumatol. 1993;20(2):331–5.
93. Waldron HA. Association between osteoarthritis of the hand and hip in a skeletal population from London, UK. J Rheumatol. 1997;24(7):1452–3.
94. Lago F, Dieguez C, Gomez-Reino J, Gualillo O. The emerging role of adipokines as mediators of inflammation and immune responses. Cytokine Growth Factor Rev. 2007;18(3–4):313–25.
95. Abella V, Scotece M, Conde J. Adipokines, metabolic syndrome and rheumatic diseases. J Immunol Res. 2014;2014:343746.
96. Gosset M, Berenbaum F, Salvat C, Sautet A, Pigenet A, Tahiri K, Jacques C. Crucial role of visfatin/pre-B cell colony-enhancing factor in matrix degradation and prostaglandin E2 synthesis in chondrocytes: possible influence on osteoarthritis. Arthritis Rheum. 2008;58(5):1399–409.
97. Holm S. Pathophysiology of disc degeneration. Acta Orthop Scand Suppl. 1993;251:13–5.
98. King AI, Prasad P, Ewing CL. Mechanism of spinal injury due to caudocephalad acceleration. Orthop Clin North Am. 1975;6(1):19–31.
99. Nachemson A. Lumbar intradiscal pressure. Experimental studies on post-mortem material. Acta Orthop Scand Suppl. 1960;43:1–104.
100. Adams MA, Hutton WC. The mechanical function of the lumbar apophyseal joints. Spine. 1983;8(3):327–30.
101. Sellam J, Berenbaum F. The role of synovitis in pathophysiology and clinical symptoms of osteoarthritis. Nat Rev Rheumatol. 2010;6(11):625–35.
102. Igarashi A, Kikuchi S, Konno S. Correlation between inflammatory cytokines released from the lumbar facet joint tissue and symptoms in degenerative lumbar spinal disorders. J Orthop Sci. 2007;12(2):154–60.
103. Xu D, Sun Y, Bao G, Liu W, Zhu X, Cui S, Fan J, Cui Z. MMP-1 overexpression induced by IL-1beta: possible mechanism for inflammation in degenerative lumbar facet joint. J Orthop Sci. 2013;18(6):1012–9.
104. Williams CM, Maher CG, Latimer J, McLachlan AJ, Hancock MJ, Day RO, Lin CW. Efficacy of paracetamol for acute low-back pain: a double-blind, randomised controlled trial. Lancet. 2014;384(9954):1586–96.
105. Chou R, Huffman LH. Medications for acute and chronic low back pain: a review of the evidence for an American Pain Society/American College of Physicians clinical practice guideline. Ann Intern Med. 2007;147(7):505–14.
106. van Tulder MW, Touray T, Furlan AD, Solway S, Bouter LM. Muscle relaxants for nonspecific low back pain. Cochrane Database Syst Rev. 2003;(2):Cd004252.
107. Martell BA, O'Connor PG, Kerns RD, Becker WC, Morales KH, Kosten TR, Fiellin DA. Systematic review: opioid treatment for chronic back pain: prevalence, efficacy, and association with addiction. Ann Intern Med. 2007;146(2):116–27.
108. Staiger TO, Gaster B, Sullivan MD, Deyo RA. Systematic review of antidepressants in the treatment of chronic low back pain. Spine. 2003;28(22):2540–5.
109. Chou R, Loeser JD, Owens DK, Rosenquist RW, Atlas SJ, Baisden J, Carragee EJ, Grabois M, Murphy DR, Resnick DK, et al. Interventional therapies, surgery, and interdisciplinary rehabilitation for low back pain: an evidence-based clinical practice guideline from the American Pain Society. Spine. 2009;34(10):1066–77.
110. Staal JB, de Bie R, de Vet HC, Hildebrandt J, Nelemans P. Injection therapy for subacute and chronic low-back pain. Cochrane Database Syst Rev. 2008;(3):Cd001824.
111. Benoist M, Boulu P, Hayem G. Epidural steroid injections in the management of low-back pain with radiculopathy: an update of their efficacy and safety. Eur Spine J. 2012;21(2):204–13.

112. Choi HJ, Hahn S, Kim CH, Jang BH, Park S, Lee SM, Park JY, Chung CK, Park BJ. Epidural steroid injection therapy for low back pain: a meta-analysis. Int J Technol Assess Health Care. 2013;29(3):244–53.
113. Bresnahan BW, Rundell SD, Dagadakis MC, Sullivan SD, Jarvik JG, Nguyen H, Friedly JL. A systematic review to assess comparative effectiveness studies in epidural steroid injections for lumbar spinal stenosis and to estimate reimbursement amounts. PM R. 2013;5(8):705–14.
114. Shamliyan TA, Staal JB, Goldmann D, Sands-Lincoln M. Epidural steroid injections for radicular lumbosacral pain: a systematic review. Phys Med Rehabil Clin N Am. 2014;25(2):471–489.e471-450.
115. Poetscher AW, Gentil AF, Lenza M, Ferretti M. Radiofrequency denervation for facet joint low back pain: a systematic review. Spine. 2014;39(14):E842–9.
116. Falco FJ, Manchikanti L, Datta S, Sehgal N, Geffert S, Onyewu O, Zhu J, Coubarous S, Hameed M, Ward SP, et al. An update of the effectiveness of therapeutic lumbar facet joint interventions. Pain Physician. 2012;15(6):E909–53.
117. Ammendolia C, Stuber K, de Bruin LK, Furlan AD, Kennedy CA, Rampersaud YR, Steenstra IA, Pennick V. Nonoperative treatment of lumbar spinal stenosis with neurogenic claudication: a systematic review. Spine. 2012;37(10):E609–16.
118. Deyo RA. Back surgery – who needs it? N Engl J Med. 2007;356(22):2239–43.
119. Weinstein JN, Tosteson TD, Lurie JD, Tosteson AN, Blood E, Hanscom B, Herkowitz H, Cammisa F, Albert T, Boden SD, et al. Surgical versus nonsurgical therapy for lumbar spinal stenosis. N Engl J Med. 2008;358(8):794–810.
120. Tosteson AN, Tosteson TD, Lurie JD, Abdu W, Herkowitz H, Andersson G, Albert T, Bridwell K, Zhao W, Grove MR, et al. Comparative effectiveness evidence from the spine patient outcomes research trial: surgical versus nonoperative care for spinal stenosis, degenerative spondylolisthesis, and intervertebral disc herniation. Spine. 2011;36(24):2061–8.
121. Pearson A, Blood E, Lurie J, Abdu W, Sengupta D, Frymoyer JW, Weinstein J. Predominant leg pain is associated with better surgical outcomes in degenerative spondylolisthesis and spinal stenosis: results from the Spine Patient Outcomes Research Trial (SPORT). Spine. 2011;36(3):219–29.
122. Rampersaud YR, Tso P, Walker KR, Lewis SJ, Davey JR, Mahomed NN, Coyte PC. Comparative outcomes and cost-utility following surgical treatment of focal lumbar spinal stenosis compared with osteoarthritis of the hip or knee: part 2 – estimated lifetime incremental cost-utility ratios. Spine J. 2014;14(2):244–54.
123. Rampersaud YR, Lewis SJ, Davey JR, Gandhi R, Mahomed NN. Comparative outcomes and cost-utility after surgical treatment of focal lumbar spinal stenosis compared with osteoarthritis of the hip or knee – part 1: long-term change in health-related quality of life. Spine J. 2014;14(2):234–43.
124. Weinstein JN, Lurie JD, Tosteson TD, Zhao W, Blood EA, Tosteson AN, Birkmeyer N, Herkowitz H, Longley M, Lenke L, et al. Surgical compared with nonoperative treatment for lumbar degenerative spondylolisthesis. four-year results in the Spine Patient Outcomes Research Trial (SPORT) randomized and observational cohorts. J Bone Joint Surg Am. 2009;91(6):1295–304.
125. Weinstein JN, Tosteson TD, Lurie JD, Tosteson A, Blood E, Herkowitz H, Cammisa F, Albert T, Boden SD, Hilibrand A, et al. Surgical versus nonoperative treatment for lumbar spinal stenosis four-year results of the Spine Patient Outcomes Research Trial. Spine. 2010;35(14):1329–38.
126. Weinstein JN, Lurie JD, Tosteson TD, Hanscom B, Tosteson AN, Blood EA, Birkmeyer NJ, Hilibrand AS, Herkowitz H, Cammisa FP, et al. Surgical versus nonsurgical treatment for lumbar degenerative spondylolisthesis. N Engl J Med. 2007;356(22):2257–70.
127. Jacobsen S, Sonne-Holm S, Rovsing H, Monrad H, Gebuhr P. Degenerative lumbar spondylolisthesis: an epidemiological perspective: the Copenhagen Osteoarthritis Study. Spine. 2007;32(1):120–5.
128. Kalichman L, Kim DH, Li L, Guermazi A, Berkin V, Hunter DJ. Spondylolysis and spondylolisthesis: prevalence and association with low back pain in the adult community-based population. Spine. 2009;34(2):199–205.

129. Aono K, Kobayashi T, Jimbo S, Atsuta Y, Matsuno T. Radiographic analysis of newly developed degenerative spondylolisthesis in a mean twelve-year prospective study. Spine. 2010;35(8):887–91.
130. Barrey C, Jund J, Perrin G, Roussouly P. Spinopelvic alignment of patients with degenerative spondylolisthesis. Neurosurgery. 2007;61(5):981–6; discussion 986.
131. Huang RP, Bohlman HH, Thompson GH, Poe-Kochert C. Predictive value of pelvic incidence in progression of spondylolisthesis. Spine. 2003;28(20):2381–5; discussion 2385.
132. Kelleher MO, Timlin M, Persaud O, Rampersaud YR. Success and failure of minimally invasive decompression for focal lumbar spinal stenosis in patients with and without deformity. Spine. 2010;35(19):E981–7.
133. Sasai K, Umeda M, Maruyama T, Wakabayashi E, Iida H. Microsurgical bilateral decompression via a unilateral approach for lumbar spinal canal stenosis including degenerative spondylolisthesis. J Neurosurg Spine. 2008;9(6):554–9.
134. Matsudaira K, Yamazaki T, Seichi A, Takeshita K, Hoshi K, Kishimoto J, Nakamura K. Spinal stenosis in grade I degenerative lumbar spondylolisthesis: a comparative study of outcomes following laminoplasty and laminectomy with instrumented spinal fusion. J Orthop Sci. 2005;10(3):270–6.
135. Schwab FJ, Smith VA, Biserni M, Gamez L, Farcy JP, Pagala M. Adult scoliosis: a quantitative radiographic and clinical analysis. Spine. 2002;27(4):387–92.
136. Faldini C, Di Martino A, De Fine M, Miscione MT, Calamelli C, Mazzotti A, Perna F. Current classification systems for adult degenerative scoliosis. Musculoskelet Surg. 2013;97(1):1–8.
137. de Vries AA, Mullender MG, Pluymakers WJ, Castelein RM, van Royen BJ. Spinal decompensation in degenerative lumbar scoliosis. Eur Spine J. 2010;19(9):1540–4.
138. Silva FE, Lenke LG. Adult degenerative scoliosis: evaluation and management. Neurosurg Focus. 2010;28(3), E1.
139. Pritchett JW, Bortel DT. Degenerative symptomatic lumbar scoliosis. Spine. 1993;18(6):700–3.
140. Tribus CB. Degenerative lumbar scoliosis: evaluation and management. J Am Acad Orthop Surg. 2003;11(3):174–83.
141. Grubb SA, Lipscomb HJ, Coonrad RW. Degenerative adult onset scoliosis. Spine. 1988;13(3):241–5.
142. Kotwal S, Pumberger M, Hughes A, Girardi F. Degenerative scoliosis: a review. HSS J. 2011;7(3):257–64.
143. Savage RA, Whitehouse GH, Roberts N. The relationship between the magnetic resonance imaging appearance of the lumbar spine and low back pain, age and occupation in males. Eur Spine J. 1997;6(2):106–14.
144. Pye SR, Reid DM, Smith R, Adams JE, Nelson K, Silman AJ, O'Neill TW. Radiographic features of lumbar disc degeneration and self-reported back pain. J Rheumatol. 2004;31(4):753–8.
145. Muraki S, Oka H, Akune T, Mabuchi A, En-Yo Y, Yoshida M, Saika A, Suzuki T, Yoshida H, Ishibashi H, et al. Prevalence of radiographic lumbar spondylosis and its association with low back pain in elderly subjects of population-based cohorts: the ROAD study. Ann Rheum Dis. 2009;68(9):1401–6.
146. de Schepper EI, Damen J, van Meurs JB, Ginai AZ, Popham M, Hofman A, Koes BW, Bierma-Zeinstra SM. The association between lumbar disc degeneration and low back pain: the influence of age, gender, and individual radiographic features. Spine. 2010;35(5):531–6.
147. Kalichman L, Guermazi A, Li L, Hunter DJ, Suri P. Facet orientation and tropism: associations with spondylolysis. J Spinal Disord Tech. 2010;23(2):101–5.

Chapter 5
Ankle Osteoarthritis

Johnny Lau, Andrea N. Veljkovic, and Patricia Farrugia

Key Points

- Ankle Osteoarthritis (OA) arthritis usually results from posttraumatic arthritis.
- Patients with ankle OA are usually younger than those individuals with hip and knee OA but are equally disabled.
- Common traumatic injuries to the ankle include ankle fractures and sprains.
- Ankle fractures are common in young and old adult populations and are one of the most common orthopedic injuries.
- Ankle OA has a specific pathology in cartilage load bearing and injury compared to OA of the knee and hip.
- Injuries to the ankle may predispose to an altered gait cycle and weight-bearing process in the lower extremity.
- Treatment for ankle injuries can be nonoperative or operative depending on the severity of trauma, involved soft tissue, and bony anatomy.
- OA of the ankle can be treated conservatively with anti-inflammatory medications and therapy. Surgical treatments include joint-sparing procedures, joint fusions, or total ankle replacements.
- Research related to the biomechanics of trauma and ankle OA remains an area of focus.

J. Lau, MD (✉) • A.N. Veljkovic, MD • P. Farrugia, MD
Division of Orthopedic Surgery, Toronto Western Hospital, University Health Network, Toronto, ON, Canada
e-mail: drjohnnylau@gmail.com

M. Kapoor, N.N. Mahomed (eds.), *Osteoarthritis: Pathogenesis, Diagnosis, Available Treatments, Drug Safety, Regenerative and Precision Medicine*,
DOI 10.1007/978-3-319-19560-5_5

Introduction

The ankle joint is one of the major weight-bearing joints in the body. Unlike the common degenerative pathology in hip and knee arthritis related to aging, arthritis in the ankle usually results from posttraumatic causes [1]. Ankle arthritis can affect both young and older populations, resulting in pain, limited mobility, and decreased quality of life [2]. Combination of both bony and ligamentous issues related to trauma and aging may play a role in accelerating the quality and viability of the cartilage, ligaments, and tendons of the ankle [3]. Alterations to the unique biomechanical properties of the ankle which are involved in the gait cycle can create issues with mobility and stability of the lower limbs. There are many different treatment options, both surgical and nonsurgical, which have been developed. Potential treatment options for ankle arthritis continue to be a dedicated focus for clinical research, with an aim to better address the symptoms and pathologies involved in ankle degeneration.

Incidence

The common pathology of arthritis can have many causes including trauma, infection, and inflammatory and systemic disorders. Primary OA has been defined as an idiopathic condition developing in previously undamaged joints in the absence of an obvious causative mechanism [4]. Secondary arthritis can be caused by an underlying condition, such as a joint injury, accumulation of calcium inside the joint, other inflammatory bone and joint conditions (e.g., rheumatoid arthritis (RA)), or a medical condition, such as diabetes. Rheumatoid and psoriatic arthritis, as well as gout, neuromuscular disorders, and infection, can contribute to degeneration of a joint. However, in the ankle, posttraumatic arthritis is the most common cause of OA.

The most common etiological factor in the development of OA of the ankle is posttraumatic following fractures and severe sprains of the ankle [5]. Injuries to the ankle have a bimodal population distribution among young, active, risk-taking individuals and middle-aged individuals with sprains or work-related injuries. Foot and ankle fractures were most common presentations seen at major trauma hospitals in the United States [6], with a majority of the posttraumatic ankle arthritis resulting from rotational ankle fractures. While the reported prevalence of posttraumatic arthritis in the ankle has been variable, an important predictor is the severity of the injury to the articular cartilage [7].

Ankle Anatomy and Osteoarthritis

The ankle joint provides a combination of the ability to serve as a weight-bearing surface with the ability to permit motion and force alterations in a normal gait cycle. In order to address the complex changes which can occur in this joint due to injury and resultant pathology, a basic understanding of the anatomical structure of the ankle is paramount.

The ankle joint is comprised of three bony surfaces: the distal tibia, the distal fibula, and the talus. These three surfaces articulate with each other with each step of the gait cycle. The tibiotalar joint is covered with articular cartilage that reduces the shear and compressive forces transmitted across the ankle with normal weight-bearing. The distal fibula is the central attachment point for the lateral ankle ligaments as well as the syndesmosis of the ankle. The syndesmosis complex is located 2 cm above the ankle joint and contains four ligaments, including the anterior and posterior tibiofibular ligamentous complex which helps to stabilize the mortise of the ankle. The deltoid, a primary robust stabilizer of the ankle, attaches to the medial aspect of the tibia and inserts along the medial column of the foot. Stability of the ankle is dependent on the interaction between the bony articulations of the ankle joint and ligamentous structures for balance. These ligaments ensure that the tibia and fibula, which create the primary constraints of the joint, stay in close contact while weight-bearing, and the joint remains a stable construct in the ankle mortise. Any pathology which may affect the bone [8] and soft tissue complex of the ankle can cause altered biomechanics and acceleration in degenerative changes.

The ankle–foot mechanism is a critical component of gait. The gait cycle is a complex of interdependent physiological interactions between the bony and soft tissue components of the foot and ankle, and the surrounding environment. The gait cycle has two phases – the stance phase and the swing phase. During the stance phase, bony articulations of the foot and ankle lock together to provide a platform for weight-bearing, whereas in the swing phase, the bony and soft tissue articulations unlock to allow for push-off of the foot to follow with an additional step, which creates the cycle again. The joints that comprise the ankle and the foot allow for full weight-bearing through the stance phase while at the same time dynamically adjusting to any alterations in terrain. The ability of the foot to adjust and respond to terrain variability optimizes people's ability to mobilize. Unfortunately, it also increases the risk of trauma to the ankle/foot mechanism [9].

Pathogenesis

The process of cartilage degeneration can vary among different joints in the body. Primary and progressive OA is not common in the ankle compared to other joints, such as the hip and knee [10]. Cartilage in the ankle, with its terminal weight-bearing properties and smaller joint surface area compared to the knee and hip, has unique features to allow these functions. Basic science research has dedicated a focus to determining specific biochemical and mechanical properties following traumatic injuries which may explain this phenomenon. Although the exact mechanisms underlying the pathogenesis of posttraumatic OA have not yet been fully established, inflammatory responses within the joint, direct impact of the articular cartilage, and early changes in subchondral bone have all been implicated as potentially deleterious processes predisposing to OA development over the long term [11]. Nakasa et al. [12] studied these differences between the ankle and other joints and concluded a strong relationship between the subchondral bone plate and cartilage degeneration in the progression of OA in the ankle. Cartilage in the ankle joint differs from other joints of the body due to the unique properties with weight-bearing and gait. Interestingly, the articular cartilage of the ankle is one of the thinnest of the weight-bearing joints and ranges from 1 to 1.7 mm [13]. In addition, ankle cartilage shows a higher compressive stiffness and proteoglycan density, lower matrix degradation, and decreased response to catabolic stimulations [14].

Compared to other smaller joints in the body, such as the elbow and wrist, the ankle joint maintains a flexible range of motion (ROM). However, in the ankle as a weight-bearing joint, the osteoarthritic process of degeneration and biomechanics are strongly linked: altered loading patterns, micro-ligamentous instability, increased intra-articular and periarticular mechanical forces, and changed biomechanics are substantial contributing factors in the initiation and progression of ankle OA [15]. This is illustrated in the fact that 1 mm of lateral displacement of the fibula post fracture can result in significantly diminished joint contact area and increased joint reactive forces on the talus that result in accelerated abnormal wear patterns [16].

Structural/Biomechanical Alterations

During normal walking, forces up to five times the body weight are transferred through the ankle, and this increases with running and other strenuous exercise [17]. The cartilage of the ankle joint possesses unique physical and biomechanics characteristics which allow adaption to weight-bearing stressors. The cartilage in the ankle is stiffer and more resistant to deformation than other weight-bearing joints, allowing it to support these increased loads [18]. In the setting of OA, the cartilage of the ankle joint degenerates, which may negatively impact the weight-bearing properties and mobility of the ankle during the gait cycle.

Changes in gait patterns are common complaints in patients with ankle OA. Quality and quantity of distance walking ability, usually diminish as the disease progresses. Patients with restricted ankle function due to OA generally walk slower than normal [19], which has been shown to mediate joint load reduction [20].

In addition to changes in gait, other factors may predispose individuals with previous ankle trauma to an accelerated process of cartilage and joint degeneration. The circumstances and timeline surrounding acute treatment of ankle injuries have been shown to be a critical factor in increased risk of developing OA. The more severe the fracture, the more likely a patient develops degenerative joint disease [21]. Several conditions have been associated with an increased risk of developing radiographic ankle OA or end-stage OA following a malleolar fracture. These include increasing age, female gender, fracture severity, location and extent of cartilage lesions (especially of the medial malleolus), quality of fracture reduction, and presence of a fracture dislocation [22]. Goals of acute operative fracture treatment, include, anatomic restoration of the joint; adequate reduction is critical, with reduction of the lateral malleolus to restore normal length, and produce correct alignment of the talus within the mortise being most important [23]. A mere 1 mm of lateral displacement of the talus, the combination of decreased surface area and increased contact pressures across the ankle joint articular cartilage, if left unaddressed, results in cartilage wear and arthritis [24].

There are other factors that can increase the likelihood of complications and predispose one to the development of ankle OA. Patients with a body mass index (BMI) greater than 25 have a 1.5 times higher risk for the diagnosis of foot and ankle OA [25], with the risk increasing in people with rising BMI and in patients over 30 years of age at the time of injury and with increasing length of time since surgery. The probability of developing posttraumatic ankle OA among patients having three or more risk factors was 60–70 % in an 18-year follow-up study [22]. In general, a higher risk for ankle fractures in overweight and obese persons has been suggested [26]. Additionally, overweight and obese subjects seem to sustain more severe types of ankle fractures [27].

Stufkens et al. [28] performed a long-term follow-up study of a prospective cohort of 288 ankle fractures that were treated operatively between 1993 and 1997. In the initial study, arthroscopy was performed in all cases to assess the extent and location of intra-articular cartilage damage. In a follow-up study, a total of 109 patients were available for clinical and radiographic assessment. Deep cartilage lesions on the anterior and lateral aspect of the talus and on the medial malleolus with odds ratios of 12.3, 5.4, and 5.2, respectively, were identified as independent predictors of the development of posttraumatic ankle OA [29]. Traumatic injuries to the ankle joint can accelerate the process of OA. Although this may not occur as an acute process in all individuals with ankle injuries, it may accelerate osteoarthritic symptoms and cartilage quality of the ankle joint. Traumatic ankle injuries that may result in OA, include, fractures of the malleoli, tibial plafond, talus, isolated osteochondral damage of the talar dome secondary to ankle sprain, and ankle ligament injury. The fact that primary injuries are more likely to be sustained by younger individuals indicates that posttraumatic OA develops earlier than other forms of OA, with a recent study finding that individuals with ankle and knee posttraumatic OA were approximately 14 and 10.4 years younger, respectively, than their counterparts with other forms of OA [30].

Clinical Presentation/Risk Factors

Clinical history is of uttermost importance in patients presenting with ankle OA. Due to the nature of causes of OA in the ankle, commonly being a result of injury, information about the timeline since injury, method of treatment, and location of symptoms can assist with clinical decision making. Gathering information regarding duration and specificity of symptoms, in conjunction with complete physical exam of the ankle, including, gait analysis, can help to identify issues of concern specific to each patient.

Patients with ankle OA usually present with gait abnormalities and decreased ROM of the affected ankle. These abnormalities may affect simple daily functions of living, such as, walking upstairs, and tolerating inclines and uneven surfaces. Clinical examination should include, observation of gait, and stance of the lower extremities. In general, gait analyses in patients with ankle OA revealed a lower walking speed, cadence, step length, and stride length compared to healthy people of a similar age [19]. Individuals may be able to specify the exact location of their discomfort with a related activity, whereas others may complain of overall ankle pain. It is common for patients with ankle OA to have small to moderate joint effusions and crepitus of the affected ankle. Patients may complain of symptoms related to impingement, secondary to osteophyte and degenerative bony changes, and hypertrophied soft tissues with stair climbing, with walking on uneven surfaces, or with prolonged activity. Specifying the location and distinguishing features of ankle-related pain can help direct clinical testing and radiographic investigations.

Identification of the position of the ankle, hind foot, and forefoot during weight-bearing and phases of the gait cycle can help identify primary or secondary structural abnormalities. Altered positions of the ankle and foot may reflect underlying soft tissue pathologies such as tenosynovitis, tendon dysfunction, incompetent ligaments, neurological abnormalities, or associated degenerative joints of the ankle and foot. These structural differences may be unilateral or bilateral and should be explored as possible contributors to the patients' spectrum, dysfunction, and presentation of ankle OA.

Tendons and ligaments of the affected ankle and foot should be examined for excursion, strength, and fatigue. Specific structures to examine on the lateral side of the ankle include, the peroneus longus and brevis, the lateral ankle ligamentous complex, and the syndesmosis. On the medial side, specific attention should be directed to the deltoid ligament, the tibialis posterior tendon, and the spring ligament. It is important to determine whether the interplay of ligament or tendon pathology is functional or mechanical in nature. Quality of the ligaments and tendons as well as ROM of the affected side should be compared to the contralateral side.

A complete neurological as well as a vascular exam should accompany any physical exam of the lower extremities. Patients with underlying systemic conditions, such as, diabetes mellitus or vascular insufficiency may be at an increased risk for complications such as, infection, nonunion, and wound healing issues. Identifying these potential risk factors may guide decision making for specific treatments in joint-preserving versus joint-sacrificing procedures within the ankle.

Although it is not always feasible, reviewing previous imaging and identification of possible complications and treatments to date can guide ongoing treatment decisions. Review of imaging with evolving symptoms and complaints is important to determine which structures of the ankle joint may be involved or becoming progressively involved.

Diagnosis

There are many facets to the clinical diagnosis of OA: clinical exam, patient complaints, and history can help point to the diagnosis. With the adjuncts of radiographic imaging and application to research-based ankle OA scales, treatment-specific goals can help address the underlying stage of OA of the ankle.

Radiographic evaluation should begin with weight-bearing anteroposterior, lateral, and mortise (oblique) views of the ankle (Fig. 5.1a–c). Weight-bearing radiographs of the ankle are essential to observe the natural joint reference contact relationships of the ankle and supporting hind and midfoot joints. The Saltzman hind foot alignment view is helpful for the evaluation of hind foot deformity. Standing AP hip to ankle views (4 ft standing) can also be helpful in assessing generalized limb alignment. Additional imaging studies, such as, computed tomography

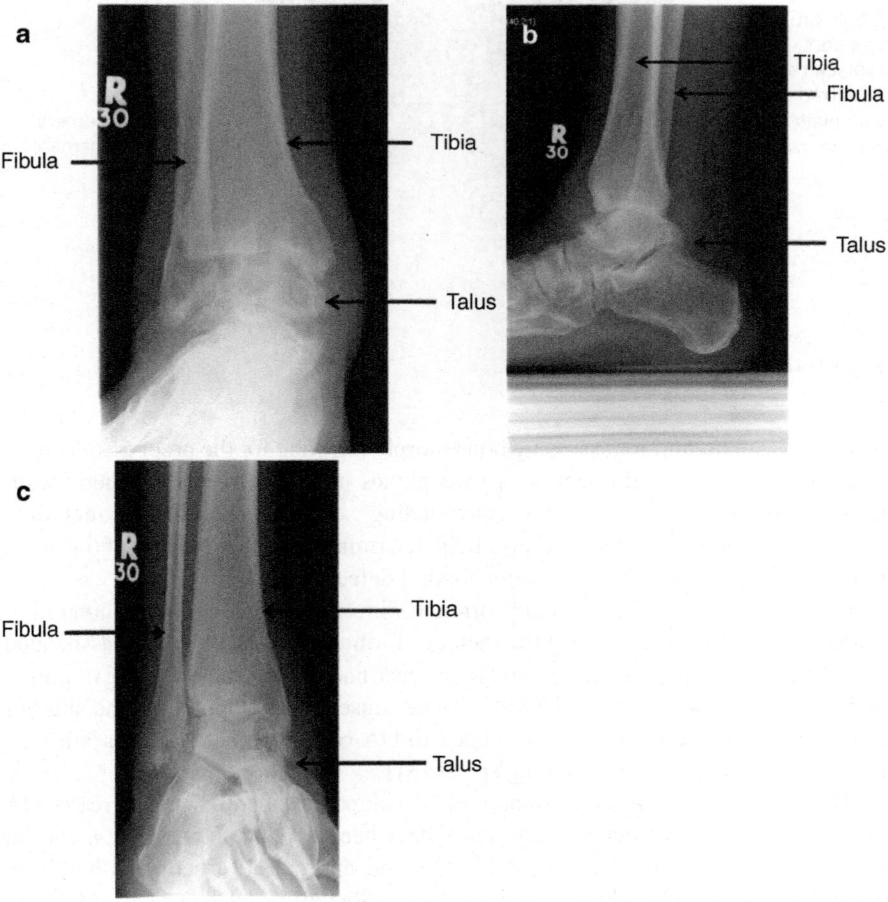

Fig. 5.1 Radiographic images showing (**a**) anterior–posterior, (**b**) lateral, and (**c**) oblique views of the right ankle. Radiographs showing right (**d**) lateral and (**e**) oblique views of a total ankle replacement

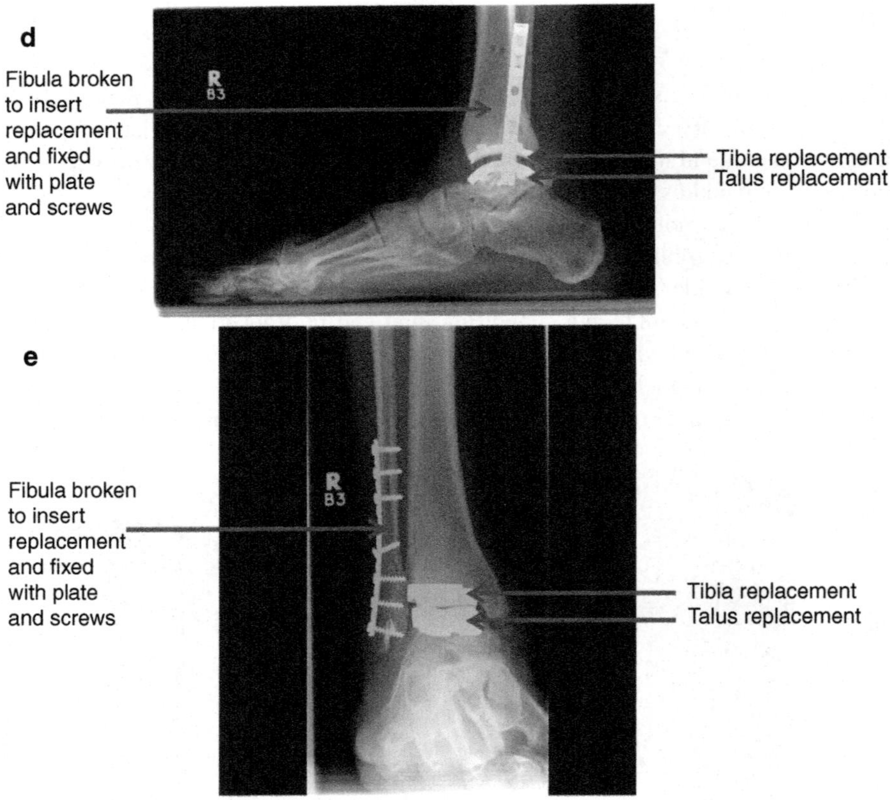

Fig. 5.1 (continued)

(CT) scans are helpful for assessing bone morphology and for the preoperative mapping of size, shape, and quantity of osteophytes or loose bodies. Magnetic resonance imaging (MRI) can define surrounding soft tissue structures, including tendons and ligaments. MRIs can also help determine cartilage quantity of the ankle joint, including the presence of osteochondral defects.

Positive imaging findings should correlate with clinical findings. Common radiographic signs associated with OA, include, formation of osteophytes, associated bone cysts, subchondral sclerosis, and joint space narrowing (JSN). Painful impingement at the ankle joint on dorsiflexion can be caused by osteophytes at the anterior joint margin. These spurs may be related to OA but can also be seen in athletes, especially those involved in kicking sports [31].

There have been many scales and tools developed to quantify the degree of OA of the ankle. Although many of the scales have been applied and revised, a current scale to determine the stages of ankle OA and appropriate treatments has been developed by the Canadian Foot and Ankle Society (COFAS). This tool was designed to be a simple and reliable tool to be used for arthritis stratification and outcome comparison in research, being a representation of the local anatomic con-

Table. 5.1 The COFAS Preoperative and Postoperative Classification System for End-Stage Ankle Arthritis

Type I	Type 2	Type 3	Type 4
Isolated ankle arthritis	Ankle arthritis with intra-articular varus/valgus deformity or a tight heel cord, or both	Ankle arthritis with hind foot deformity, tibial malunion, midfoot abductus or adductus, supinated midfoot, plantar flexed first ray, etc.	Types I–3 plus subtalar, calcaneocuboid, or talonavicular arthritis

ditions that may affect outcome and surgical decisions, not applicable to patients who are not eligible for a joint replacement [32]. Although it does not take into account patient factors, it is a valuable and useful tool for surgeons to utilize as a platform for decision making for nonsurgical and surgical treatment options for the patient with ankle OA (Table 5.1).

Nonsurgical Treatment/Foot and Ankle Care

First-line treatment in many orthopedic conditions is nonsurgical treatment. Due to the pathologies involved in the development of ankle OA, different populations may require different nonoperative treatment options; they should be offered for a minimum of 6 months for all older patients. However, early discussions among young and active patients with mild, moderate, and occasionally even advanced asymmetric ankle OA should occur more expediently, as certain joint-preserving treatment may help delay the progression of joint degeneration [33].

Successful conservative care is dependent on the stage of the ankle OA and the patients' age and motivation. When choosing between conservative and joint-sparing/joint-sacrificing treatment, the extent of subchondral bone exposed and the time over which the OA has advanced are factors that should be considered. Patients with only little exposure of subchondral bone and slow OA progression will likely respond better to conservative treatment.

There are several modes of nonoperative and conservative treatment. Some options have research examined benefits, while others are newer therapies that lack concrete evidence of the benefits. Therapies include activity modification, shoe wear modification, weight loss, the use of anti-inflammatories, bracing, and physical therapy. These nonoperative treatments immobilize or off-load the joint to improve symptoms. Newer modalities include intra-articular injections, such as, hyaluronate viscosupplementation to help reduce joint inflammation and pain and assist in lubrication.

These newer modalities remain popular in the orthopedic literature as a clear determination of efficacy remains undefined. Clinically, a benefit of chondroitin or glucosamine for ankle OA has not yet been proven. In ankle OA, viscosupplementation demonstrated evidence for significant improvement after 1 and 6 months of five weekly injections in a prospective randomized double-blind trial [34]. A randomized control trial (RCT) was done by Witteveen et al. [35] of 70 patients who received HA injection into the joint under fluoroscopy versus distraction in patients with severe OA. There is no significant difference between the two injection methods regarding any of our formulated outcome measures. Considering the substantial amount of possible extra-articular injections prior to fluoroscopic control with both techniques, the use of contrast-aided fluoroscopy for injecting the ankle with severe OA, anterolateral or anteromedial osteophytes, is advisable.

There is no evidence of the efficacy of protein-rich plasma for ankle OA in the literature. Furthermore, the efficacy of intra-articular corticosteroid injections in the osteoarthritic ankle has not been studied; most clinical studies have involved knee OA.

Additional oral conservative treatment for OA includes the use of nonsteroidal anti-inflammatory medications or drugs (NSAIDs) [36]. They can be used as a temporary measure for control of intermittent pain, inflammation, and symptoms. However, many older individuals may have other medical conditions, such as, cardiac and respiratory disorders, that may interact with these medications and preclude their use.

Physical therapy and activity modification can be effective in addressing the loss of mobility in ankle OA; muscle strength during dorsiflexion and plantar flexion in individuals with ankle arthritis has been found to be decreased [37]. Therapy programs for the nonoperative management of ankle arthritis should have a focus on lower extremity strengthening, proprioception, and gait training.

Orthoses and shoe modifications can provide effective pain alleviation, improve quality of life, and postpone total ankle replacement or ankle arthrodesis in patients affected by advanced ankle arthritis with or without deformity [38]. The Ankle Foot Orthosis (AFO) is used to address pathology at the level of the ankle joint during the stance phase of gait [39].

Surgical Treatments

Conservative treatment should be the first-line treatment in ankle OA. However, many individuals fail to alleviate their symptoms of pain and limited mobility despite their best efforts. Although conservative treatment should be attempted, there may be a limit to its efficacy, and surgical management of ankle OA may be considered.

The goals of surgical management remain directed toward a pain-free ankle joint. Although in many of the surgical options, joint motion may be sacrificed to achieve this goal; joint-sparing procedures may provide options for sufficient pain relief while allowing ankle motion to remain. Treatment, joint-sparing versus joint-sacrificing, depends on many factors including patient age, patient preference, cartilage quality and quantity, and other systemic conditions.

Severe ankle OA treatments are usually joint sacrificing in nature, including total ankle arthroplasty and ankle arthrodesis. Mild to moderate OA in a younger patient may be treated by joint-preserving surgery, such as arthroscopic debridement, osteochondral repair, ligament and tendon reconstruction, and osteotomies.

Arthroscopic Debridement/Osteophyte Resection

With any injury, the cartilage of the ankle joint may be affected. Radiographic investigations, such as, MRIs can help to provide information about the cartilage of the ankle joint. Despite the emerging role of three-dimensional imaging studies, ankle arthroscopy is considered the gold standard in determining the true extent of cartilage damage in the ankle joint [40].

Diagnostic arthroscopy also has a role in the prognostication of OA development as a result of trauma [41]. Glazebrook [42] and colleagues performed a systematic review of the benefits of ankle arthroscopy treatment in ankle injuries and posttraumatic arthritis. This systematic review found a general trend of improved postoperative outcomes in these case series in patients with soft tissue impingement compared with bony impingement and increasingly poor results with increasing degree of ankle OA. Although evidence is limited, arthroscopic debridement has shown benefits in the treatment of arthritic disorders that primarily involve synovium of the ankle joint including RA, localized pigmented villonodular synovitis, and hemophilic arthropathy [41]. It is, however, important to assess alignment prior to arthroscopy, as this may need to be additionally addressed so that the mechanical forces for creating osteophytes may be altered.

Indications for ankle arthroscopy for ankle OA include diagnostic arthroscopy and loose body removal, anterior ankle impingement, and early stage ankle OA with intact joint space.

With any surgical procedure, there are postoperative risks and complications. Review of ankle arthroscopy complications by Deng et al. [43] revealed that the most common complication was cutaneous nerve injury, which involved nine cases (3.46 %), and localized superficial infection, which involved eight cases (3.08 %). Injury to the superficial peroneal nerve accounted for five of the cutaneous nerve injuries.

Allograft Resurfacing

Osteochondral lesions can be seen as a local degeneration of the ankle joint, can be the result of injury to the tibiotalar joint from direct trauma, or can be seen as a secondary injury due to a severe ankle sprain. Within the foot and ankle, the talar dome is the most common location for development of an osteochondral lesion [44], termed an osteochondral lesion of the talus, and can be degenerative or posttraumatic. Surgical treatment techniques can be categorized into non-tissue transplantation and tissue transplantation methods. Potential options for repair or reconstruction, include, procedures such as arthroscopic debridement combined with microfracture and/or drilling, autologous chondrocyte implantation, and the osteochondral autograft transplant system (OATS)/mosaicplasty. However, each of these has limitations in the treatment of large lesions for which the success rates are poor and tissue available for harvest and implantation is limited by risk of harvest-site morbidity [44].

Treatment of osteochondral lesions may be a temporary measure to prevent further joint degeneration, although most studies demonstrate little long-term success. Despite the fact that in theory, this procedure is a potentially desirable option for a young patient with advanced ankle arthritis, it has a high level of technical difficulty and complications with the reported results showing a high failure rate [44].

Supramalleolar Osteotomy

In younger patients with mild to moderate ankle OA, goals of treatment include preserving the joint while addressing altered joint mechanics as a result of injury. Supramalleolar osteotomy (SMO), reported to be an effective realignment surgery in patients with varus ankle OA, is performed to restore orientation and axial alignment of the ankle. It has been shown to reduce pain and improve function and radiological signs of arthritis, as well as postpone fusion and replacement surgery in these patients [45].

The main indication for SMOs is asymmetric ankle OA with concomitant valgus or varus deformities and a partially (at least 50 %) preserved tibiotalar joint surface [46].

SMO is an option for some surgeons to consider but is based on surgeon experience. In patients with supramalleolar valgus or varus deformities, the surgeon can choose from four surgical options: medial closing wedge osteotomy (anti-valgus osteotomy), medial opening wedge osteotomy, lateral closing wedge osteotomy (anti-varus osteotomy), and dome osteotomy. Rotational and translational osteotomies can also be performed where necessary. In some cases where there is a sagittal (anterior–posterior) deformity, various osteotomies can be performed to correct the deformity at the center of rotation and angulation [47].

The clinical effectiveness of SMOs can vary from patient to patient. A study by Egloof et al. demonstrated a decrease in tibial and talar subchondral bone plate density distribution after supramalleolar medial closing wedge osteotomy in patients with valgus ankle OA; our patients reported a decrease in pain and most of them were satisfied with the procedure. SMO should be considered a surgical treatment option for ankle OA in certain patients with remaining joint space.

Total Ankle Arthroplasty

Total ankle arthroplasty was designed as an alternative to arthrodesis of the ankle joint in the treatment of OA. The design of this prosthetic joint implant has continued to develop since its inception in the early 1970s, with several generations of prosthetic templates continuing to evolve (Fig. 5.1d, e).

Total ankle arthroplasty was developed to reduce pain and retain motion of the ankle joint in patients with OA, much like its total hip and knee counterparts. Total knee and hip arthroplasties remain one of the most common surgical procedures in the modern orthopedic theater. While arthrodesis is still considered the "gold standard" for treatment of end-stage ankle arthritis, progression of adjacent joint arthrosis and diminished gait efficiency has led to a resurgence of interest in ankle arthroplasty. Long-term outcome studies for total ankle replacement found excellent or good results in 82 % of patients who received a newer generation ankle device compared with 72 % if undergoing ankle fusion [48].

The optimal patient is older (>50 years old), with end-stage ankle arthrosis, non-obese, and with low physical demands [49]. Patients with posttraumatic ankle arthrosis, especially younger patients, seem to have worse outcomes and are more likely to undergo revision than patients with other causes of arthritis [50].

Complications, such as, infection required revision for implant failure with positive radiographical anomalies in 18 AES total ankle arthroplasties. In this study by Rodgiuez et al. [51], the most frequently encountered complication was asymptomatic osteolysis, which was best detected on CT scan compared to conventional X-rays. For now, the osteolysis leads to only a very low frequency revision. It was most frequently seen around the tibial component on X-ray and in the talar body on CT scan. Therefore, it is recommended to repeat CT scans every 6 months to monitor for osteolysis and prosthesis stability.

Symptomatic improvement can vary from patient to patient depending on preoperative symptoms. However, many patients may prefer maintaining some movement of the affected joint choosing arthroplasty versus arthrodesis. The gait patterns of patients following three-component, mobile-bearing total ankle arthroplasty more closely resembled normal gait when compared with the gait patterns of patients following arthrodesis [52].

In conclusion, the intermediate-term clinical outcomes of ankle replacement and arthrodesis in a diverse cohort of patients were comparable, even when patients who required revision ankle replacement were included; however, the rates of additional surgery and major complications were higher after ankle replacement than after arthrodesis [53].

Ankle Arthrodesis

Another treatment option for ankle OA includes ankle arthrodesis. Debilitating posttraumatic arthritis is the most common indication for arthrodesis and is widely considered the gold standard. It is also indicated for pain and deformity secondary to previous infection, osteochondral defects, osteonecrosis of the talus, OA, inflammatory arthropathies, and RA [48].

While ankle arthrodesis, otherwise known as ankle fusion, sacrifices any remaining ankle joint motion, the results are predictable with regard to consistent pain relief once fusion is achieved. Assessment of postoperative fusion is based on clinical and radiographic means, such as, CT.

In most cases, good and excellent intermediate-term results are reported for modern arthrodesis techniques. Long-term reliability, however, is questioned because ankle fusion has been associated with premature arthritis, pain, and dysfunction of the adjacent hind foot joints. Waters and coworkers reported a 16 % decrease in gait velocity, 3 % increase in oxygen consumption, and 10 % decrease in gait efficiency after ankle fusion [54]. In a long-term follow-up study of 23 patients evaluated over an average of 22 years after tibiotalar arthrodesis, Coester and associates [55] demonstrated progressive degenerative changes of ipsilateral subtalar (91 %), talonavicular (57 %), and tarsometatarsal (41 %) joints. The progressive arthritis in these joints led to ipsilateral foot pain and limitations in ambulation and activities of daily living. Pseudoarthrosis rates approach 50 % in some studies, and appropriate position for fusion is often difficult to obtain in cases with bone loss. With the advent of arthroscopic ankle fusion, there are the potential benefits of improved wound and bony healing, due to preservation of the soft tissue envelope and diminished soft tissue stripping, and potential improved outcomes.

Several patient factors can contribute to post-op complications including nonunion. Factors associated with nonunion, included, fracture type, evidence of avascular necrosis, infection, major medical problems, and open injuries. Factors that were not associated with nonunion, included, age, past history of subtalar or triple arthrodesis, and technique [56].

Joint fusion in foot and ankle surgery may allow a high activity level, but degeneration of the neighboring joints occurs in up to 50 % of cases after 7–8 years and up to 100 % of cases after 22 years [57].

The debate continues over which joint-sacrificing procedure – total ankle arthroplasty or ankle arthrodesis – is best to address ankle OA. A recent systematic review was done by Jordon et al. [58] to determine how end-stage ankle OA should be managed. Although half of the reviewed studies report some functional improvement following total ankle replacement, the lack of high quality evidence limits a definitive conclusion being drawn. Insufficient evidence is available to decide whether total ankle replacement or ankle arthrodesis improves functional outcomes and further research in the form of robust RCTs is indicated.

Conclusions

Ankle OA is a common pathology among young adults and older populations. There are many etiologies contributing to the prevalence of this disease, although posttraumatic OA is the primary cause. Recognizing the uniqueness of the properties of the ankle joint, both biology and biomechanics, is important for determination of nonoperative versus operative treatment. Many nonoperative treatments may be applicable to particular populations; however, many still lack evidence for efficacy. Operative therapies should be attempted after a trial of conservative therapy, although conversations with younger patients about joint-sparing procedures should take place early. Joint-preserving and sacrificing procedures may offer symptom relief but are associated with increased risks and complications. Pathogenesis and associated treatments of ankle OA remains a topic of interest in orthopedic research and will continue to provide additional information to address this common disease. Patient-tailored approaches with biologics and mechanical realignment may be the key focus for future research, as it may allow for patient-specific joint-preserving modalities.

References

1. Saltzman CL SM, Blanchard GM, Huff T, Hayes A, Buckwalter JA, Amendola A. Epidemiology of ankle arthritis: report of a consecutive series of 639 patients from a tertiary orthopaedic center. Iowa Orthop J. 2005;25:44–6.
2. Glazebrook MP, Daniels T, Younger A, Foote CJ, Penner M, Wing K, Lau J, Leighton R, Dunbar M. Comparison of health-related quality of life between patients with end-stage ankle and hip arthrosis. J Bone Joint Surg Am. 2008;90(3):499–505.
3. Snedeker JG, Wirth SH, Espinosa N. Biomechanics of the normal and arthritic ankle joint. Foot Ankle Clin. 2012;17(4):517–28.
4. Herrero-Beaumont G, Roman-Blas JA, Castañeda S, Jimenez SA. Primary osteoarthritis no longer primary: three subsets with distinct etiological, clinical, and therapeutic characteristics. Semin Arthritis Rheum. 2009;39(2):71–80.
5. Zaidi R, Cro S, Gurusamy K, Siva N, Macgregor A, Henricson A, Goldberg A. The outcome of total ankle replacement: a systematic review and meta-analysis. Bone Joint J. 2013;95(11):1500–7.
6. Shibuya N, Davis M, Jupiter DC. Epidemiology of foot and ankle fractures in the United States: an analysis of the National Trauma Data Bank (2007 to 2011). J Foot Ankle Surg. 2014;53(5):606–8.
7. Thomas RH, Daniels TR. Ankle arthritis. J Bone Joint Surg Am. 2003;85(5):923–36.
8. Bartonícek J. Anatomy of the tibiofibular syndesmosis and its clinical relevance. Surg Radiol Anat. 2003;25(5–6):379–86.
9. Dubin A. Gait: the role of the ankle and foot in walking. Med Clin North Am. 2014;98(2):205–11.
10. Coughlin MJ, Saltzman CL, Roger A. Mann, Mann's surgery of the foot and ankle. Philadelphia: Elsevier Saunders; 2014.
11. Riordan E, Little C, Hunter D. Pathogenesis of post-traumatic OA with a view to intervention. Best Pract Res Clin Rheumatol. 2014;28(1):17–30.
12. Nakasa T, Adachi N, Kato T, Ochi M. Correlation between subchondral bone plate thickness and cartilage degeneration in osteoarthritis of the ankle. Foot Ankle Int. 2014;35(12):1341–9.
13. Simon TM, Jackson D. Articular cartilage: injury pathways and treatment options. Sports Med Arthrosc. 2006;14(3):146–54.
14. Eger W, Schumacher B, Mollenhauer J, Kuettner KE, Cole AA. Human knee and ankle cartilage explants: catabolic differences. J Orthop Res. 2002;20(3):526–34.
15. Egloff C, Hügle T, Valderrabano V. Biomechanics and pathomechanisms of osteoarthritis. Swiss Med Wkly. 2012;19(July):142.
16. Dattani R, Patnaik S, Kantak A, Srikanth B, Selvan TP. Injuries to the tibiofibular syndesmosis. J Bone Joint Surg Br. 2008;90(4):405–10.
17. Rodgers MM. Dynamic biomechanics of the normal foot and ankle during walking and running. Phys Ther. 1998;68(12):1822–30.
18. Ritterman SA, Fellars T, Digiovanni CW. Current thoughts on ankle arthritis. R I Med J. 2013;96(3):30–3.
19. Valderrabano V, Horisberger M, Russell I, Dougall H, Hintermann B. Etiology of ankle osteoarthritis. Clin Orthop Relat Res. 2009;467(7):1800–6.

20. Mündermann A, Dyrby CO, Andriacchi TP. Secondary gait changes in patients with medial compartment knee osteoarthritis: increased load at the ankle, knee, and hip during walking. Arthritis Rheum. 2005;52(9):2835–44.
21. Broos PL, Bisschop A. Operative treatment of ankle fractures in adults: correlation between types of fracture and final results. Injury. 1991;22:403–6.
22. Lübbeke A, Salvo D, Stern R, Hoffmeyer P, Holzer N, Assal M. Risk factors for post-traumatic osteoarthritis of the ankle: an eighteen year follow-up study. Int Orthop. 2012;36(7):1403–10.
23. Yablon I. The key role of the lateral malleolous in displaced fractures of the ankle. J Bone Joint Surg Am. 1977;59(2):69–73.
24. Mandi D. Ankle fractures. Clin Podiatr Med Surg. 2012;29(2):155–86.
25. Schmid T. Conservative treatment of asymmetric ankle arthritis. Foot Ankle Clin. 2013;18(3):437–48.
26. Bergkvist D. Obesity in orthopedic patients. Surg Obes Relat Dis. 2009;5(6):670–2.
27. Bostman O. Body mass index of patients with elbow and ankle fractures requiring surgical treatment. J Trauma. 1994;37(1):62–5.
28. Stufkens SA, Knupp MM, Horisberger M, Lampert C, Hintermann B. Cartilage lesions and the development of osteoarthritis after internal fixation of ankle fractures. J Bone Joint Surg Am. 2010;92(2):279–86.
29. Hintermann MB, Boss A, Schäfer D. Arthroscopic findings in patients with chronic ankle instability. Am J Sports Med. 2002;30(3):402–9.
30. Brown TD, Johnston R, Saltzman CL, Marsh JL, Buckwalter JA. Posttraumatic osteoarthritis: a first estimate of incidence, prevalence, and burden of disease. J Orthop Trauma. 2006;20(10):739–44.
31. Koulouris MG, Morrison WB. Foot and ankle disorders: radiographic signs. Semin Roentgenol. 2005;40(4):358–79. Elsevier Inc.
32. Krause FG, Di Silvestro M, Penner MJ, Wing KJ, Glazebrook MA, Daniels TR, Lau JT, Younger AS. The postoperative COFAS end-stage ankle arthritis classification system: interobserver and intraobserver reliability. Foot Ankle Spec. 2012;5(1):31–6.
33. Van Valburg AA, Van Roermund PM, Marijnissen ACA, Van Melkebeek J, Lammens J, Verbout AJ, Bijlsma JWJ. Joint distraction in treatment of osteoarthritis: a two-year follow-up of the ankle. Osteoarthritis Cartilage. 1999;7(5):474–9.
34. Salk RS, Chang TJ, D'Costa WF, Soomekh DJ, Grogan KA. Sodium hyaluronate in the treatment of osteoarthritis of the ankle: a controlled, randomized, double-blind pilot study. J Bone Joint Surg Am. 2006;88(2):295–302.
35. Witteveen AG, Sierevelt IN, Blankevoort L, Kerkhoffs GM, van Dijk CN. Intra-articular sodium hyaluronate injections in the osteoarthritic ankle joint: effects, safety and dose dependency. Foot Ankle Surg. 2010;16(4):159–63.
36. Bijlsma JW, Berenbaum F, Lafeber FP. Osteoarthritis: an update with relevance for clinical practice. Lancet. 2011;377(9783):2115–26.
37. Shih LY, Wu JJ, Lo WH. Changes in gait and maximum ankle torque in patients with ankle arthritis. Foot Ankle Int. 1993;14(2):97–103.
38. John S, Bongiovanni F. Brace management for ankle arthritis. Clin Podiatr Med Surg. 2009;26(2):93–7.
39. Lin RS, Gage JR. The neurological control system for normal gait. J Prosthetics Orthot. 1989;2(1):1–13.
40. Sugimoto K, Takakura Y, Okahashi K, Samoto N, Kawate K, Iwai M. Chondral injuries of the ankle with recurrent lateral instability: an arthroscopic study. J Bone Joint Surg Am. 2009;91(1):99–106.
41. Phisitkul P, Tennant JN, Amendola A. Is there any value to arthroscopic debridement of ankle osteoarthritis and impingement? Foot Ankle Clin. 2013;18(3):449–58.
42. Glazebrook MA, Ganapathy V, Bridge MA, Stone JW, Allard JP. Evidence-based indications for ankle arthroscopy. Arthroscopy. 2009;25(12):1478–90.

43. Deng DF, Hamilton GA, Lee M, Rush S, Ford LA, Patel S. Complications associated with foot and ankle arthroscopy. J Foot Ankle Surg. 2012;51(3):281–4.
44. Winters BS, Raikin SM. The use of allograft in joint-preserving surgery for ankle osteochondral lesions and osteoarthritis. Foot Ankle Clin. 2013;18(3):529–42.
45. Kim YS, Youn HK, Kim BS, Choi YJ, Koh YG. Arthroscopic evaluation of persistent pain following supramalleolar osteotomy for varus ankle osteoarthritis. Knee Surg Sports Traumatol Arthrosc. 2014;1(8).
46. Barg A, Pagenstert GI, Horisberger M, Paul J, Gloyer M, Henninger HB, Valderrabano V. Supramalleolar osteotomies for degenerative joint disease of the ankle joint: indication, technique and results. Int Orthop. 2013;37(9):1683–95.
47. Wukich DK, Belczyk RJ. An introduction to the Taylor spatial frame for foot and ankle applications. Oper Tech Orthop. 2006;16(1):2–9.
48. John JY, Sheskier S. Total ankle replacement. Bull Hosp Joint Dis. 2014;72(1):120–8.
49. Saltzman C. Total ankle replacement – State of art. Instr Course Lect. 1999;49:263–8.
50. Easley ME, Vertullo CJ, Urban WC, Nunley JA. Total ankle arthroplasty. J Am Acad Orthop Surg. 2002;10(3):157–67.
51. Rodriguez D, Bevernage BD, Maldague P, Deleu PA, Tribak K, Leemrijse T. Medium term follow-up of the AES ankle prosthesis: high rate of asymptomatic osteolysis. Foot Ankle Surg. 2010;16(2):54–60.
52. Singer S, Klejman S, Pinsker E, Houck J, Daniels T. Ankle arthroplasty and ankle arthrodesis: gait analysis compared with normal controls. J Bone Joint Surg Am. 2013;95(24):e191–1.
53. Daniels TR, Younger AS, Penner M, Wing K, Dryden PJ, Wong H, Glazebrook M. Intermediate-term results of total ankle replacement and ankle arthrodesis: a COFAS multicenter study. J Bone Joint Surg Am. 2014;96(2):135–42.
54. Waters RL, Barnes G, Husserl T, Silver L, Liss R. Comparable energy expenditure after arthrodesis of the hip and ankle. J Bone Joint Surg Am. 1998;70(7):1032–7.
55. Coester LM, Saltzman CL, Leupold J, Pontarelli W. Long-term results following ankle arthrodesis for post-traumatic arthritis. J Bone Joint Surg Am. 2001;83(2):219.
56. Frey C, Halikus NM, Vu-Rose T, Ebramzadeh E. A review of ankle arthrodesis: predisposing factors to nonunion. Foot Ankle Int. 1994;15(11):581–4.
57. Takakura Y, Tanaka Y, Sugimoto K, Akiyama K, Tamai S. Long term results of arthrodesis for osteoarthritis of the ankle. Clin Orthop Relat Res. 1999;361:178–85.
58. Jordan RW, Chahal GS, Chapman A, Jordan RW, Chahal GS, Chapman A. Is end-stage ankle arthrosis best managed with total ankle replacement or arthrodesis? a systematic review. Advances in orthopedics. 2014.

Chapter 6
Hand and Wrist Osteoarthritis

Herbert P. von Schroeder and Steven J. McCabe

Key Points

- Hand and wrist osteoarthritis (OA) affects almost every individual as they age. It is painful and results in profound weakness of pinch and grip strength as more joints are involved. It can result in profound functional limitations.
- The distal interphalangeal joints of the fingers and interphalangeal joint of the thumb are the most commonly involved when assessed on physical examination. Osteophytes, mucus cysts (with nail deformities), and progressive deformity are some of the physical characteristics of hand OA. Patients often complain that their arthritic fingers are unsightly.
- Other common sites of OA include the carpometacarpal joint of the thumb and the scaphotrapeziotrapezoid of the wrist. Chronic scaphoid fracture nonunions and scapholunate ligament tears lead to characteristic arthritic patterns.
- The diagnosis of OA in any joint of the hand is usually made by history and physical examination. Radiographs are useful to confirm the diagnosis; to evaluate the severity of joint changes, for the purposes of discussion with the patient; and to assist in surgical planning.
- Medical management of OA commonly includes oral acetaminophen, oral or topical nonsteroidal anti-inflammatory drugs (NSAIDs), corticosteroid injections, and the use of splints.
- Surgical arthrodesis (joint fusion) or arthroplasty (joint replacement) can be useful in controlling pain, improving stability, and, in some cases, maintaining motion to improve function and appearance of the hand.

H.P. von Schroeder, MD, MSc, FRCSC (✉) • S.J. McCabe, MD, MSc, FRCSC
The University of Toronto Hand Program, University Health Network, Altum Health, Toronto Western Hospital, 399 Bathurst Street, Toronto, ON M5T 2S8, Canada
e-mail: herb.vonschroeder@uhn.ca

M. Kapoor, N.N. Mahomed (eds.), *Osteoarthritis: Pathogenesis, Diagnosis, Available Treatments, Drug Safety, Regenerative and Precision Medicine*,
DOI 10.1007/978-3-319-19560-5_6

Introduction

OA of the hand and wrist is a ubiquitous condition that eventually affects virtually everyone. It is painful and results in profound weakness of the hands as well as progressive deformity that we associate with aging. The severity of hand OA is related to hand dysfunction. Weakness of pinch and grip strength is more profound with more joints involved, and pain and tenderness have significant effects on hand function [1].

OA is one the most common diagnoses treated by hand surgeons. It can occur de novo or can be the long-term sequelae following a fracture or ligament injury. It may also represent the final stage of osteonecrosis. The diagnosis of OA in any joint of the hand can typically be made by history and physical examination. Radiographs are useful to confirm the diagnosis; to evaluate the severity of joint changes, for the purposes of discussion with the patient; and to assist in surgical planning.

Medical management of OA commonly includes oral acetaminophen, oral or topical nonsteroidal anti-inflammatory drugs (NSAIDs), corticosteroid injections, and the use of splints. There has been increased awareness of the adverse events associated with nonsteroidal anti-inflammatory drugs beyond gastrointestinal bleeding. In a systematic review of cost-effectiveness analysis, Wielage has reviewed the evolution in the care and evaluation of patients with OA. There has been a shift to improved research methods, evaluation of multiple oral agents, and inclusion of cardiovascular and neurologic outcomes [2]. Recently, topical NSAIDs have become an alternative to oral agents. In a comprehensive review of the effectiveness and safety of topical versus oral NSAID drugs, Klinge and Sawyer found that both topical and oral agents performed better than placebo and were similar in efficacy. As might be expected, there are less serious adverse events but more skin reactions with topical agents [3]. It is noted that topical salicylates and capsaicin have not shown substantial efficacy in clinical trials [4].

Occupational therapists help to improve patients' daily function. Surgical arthrodesis (joint fusion) or arthroplasty (joint replacement) can be useful in controlling pain, improving stability, and, in some cases, maintaining motion to improve function and appearance of the hand. Denervation of the wrist is also possible as an attempt to control pain in some cases.

Distal Interphalangeal (DIP) Joints of the Fingers and Interphalangeal (IP) Joint of the Thumb OA

OA at the DIP joints (Fig. 6.1) is the most common location in the body, found in 70 % of a large cohort of 61–63-year-olds. This was compared to 23 % at the proximal interphalangeal joints, 10 % at the metacarpal phalangeal joints, and 41 % at the basal (carpometacarpal) joint of the thumb [5]. The DIP joints and the IP joint of the thumb are also the most commonly involved when assessed on physical examination. Osteophytes (traditionally called Heberden nodes in this location), mucus cysts

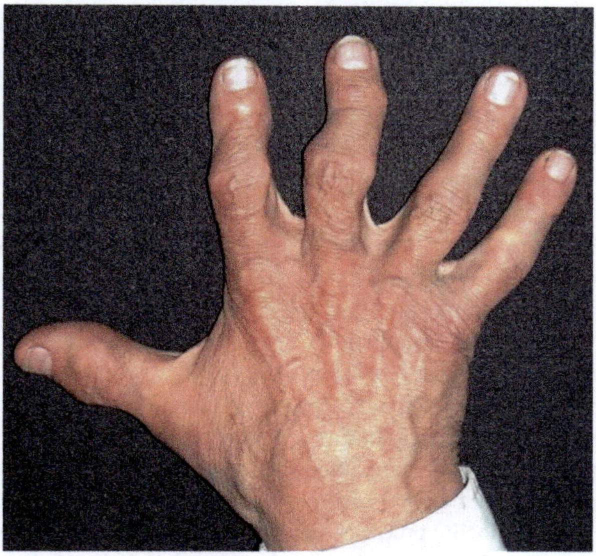

Fig. 6.1 Photograph of an 82-year-old man's hand with severe osteoarthritis and deformity of the small joints of the hand

(with nail deformities), and progressive deformity are noted. The joints may become unstable and angulated. Patients complain that their arthritic fingers are unsightly. Painful arthritis in the distal or proximal interphalangeal joints is associated with worse health status when measured by patient-reported outcome measures [6].

Splinting can be used to immobilize painful joints and is almost always indicated as initial treatment of OA of the DIP joint. In a small non-randomized study, DIP joints splinted at night were less painful at 6 months compared to joints without nighttime splinting. There was decreased extensor lag in the treated group without increased stiffness of the joint [7]. In another study of 25 patients splinted for 6 months, pain scores measured on a visual analog scale decreased from 100 to 34 %, and DASH scores improved from 28 to 17. The change in DASH score was not significant [8].

The primary indication for surgery to treat OA of the distal interphalangeal joints is pain, but surgery is sometimes done for dysfunction or cosmesis. Several surgical approaches have been evaluated; however, since the mainstay for surgical treatment is arthrodesis, a patient with a cosmetic concern would need to give up all motion of the joint for the sake of appearance.

Arthrodesis is the primary surgical option for OA of the distal interphalangeal joint. This procedure is indicated for severe pain that is not controlled adequately by splinting and medication. A variety of methods have been used to achieve fusion of the DIP joint. These include K wires alone or in combination with an interosseous cerclage wire, or headless compression screw techniques.

Using evidence from a splinting study, it was found that fusion of the index finger in 20° of flexion resulted in higher grip strength and improved dexterity compared to zero degrees. Position of the middle finger at one of these two angles did not affect dexterity or grip strength [9]. One concern about studies that use splinting to simulate arthrodesis is the negation of shortening that must occur with fusion but not splinting. As flexion functionally shortens the digit, this would suggest that splinting experiments might overestimate the degree of flexion recommended. In addition, tip and key pinch are perhaps the most important functions for the index. Our personal preference is to fuse the DIP joint in zero degrees of flexion.

A systematic review of the English language literature revealed that most studies are evidence level IV. The most common techniques were K wires, headless compression screws, and cerclage wires. The headless screws appeared to have higher union rates but introduced negative events otherwise not seen [10]. Stern found the same nonunion rates for fusions using either crossed K wires, an interfragmentary wire plus a longitudinal K wire, or a Herbert screw at 12 %, 12 %, and 11 %, respectively. Major complications occurred in 20 %. Stern prefers "Herbert screw fixation when there is adequate bone stock and sufficient cross-sectional area to contain the screw" [11]. Other authors report arthrodesis of the DIP joint using a headless compression screw has resulted in high union rates around 95 %. Cox had a union rate of 94 % with a complication rate of 9 % [12].

One specific problem that can occur with screw fixation is penetration of the cortex. One study noted the distal phalanx shaft as measured on the lateral view is the narrowest determinant of fit and that most commercially available screws were too large [13]. Iwamoto placed the screw in a proximal to distal direction in an oblique fashion to avoid invasion of the nail bed. They report a union rate of 96 % [14].

In an interesting approach, Renfree compared the standard use of the headless compression screw with an in situ group where there was no preparation of the articular surfaces. Interestingly, ten of 17 joints fused with no preparation of the surfaces compared to 11 of 12 with the standard technique [15]. Despite the finding that fusion can be successful without joint surface preparation, the rate was lower, and therefore this procedure is not recommended. These studies have typically included a heterogeneous population of patients with a variety of pathology, not just osteoarthritis.

Authors' Technique

We favor a traditional technique for DIP joint fusion using a longitudinal K wire and a transverse cerclage wire. This is a quick, low-cost, and reliable method.

The procedure is performed using local anesthetic and a digital tourniquet. A curved incision is made in a transverse direction at the DIP joint dorsally, proximal and parallel to the nail margin. This must be proximal to the most proximal extent of the nail bed. In addition, the incision can be scythed proximally to avoid the nail bed. A longitudinal incision is made proximal to this along the central dorsal axis of the middle phalanx. This incision is made directly onto the bone of the middle phalanx, and using a skin hook to hold the now split extensor apparatus, the extensor insertion on the base of the distal phalanx is elevated, continuing around to elevate the collateral ligaments from both sides of the DIP joint. At this time, the joint can be hyperflexed. If this is not possible, the collateral ligaments would require further release from the distal aspect of the middle phalanx. The power saw is used to make a cut just proximal to the articular surface of the middle phalanx. This is cut first as it is accessible and once accomplished allows more space to work on the base of the distal phalanx. We attempt to preserve cortical bone on the lateral margins of both opposing surfaces as this will be required to hold the interosseous wire loop. The soft tissue is dissected off the circumference of the distal phalanx for a few millimeters dorsally and palmarly and for about 5 mm laterally. The saw is then used to make a parallel transverse cut in the distal phalanx. We typically fuse the DIP joints in 0° of flexion. A 0.35″ K wire is used to drill a hole transversely in the middle and distal phalanx and pass a cerclage wire through each. The same K wire is then passed through the base of the distal phalanx to exit the tip of the finger just palmar to the nail. This is passed all the way until the proximal pin is at the osteosynthesis site. The joint is reduced and the pin is passed into the middle phalanx. Intraoperative X-rays are used to confirm the reduction and hardware placement, and the cerclage wire is tightened. A small dressing and splint are then applied. The K wire is protected and is left in place for 6–8 weeks. X-rays are taken at the first postoperative visit and at 6 weeks post-op. A splint is always worn when the K wire is in place and can be continued as needed.

As an alternative to surgical arthrodesis, flexible implant arthroplasty has been reported and has the advantage of preservation of motion when compared to fusion. In comparison to the proximal interphalangeal joint and the metacarpal phalangeal joint however, its use is less common in the distal interphalangeal joint. The procedure mimics implant arthroplasty of the PIP joint with division of the extensor tendon, preparation of the proximal joint articular surface and canals, and fitting of the implant. Although few cases have been reported, the results seem reasonable [16, 17].

As an innovative strategy, we have observed Dr. Harold Kleinert perform surgical debridement and extensor tendon plication and re-balancing at the DIP joints. He then distracted the joints over a K wire for a period of time. This allowed the preservation of motion with the intention of pain relief.

Proximal Interphalangeal (PIP) Joints of the Fingers OA

The proximal interphalangeal (PIP) joint is a common site for OA. Joint pain, deformity, and stiffness are common presenting features (Fig. 6.2). Osteophytes in this location are termed Bouchard nodes. As with DIP joints, the same nonsurgical care is available for the PIP joints including medication, the application of hand therapy modalities, and splinting. The role of the PIP joints is to bring the fingers into the palm, and motion is therefore more important at the PIP than the DIP joint, and hence arthroplasty has a large role in the surgical management of PIP arthritis. Ironically, it has been shown that arthroplasty preserves but does not improve motion at the PIP joint. Both arthrodesis and arthroplasty have been shown to reduce pain.

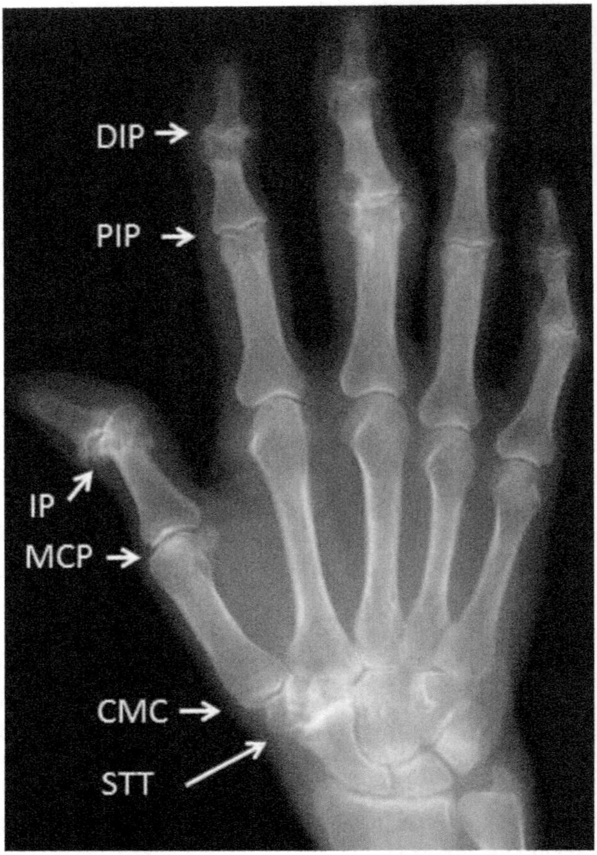

Fig. 6.2 DIP joint OA seen on a radiograph with typical joint space narrowing, osteophytes, and angular deformity at the index finger and at the thumb IP joint. PIP joint OA seen clearly on the long finger. The STT joint of the wrist is also arthritic

The index and small fingers can retain good function following joint arthrodesis. The small finger has motion at the CMC joint and can hyperextend at the MCP joint which compensates for a fused PIP joint. The index finger is functional with a fused PIP joint primarily because the other fingers will provide good grip strength and the presence of the bulk of the thenar muscles makes incomplete flexion of the PIP joint less important for gripping. In contrast, the long and ring fingers tolerate arthrodesis poorly. The long and ring finger with a fused PIP joint can neither flex nor extend adequately.

In our opinion, fusion of the PIP joint of the index finger should be in slight flexion. Once again, splinting experiments overestimate the degree of flexion that results in the best function because they fail to account for the shortening of the finger caused by the surgery. The ideal angle of fusion of the PIP joints is likely less than advocated in most texts. The small finger PIP joint can be fused in 30–35°. This will allow the hand to lie "flat" on a table and to have good grip of small objects.

In cadaveric testing of the stiffness of PIP joint fusion techniques, the intramedullary linked screw method had higher stiffness than 90/90 wiring, tension band wiring, and cerclage wire with an oblique K wire in all planes of motion and greater stiffness than a dorsal plate in extension [18]. In a study comparing fusions of the MP and PIP joints using tension band arthrodesis versus a compression screw, both had similar healing times and complications. Removal of hardware was required more often following tension band arthrodesis [19].

Authors' Technique

For arthrodesis of a joint in flexion (always for the PIP joints), we use a tension band technique. A straight dorsal incision is made over the PIP joint and taken straight through the extensor mechanism. The tendon is retracted with skin hooks and sharply dissected from the base of the middle phalanx. The sharp dissection is continued releasing the collateral ligaments. This allows the joint to be flexed to almost 180°. The collateral ligaments are dissected from the distal aspect of the proximal phalanx, and the power saw is used to remove the articular surface with a slight proximal palmar angle. This angle is the angle that is anticipated for the joint upon completion of the procedure. Having removed the phalangeal head, there is more room to work on the base of the middle phalanx. The soft tissues are dissected from the base of the phalanx including enough dorsal dissection to pass a transverse pin for the tension band wire. The base of the middle phalanx is then removed with the power saw parallel to the joint surface. The joint is then reduced to test the fit and the osteosynthesis is performed. To fix the fusion, a 0.35″ K wire is used to drill a transverse hole across the dorsal aspect of the base of the middle phalanx about 5 mm distal to the bone cut. A cerclage wire is passed through this hole. This must be done before the K wires are inserted into the middle phalanx as the K wires can crimp this hole and make passage of the tension band impossible. A 0.35″ K wire is then inserted through the cut end of the proximal phalanx at the same angle as the intended fusion to exit the dorsum of the proximal phalanx 1 cm from the cut end. The second pin is placed parallel to the first. The placement of these pins is important as the surgeon must plan ahead to insure they will penetrate into the medullary canal of the middle phalanx when the fusion site is reduced. The fusion is reduced and the K wires are passed into the medullary canal of the middle phalanx. Position is checked with fluoroscopy. The cerclage wire is then crossed over the dorsum of the middle phalanx and osteosynthesis site and twisted around the pins on the dorsal surface of the proximal phalanx. The wire is tightened and the pins are bent, cut, and twisted so the bent end is at the shoulder of the phalanx. A short period of splinting is used; however, early motion creates compression and is encouraged.

The importance of motion of the PIP joint is reflected in the common use of arthroplasty to treat OA of this joint. The procedure has traditionally been performed using a dorsal approach and silicone implants; however, there are variations described in the literature. New materials have created ongoing interest in this procedure.

The techniques for flexible implant arthroplasty have been detailed including a dorsal and palmar approach [20]. The dorsal approach has the potential to disrupt the extensor mechanism although the central slip-sparing approach described by Swanson can minimize this. The palmar approach has the theoretic advantage of sparing the extensor mechanism. In a comparison of the palmar and dorsal approach, better preservation of extension was found with the palmar approach. At mean follow-up of 29 months, the PIP motion was 60/15 with the dorsal approach and 62/2 with the palmar approach [21].

New materials have been introduced for PIP arthroplasty. In a large series of pyrocarbon implants with minimum of 2-year follow-up, it was found that patients had good relief of pain but no improvement of range of motion. Thirty-six percent of patients needed repeat surgery [22]. A systematic review of studies evaluating the outcomes of silicone and pyrocarbon arthroplasties of the PIP joint revealed similar postoperative arcs of motion but higher rates of revision and salvage procedures performed secondary to pyrocarbon arthroplasty. The authors cautioned against widespread use of this implant until further evidence is developed [23]. Further evolution of PIP implants has yielded metal alloy and polyethylene anatomically based designs. These are used as total joints or as hemiarthroplasty. This method has been shown to improve pain and preserve joint motion [24].

Authors' Technique

For a PIP arthroplasty, we use the dorsal approach with a central slip-sparing method. A straight dorsal incision is made through skin and subcutaneous tissue to the plane overlying the extensor tendon. A small "entry incision" is made at the lateral margins of the extensor apparatus about 1 cm proximal to the PIP joint, and an elevator is passed under the extensor tendon on the dorsolateral aspect of the PIP joint on each side sequentially. This separates the extensor mechanism and transverse retinacular fibers from the underlying collateral ligaments. The transverse fibers are marked with a small permanent suture proximally and distally and divided a few mm from the lateral band to allow suturing at the end of the procedure. This is done on both sides of the joint. The true collateral ligaments, now under direct vision, are released from the attachment to the proximal phalanx. The central slip is intact throughout this procedure but may require sacrifice if OA is extreme. Release of the collateral ligaments allows dislocation of the joint through flexion and rotation of the joint. Working from both sides of the central slip, the proximal joint surface is prepared and resected using a power saw. Osteophytes are removed from the base of the middle phalanx but no bone is resected with the saw.

The medullary canals are prepared and the implants are fitted. The collateral ligaments are not repaired although stability is achieved by suturing the previously marked transverse retinacular ligaments. The alignment is evaluated and the wounds are closed. Since the central slip is preserved, early motion can be started with a splint used for resting.

Metacarpal Phalangeal (MCP) Joint of the Index, Long, Ring, and Small Finger OA

The MCP joint is readily accessed for steroid injection which is recommended in conjunction with the nonsurgical procedures used for the IP joints. Buddy taping can also be useful to reduce pain in the joint.

If nonsurgical treatment is not satisfactory, arthroplasty can be recommended. Compared to rheumatoid disease, OA in the MCP joint is less frequently a cause of significant problems. Additionally, OA in the MCP joints can occur in a single joint often requiring arthroplasty of one joint in contrast to rheumatoid arthritis which typically requires all joints to be replaced. Fusion of the MCP joints results in poor function so preservation of motion is desirable. The wisdom of fusion versus arthroplasty of the isolated index MP joint is often debated but not resolved. For painful OA of the long, ring, and small MCP joints, arthroplasty is preferred.

Silicone interposition arthroplasty is the traditional implant used for the MCP joint in OA. The literature shows this to be effective in pain reduction, increasing motion, and providing patient satisfaction [25]. Pyrocarbon implants seem to perform well at the MCP location. Wall and Stern have shown good results at 2-year follow-up with good pain relief, improved motion, strong patient satisfaction, and few complications [26]. Both materials seem to provide similar clinical results at the MCP joints. Further evaluation of survival of the implants and cost may clarify their respective roles in the future.

Following replacement arthroplasty of the MCP joint, protection of the extensor apparatus is required. The care of a hand therapist is extremely valuable following arthroplasty of IP and MCP joints. Protection of the extensor apparatus can be done with resting splints that are removed for appropriate range of motion exercises or with splints designed with traction to position the finger to control alignment and allow flexion against elastic traction.

Metacarpal Phalangeal (MCP) Joint of the Thumb OA

OA of the thumb MCP occurs with chronic ligament injury (ulnar collateral (gamekeeper thumb) or less commonly radial collateral ligament or volar plate). OA can also occur de novo at this joint or in association with OA at the carpometacarpal (CMC) joint of the thumb. Splinting and corticosteroid injections are useful. Arthrodesis of the joint provides stability and pain control. The technique is most commonly performed in the neutral position with cerclage and K wires similar to the description for DIP joint arthrodesis. Compression screws or plate and screw fixation are also used. Regardless of surgical detail, the procedure is reliable with high patient satisfaction and requires only a brief period of immobilization.

Carpometacarpal (CMC) Joint of the Thumb OA

The CMC joint at the base of the thumb has a wide arc of motion, and radiographic OA changes are exceptionally common and increase with age (Fig. 6.3). The metacarpal bone subluxes out of the joint to create a characteristic deformity. There is prominence of the base of the metacarpal which is commonly accompanied by hyperextension of the MP joint and eventual adduction of the thumb toward the palm. Patients can have pain directly over the dorsum of the CMC joint but often complain of pain at the base of the thenar muscles. Active circular motion of the joint will often reveal crepitus. The history and physical findings are so characteristic that the grind test is not usually performed. It can be quite painful and adds little information when the findings are obvious. X-rays are done to evaluate the CMC and the STT joints and to look for other pathology that might influence treatment. X-ray staging of the severity of the disease does not strongly correlate with symptom severity. X-rays provide useful information if they are normal in the face of severe symptoms.

Nonsurgical management consisting of splinting, oral NSAIDs, and injection of corticosteroids is found to be beneficial in the management of first CMC OA. In a randomized trial, it was found that wearing an orthosis provided pain relief but no change in the function of symptomatology over time when the orthosis was not

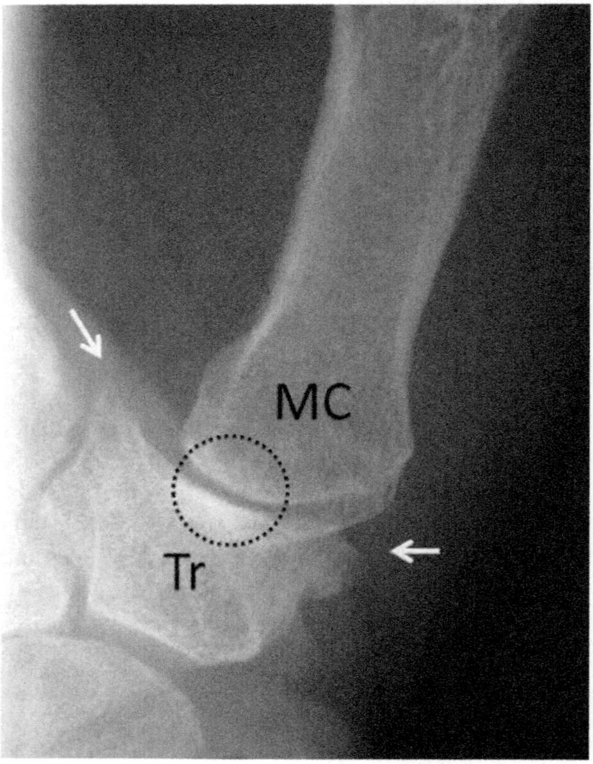

Fig. 6.3 CMC OA at the base of the thumb. Joint space narrowing and subchondral sclerosis between the thumb metacarpal (*MC*) and the triquetrum (*Tr*) are noted (*circle*) as well as osteophytes (*arrows*) at the trapezium. The thumb is subluxed off of the central axis

worn [27]. In contrast, Bani found that custom-made splints improved pain, grip, and pinch strength and function [28].

A single steroid injection into the thumb CMC joint has been found to reduce pain and increase function [29]. This confirmed a study by Day that showed "Steroid injection with splinting for the treatment of basal joint arthritis of the thumb provided reliable long-term relief in thumbs with Eaton stage 1 disease but provided long-term relief in only 7 of 17 thumbs with Eaton stage 2 and stage 3 basal joint arthritis" [30]. Interestingly, both of these studies showed that the effect of steroid injection is related to the Eaton stage of arthritis. This is in contrast to a randomized trial that showed no benefit following a steroid injection [31]. In spite of this, however, we recommend an initial trial of splinting and injection for all new patients presenting with this problem.

Common surgical procedures include excision of the trapezium with interposition of tendon or other material, other forms of arthroplasty or fusion of the joint. The CMC is a fertile ground for innovation of new surgical procedures. Various materials have been used as interpositions, a wide variety of implants have been developed, and new methods continue to be employed and advocated. Typically, these are based on products available on the marketplace and have little evidence to support their use. A Cochrane review revealed, "We were unable to demonstrate that any technique confers a benefit over another technique in terms of pain and physical function. Furthermore, the included studies were not of high enough quality to provide conclusive evidence that the compared techniques provided equivalent outcomes" [32]. Without clear evidence of superiority of alternatives, our philosophy is that autogenous tissue is always preferred for the reconstruction. The most common surgical procedure involves excision on the trapezium, ligament reconstruction with a local tendon graft, and interposition of the graft into the joint.

Arthritis in this joint is frequently associated with OA at the scaphotrapeziotrapezoid (STT) joint. Excision of the trapezium for the CMC OA will also eliminate the arthritic scaphotrapezoid pain, but the scaphoid articulation with the trapezoid should also be inspected and aggressively debrided if OA is present. The presence of STT arthritis in a percentage of patients with CMC arthritis is a common argument against fusion of the CMC joint. Despite this, however, arthrodesis continues to have support. One author found 17 nonunions of 249 thumb CMC fusions. The results showed improved pain, increased function, and excellent patient satisfaction with the procedure [33].

Carpometacarpal (CMC) Joints of the Index and Long Fingers OA

Carpal bossing is the term used to describe the deformity caused by osteophyte formation at the second and third CMC joints at the index and long fingers. It occurs with age and may be associated with tendonitis of the extensor carpi radialis tendon insertions. The boss can be excised but may recur. The joints can also be fused.

Carpometacarpal (CMC) Joints of Ring and Small Finger OA

OA of the fourth and fifth CMC joints is generally posttraumatic following fracture at the metacarpal bases or fracture-dislocation of the joints. The joints are more mobile than the second and third CMC joints, and this motion is important during gripping activities. Fusion or interposition with soft tissue can be considered in the rare cases that these joints require surgery.

Scaphotrapeziotrapezoid (STT) OA

OA of the STT (scaphotrapeziotrapezoid) joint on the radial aspect of the wrist occurs with age and is more common in women. It is a common radiographic finding (Fig. 6.4) in people over the age of 60 years and is the second most frequent OA in the wrist, but it may not be symptomatic [34]. When symptoms do occur, the pain can be localized in the distal part of the anatomic snuff box and proximal to the thumb CMC joint. Pain also occurs around the scaphoid tubercle in the thenar region and is worse with gripping and radial deviation. Progressive loss of wrist motion typically ensues. STT OA may occur in conjunction with OA of the thumb CMC joint or with chronic tears of the scapholunate ligament [35]. With disruption of all of the ligaments around the scaphoid, rotation and subluxation of the scaphoid result in increased pressure at the STT joint and local arthritic changes [36]. As with most types of OA, medical management is helpful, and when these fail, surgical options must take other regional OA into account. For isolated STT OA, excision of the distal scaphoid and soft tissue interposition is a useful motion-sparing procedure. Fusion of the joint is useful for pain control but will limit wrist motion

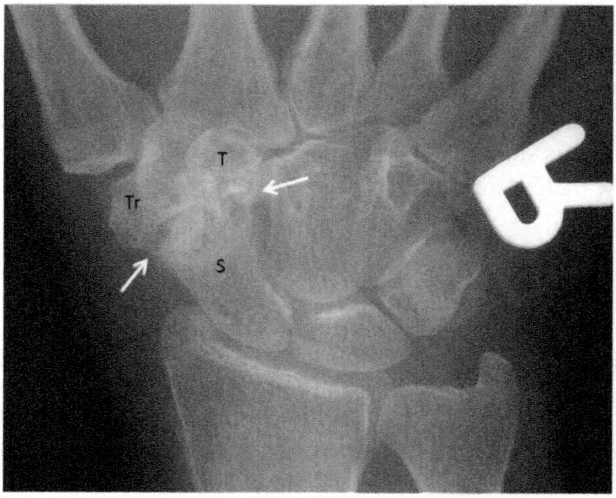

Fig. 6.4 STT joint OA (*arrows*) seen on a radiograph of a right wrist between the scaphoid (*S*), the trapezium (*Tr*), and the trapezoid (*T*) carpal bones. The STT joint is the second most common site of OA in the wrist, this condition has variable symptomatology

and carries with it a relatively high nonunion rate. If CMC OA is also present, excision of the trapezium and soft tissue interposition is required, but the proximal portion of the trapezoid must also be removed in order to excise all of the painful arthritis. Surgery requires 6 weeks of full immobilization, followed by the use of a splint.

Scaphoid Nonunion Advanced Collapse (SNAC) OA

The scaphoid bone is the most commonly fractured bone in the wrist and occurs most frequently in young men. The injury is often ignored or missed since the pain can resolve quickly, and initial X-rays can be read as being normal [37]. However, the fracture may not heal resulting in a pseudoarthrosis that causes abnormal mechanical wear and arthritis that begins between the scaphoid and the radial styloid (Fig. 6.5) and typically progresses to become symptomatic in midlife [38, 39]. Over time, the arthritis advances across the wrist but surprisingly spares the radiolunate articulation. Early symptoms include radial wrist pain and limited motion (particularly extension). With progression, there is further loss of motion, weakness of grip, pain with impact, and chronic radio-dorsal wrist swelling and joint effusion. As with all OA of the hand, NSAIDs, analgesics, corticosteroid injections, and splints are useful.

For early stages, with minimal arthritic changes, reconstruction of the scaphoid with bone graft and internal fixation can be considered [40]. Alternatively, only the distal scaphoid can be excised and interposed with soft tissue with favorable outcomes, but this procedure should only be considered as a stopgap or reserved for patients with limited overall function since further eventual collapse of the wrist will occur with time [41]. More commonly patients will benefit from a

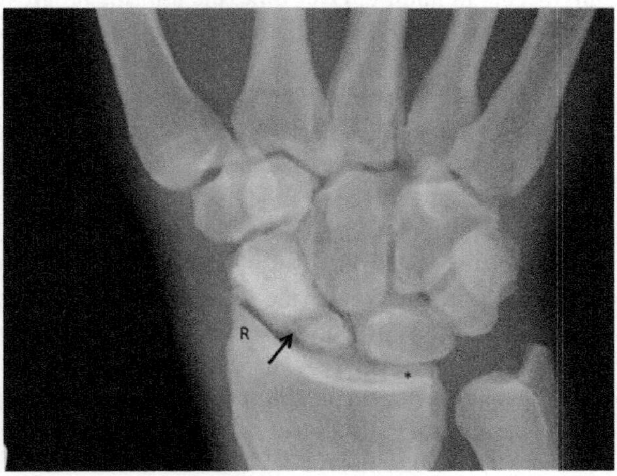

Fig. 6.5 "SNAC" OA seen on a radiograph of a right wrist resulting from a scaphoid fracture nonunion (*arrow*). A large osteophyte is present at the radial styloid (*R*). The radiolunate joint (*) is typically not arthritic and the basis for reconstructive options to allow for some motion

choice of one of the two common wrist salvage procedures [42]. A four-corner limited wrist arthrodesis fuses the lunate, capitate, hamate, and triquetrum and excises the arthritic scaphoid and often the radial styloid. The procedure has many variations and technical nuances, but all versions of the procedure capitalize on the non-arthritic radiolunate articulation. Alternatively, a proximal row carpectomy (PRC) involves complete excision of the scaphoid, lunate, and triquetrum (and often the radial styloid) and allows the capitate to articulate with the lunate fossa of the distal radius. The procedure requires that the capitate be free of arthritis. Despite the differences in the two techniques, they have similar outcomes in terms of motion and pain reduction [43]. The four-corner arthrodesis is technically more difficult and has a measurable nonunion rate. The proximal row carpectomy carries the risk of future arthritis at the radio-capitate articulation [44]. Failed procedures or heavy laborers can be given the option of a total wrist fusion which is useful for pain control but eliminates all wrist motion, leaving only pronation and supination at the forearm. Total wrist arthroplasty is a progressive alternative.

Scapholunate Advanced Collapse (SLAC) OA

Analogous in many ways to scaphoid fracture, tears of the scapholunate ligament also occur most frequently in young men. The injury is also often ignored or missed since the pain can resolve quickly and initial X-rays can be interpreted as normal. The ligament is important for maintaining the integrity of the proximal carpal row and the socket that the scaphoid and lunate come together to form for the capitate. A scapholunate ligament tear can range in severity from a partial tear to a complete tear. With the tears, the scaphoid and lunate twist and splay apart resulting in abnormal mechanical wear and arthritis that begins on the radial side of the wrist and typically occurs in midlife. Over time, the arthritis progresses across the wrist but also spares the radiolunate articulation. Early symptoms include radial wrist pain and limited motion which progresses over time resulting in chronic pain and dysfunction. For very early stages, with minimal arthritic changes, reconstruction can be considered. There are numerous reconstructive options but none can ensure full improvement of function [45]. Once the arthritis has progressed (Fig. 6.6), patients will benefit from a choice of either a four-corner limited wrist arthrodesis or a proximal row carpectomy (PRC) as noted above. The PRC procedure requires that the capitate be free of arthritis. Despite the differences in the two techniques, they have similar outcomes in terms of motion and pain reduction. The four-corner arthrodesis is technically more difficult and has a measurable nonunion rate. The proximal row carpectomy carries the risk of future arthritis at the radio-capitate articulation. Failed procedures or heavy laborers can be given the option of a total wrist fusion which is useful for pain control but eliminates all wrist motion, leaving only pronation and supination intact at the forearm. Total wrist arthroplasty is a progressive alternative that can be considered for when this type of arthritis is advanced.

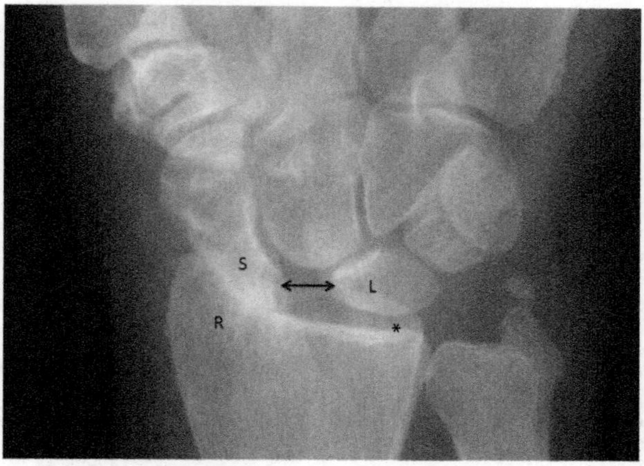

Fig. 6.6 "SLAC" OA seen on a radiograph of a right wrist resulting from a scapholunate ligament tear (double arrow) between the scaphoid (*S*) and the lunate (*L*) bones. There is complete loss of the joint space between the scaphoid (*S*) and the radius (*R*). The radiolunate joint (*) is typically not arthritic and the basis for reconstructive options to allow for some motion

Pancarpal OA

SNAC, SLAC, and other conditions, such as Kienböck's avascular necrosis of the lunate and perilunate injuries, can progress to pancarpal arthritic changes. Partial fusions and partial corpectomies are generally not satisfactory for controlling the symptoms. Instead, total wrist arthrodesis or arthroplasty can be considered. Total arthrodesis is performed with a contoured internal fixation plate from the radius to the third metacarpal to align the wrist and also to place it in slight extension for power grip. Excision of articular surfaces in the wrist, including the second and third carpometacarpal joints, and packing all debrided regions with bone graft will promote fusion rates. The proximal row can also be excised and morselized to be used as bone graft instead of using the iliac crest. Wrist arthrodesis (Fig. 6.7) does not affect pronation or supination of the forearm unless the distal radioulnar joint (DRUJ) is already arthritic. Outcomes following total fusion can be satisfactory [46].

An alternative to fusion is a total wrist arthroplasty. Several prostheses are available. The procedure and the implant allow for some, albeit not normal motion and are effective for pain relief [47, 48]. Long-term databases are not yet available to accurately predict survival, but the procedure carries risks as with all total joints which include osteolysis, loosening, and infection.

Ulnocarpal Abutment

The triangular fibrocartilage complex (TFCC) is a continuation of the articular part of the distal radius to provide a hammock for the carpus and also provides stabilization between the radius and ulna. TFCC tears themselves are not necessarily associated with arthritic changes. However, tears and degenerative changes do occur with trauma and with age. Tears and degenerative changes are more likely to occur in

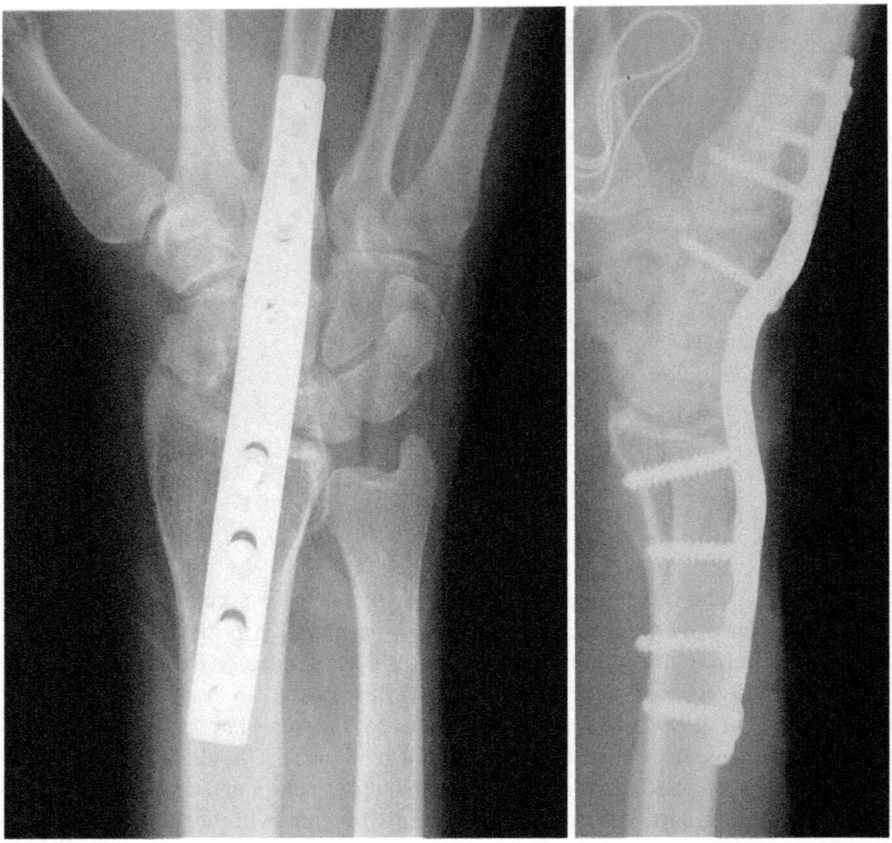

Fig. 6.7 Total wrist arthrodesis with internal fixation from the radius to the third metacarpal. The position of the wrist is in slight extension to improve gripping

conjunction with positive ulnar variance (Fig. 6.8), which is defined as an ulnar articular surface that is more distal (i.e., longer) than the radial articular surface. Under these circumstances, the TFCC is thinner and prone to injury between the ulnar head and the carpus. Changes in the ulnar corner of the lunate are the first sign of local arthritis. Ulnar shortening osteotomy is the cornerstone of treatment to mechanically reduce the forces from the carpus to the TFCC and ulna [49]. TFCC tears can be repaired in some cases either by arthroscopic or open surgery, or they can be debrided.

Distal Radioulnar Joint (DRUJ) OA

The DRUJ is responsible for stable pronation and supination of the forearm. The joint can become arthritic following injury or instability. Surgical management can include resection of the ulnar articular surface and interposition with local soft tissue. Hemi and total joint arthroplasties are also available for the joint [50, 51].

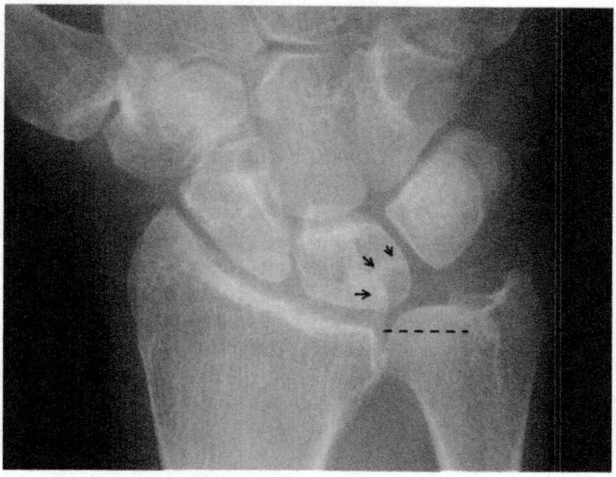

Fig. 6.8 Positive ulnar variance notes on this radiograph of a right wrist and defined by an ulna that is longer than the radius (*hashed line*). Evidence of abutment between the ulna and the lunate is seen with a large cyst at the lunate bone (*arrows*)

Summary

OA of the hand and wrist is pervasive with age and following trauma. Arthritis can cause profound functional limitations. The joints of the hand and wrist all have specific functions and all have unique surgical options to treat arthritic changes. Skilled surgical care is required to minimize complications, reduce pain, and improve or maintain hand function. In the past, there has been an emphasis on arthrodesis to control pain, but limited fusions and the advances in prosthetic arthroplasty design now provide viable options in the hand and wrist. Arthritis surgery for the hand can also result in cosmetic improvement.

References

1. Bagis S, et al. The effect of hand osteoarthritis on grip and pinch strength and hand function in postmenopausal women. Clin Rheumatol. 2003;22(6):420–4.
2. Wielage RC, et al. Cost-effectiveness analyses of osteoarthritis oral therapies: a systematic review. Appl Health Econ Health Policy. 2013;11(6):593–618.
3. Klinge SA, Sawyer GA. Effectiveness and safety of topical versus oral nonsteroidal anti-inflammatory drugs: a comprehensive review. Phys Sportsmed. 2013;41(2):64–74.
4. Altman RD, Barthel HR. Topical therapies for osteoarthritis. Drugs. 2011;71(10):1259–79.
5. Abraham AM, et al. Population prevalence of ultrasound features of osteoarthritis in the hand, knee and hip at age 63 years: the Newcastle thousand families birth cohort. BMC Musculoskelet Disord. 2014;15:162.
6. Slatkowsky-Christensen B, Haugen IK, Kvien TK. Distribution of joint involvement in women with hand osteoarthritis and associations between joint counts and patient-reported outcome measures. Ann Rheum Dis. 2010;69(1):198–201.
7. Watt FE, et al. Night-time immobilization of the distal interphalangeal joint reduces pain and extension deformity in hand osteoarthritis. Rheumatology (Oxford). 2014;53(6):1142–9.
8. Ikeda M, et al. Custom-made splint treatment for osteoarthritis of the distal interphalangeal joints. J Hand Surg Am. 2010;35(4):589–93.

9. Melamed E, et al. Simulated distal interphalangeal joint fusion of the index and middle fingers in 0 degrees and 20 degrees of flexion: a comparison of grip strength and dexterity. J Hand Surg Am. 2014;39(10):1986–91.
10. Dickson DR, et al. A systematic review of distal interphalangeal joint arthrodesis. J Hand Microsurg. 2014;6(2):74–84.
11. Stern PJ, Fulton DB. Distal interphalangeal joint arthrodesis: an analysis of complications. J Hand Surg Am. 1992;17(6):1139–45.
12. Cox C, et al. Arthrodesis of the thumb interphalangeal joint and finger distal interphalangeal joints with a headless compression screw. J Hand Surg Am. 2014;39(1):24–8.
13. Mintalucci D, et al. Distal interphalangeal joint bony dimensions related to headless compression screw sizes. J Hand Surg Am. 2014;39(6):1068–74.e1.
14. Iwamoto T, et al. An obliquely placed headless compression screw for distal interphalangeal joint arthrodesis. J Hand Surg Am. 2013;38(12):2360–4.
15. Renfree KJ. Percutaneous in situ versus open arthrodesis of the distal interphalangeal joint. J Hand Surg Eur Vol. 2015;40(4):379–83.
16. Brown LG. Distal interphalangeal joint flexible implant arthroplasty. J Hand Surg Am. 1989;14(4):653–6.
17. Zimmerman NB, et al. Silicone interpositional arthroplasty of the distal interphalangeal joint. J Hand Surg Am. 1989;14(5):882–7.
18. Capo JT, et al. Biomechanical evaluation of 5 fixation devices for proximal interphalangeal joint arthrodesis. J Hand Surg Am. 2014;39(10):1971–7.
19. Breyer JM, et al. Metacarpophalangeal and interphalangeal joint arthrodesis: a comparative study between tension band and compression screw fixation. J Hand Surg Eur Vol. 2015;40(4):374–8.
20. Swanson AB, de Groot Swanson G. Flexible implant resection arthroplasty of the proximal interphalangeal joint. Hand Clin. 1994;10(2):261–6.
21. Natera L, et al. Proximal interphalangeal joint replacement: a comparison between the volar and dorsal approach. Rev Esp Cir Ortop Traumatol. 2014;58(5):303–8.
22. Watts AC, et al. Pyrocarbon proximal interphalangeal joint arthroplasty: minimum two-year follow-up. J Hand Surg Am. 2012;37(5):882–8.
23. Chan K, et al. Pyrocarbon versus silicone proximal interphalangeal joint arthroplasty: a systematic review. Plast Reconstr Surg. 2013;131(1):114–24.
24. Murray PM, et al. Long-term outcomes of proximal interphalangeal joint surface replacement arthroplasty. J Bone Joint Surg Am. 2012;94(12):1120–8.
25. Neral MK, et al. Silicone arthroplasty for nonrheumatic metacarpophalangeal joint arthritis. J Hand Surg Am. 2013;38(12):2412–8.
26. Wall LB, Stern PJ. Clinical and radiographic outcomes of metacarpophalangeal joint pyrolytic carbon arthroplasty for osteoarthritis. J Hand Surg Am. 2013;38(3):537–43.
27. Hermann M, et al. Effects of a soft prefabricated thumb orthosis in carpometacarpal osteoarthritis. Scand J Occup Ther. 2014;21(1):31–9.
28. Bani MA, et al. The effect of custom-made splints in patients with the first carpometacarpal joint osteoarthritis. Prosthet Orthot Int. 2013;37(2):139–44.
29. Khan M, et al. Quantitative assessment of improvement with single corticosteroid injection in thumb CMC joint osteoarthritis? Open Orthop J. 2009;3:48–51.
30. Day CS, et al. Basal joint osteoarthritis of the thumb: a prospective trial of steroid injection and splinting. J Hand Surg Am. 2004;29(2):247–51.
31. Meenagh GK, et al. A randomised controlled trial of intra-articular corticosteroid injection of the carpometacarpal joint of the thumb in osteoarthritis. Ann Rheum Dis. 2004; 63(10):1260–3.
32. Wajon A, et al. Surgery for thumb (trapeziometacarpal joint) osteoarthritis. Cochrane Database Syst Rev. 2015;(2):CD004631.
33. Rizzo M, Moran SL, Shin AY. Long-term outcomes of trapeziometacarpal arthrodesis in the management of trapeziometacarpal arthritis. J Hand Surg Am. 2009;34(1):20–6.

34. Higginson AP, et al. Isolated scaphotrapeziotrapezoid osteoarthritis: prevalence, symptomatology and associated scapholunate ligament disruption in a population presenting to an accident and emergency department with acute wrist injuries. Clin Radiol. 2001;56(5):372–4.
35. Viegas SF, et al. Wrist anatomy: incidence, distribution, and correlation of anatomic variations, tears, and arthrosis. J Hand Surg Am. 1993;18(3):463–75.
36. Cope JR. Rotatory subluxation of the scaphoid. Clin Radiol. 1984;35(6):495–501.
37. Wong K, von Schroeder HP. Delays and poor management of scaphoid fractures: factors contributing to nonunion. J Hand Surg Am. 2011;36(9):1471–4.
38. Inoue G, Sakuma M. The natural history of scaphoid non-union. Radiographical and clinical analysis in 102 cases. Arch Orthop Trauma Surg. 1996;115(1):1–4.
39. Ruby LK, Leslie BM. Wrist arthritis associated with scaphoid nonunion. Hand Clin. 1987;3(4):529–39.
40. Kent ME, et al. Scaphoid nonunion in the presence of a degenerate carpus: don't rush to salvage surgery. J Hand Surg Eur Vol. 2012;37(1):56–60.
41. Malerich MM, et al. Distal scaphoid resection for degenerative arthritis secondary to scaphoid nonunion: a 20-year experience. J Hand Surg Am. 2014;39(9):1669–76.
42. Bain GI, McGuire DT. Decision making for partial carpal fusions. J Wrist Surg. 2012;1(2):103–14.
43. Saltzman BM, et al. Clinical outcomes of proximal row carpectomy versus four-corner arthrodesis for post-traumatic wrist arthropathy: a systematic review. J Hand Surg Eur Vol. 2015;9(2):52–5.
44. Wall LB, Stern PJ. Proximal row carpectomy. Hand Clin. 2013;29(1):69–78.
45. Pappou IP, Basel J, Deal DN. Scapholunate ligament injuries: a review of current concepts. Hand (N Y). 2013;8(2):146–56.
46. Wagner ER, Elhassan BT, Kakar S. Long-term functional outcomes after bilateral total wrist arthrodesis. J Hand Surg Am. 2015;40(2):224–8.e1.
47. Boeckstyns ME, Herzberg G, Merser S. Favorable results after total wrist arthroplasty: 65 wrists in 60 patients followed for 5–9 years. Acta Orthop. 2013;84(4):415–9.
48. Cooney W, et al. Total wrist replacement: a retrospective comparative study. J Wrist Surg. 2012;1(2):165–72.
49. Tatebe M, et al. Clinical, radiographic, and arthroscopic outcomes after ulnar shortening osteotomy: a long-term follow-up study. J Hand Surg Am. 2012;37(12):2468–74.
50. Sabo MT, et al. Intermediate outcomes of ulnar head arthroplasty. J Hand Surg Am. 2014;39(12):2405–11.e1.
51. Savvidou C, et al. Semiconstrained distal radioulnar joint prosthesis. J Wrist Surg. 2013;2(1):41–8.

Chapter 7
Imaging in Osteoarthritis

Peter Salat, David Salonen, and Andrea N. Veljkovic

Key Points

- Imaging of osteoarthritis (OA) can be performed with many different imaging modalities, but, in the clinical setting, the most commonly used modality is radiography.
- Radiographic manifestations of OA mirror the pathologic changes of the disease, but the technique has well-known limitations in detecting very early disease and monitoring progression.
- The limitations of radiographic assessment of OA may be one of the reasons behind the failure of many past DMOAD development trials.
- MRI allows assessment of all relevant tissues in a joint affected with OA and enables characterization of tissue changes on a biochemical level and the detection of the earliest pathologic alterations of OA.
- The clinical utility of advanced MRI techniques is limited at present with most applications being experimental and increasingly applied in DMOAD development trials.

P. Salat, MD (✉)
Joint Department of Medial Imaging (JDMI), University of Toronto, Toronto, ON, Canada
e-mail: salat.peter@gmail.com

D. Salonen, MD
Department of Medical Imaging, University of Toronto, Toronto, ON, Canada

Musculoskeletal Imaging, University Health Network, Toronto Western Hospital, Toronto, ON, Canada

A.N. Veljkovic, MD
Division of Orthopaedic Surgery, University Health Network – Toronto Western Division, Toronto, ON, Canada

M. Kapoor, N.N. Mahomed (eds.), *Osteoarthritis: Pathogenesis, Diagnosis, Available Treatments, Drug Safety, Regenerative and Precision Medicine*,
DOI 10.1007/978-3-319-19560-5_7

- Computed tomography, ultrasound, and nuclear medicine imaging have a very limited role at present in the clinical assessment of OA, but research interest in these techniques is growing and may provide additional tools in the future.

Introduction

Imaging plays a pivotal role in OA. Currently available imaging techniques enable diagnosis, grading, and monitoring of OA in the clinical setting. Research techniques can detect the earliest stages of disease and are becoming available clinically. Such advanced imaging techniques are poised to revolutionize the management of OA and will potentiate the development of effective treatments. The pathologic changes of OA in a joint mirror the imaging appearances. The final common pathway in the development of OA is cartilage damage leading to changes in the subchondral bone and growth of osteophytes. These are the cardinal features by which diagnosis of OA is confirmed on imaging. Several different imaging modalities are available for the diagnosis, staging, and monitoring of OA. The most commonly used and most important modalities for this purpose are radiography and magnetic resonance imaging (MRI).

Radiographic markers such as joint space narrowing have been the standard by which the severity and progression of OA are evaluated in clinical trials [44]. However, the use of radiography as the gold standard in clinical trials evaluating the efficacy of disease-modifying osteoarthritis drugs (DMOADs) has known limitations that may be one of the reasons why many promising DMOADs fail in human trials.

Intense research has been focused on improving the uniformity of diagnosis of OA with radiography and at increasing the sensitivity of the radiographic evaluation to progression of the disease. In addition, newer modalities such as MRI are increasingly used in experimental settings to quantify the burden of disease, to help detect OA in its earlier stages, and to monitor the progression of the disease. MRI allows the evaluation of numerous tissues that contribute to the development of OA and may more closely reflect the clinical manifestations of the disease. Some MRI techniques hold promise as markers of early OA. Other modalities such as ultrasound, computed tomography (CT), and nuclear medicine play a limited role in OA imaging; primarily restricted to a research setting at the present time. In the future, additional value in imaging OA may be realized with these modalities.

This chapter reviews the current role of imaging modalities in the evaluation of OA focusing on radiography and MRI with an overview of the ultrasound, CT, and nuclear medicine imaging. The benefits and limitations of the modalities and the implementation of each modality in the clinical and research assessment of OA are discussed, along with highlighting the current trends in imaging techniques for diagnosis and monitoring.

Radiography

The typical initial evaluation of a joint with suspected OA is radiography – the most available, inexpensive, and most widely studied imaging modality. It is based on the production of images using cathode ray tube-generated x-rays that are passed through the body part of interest and captured with a detector. This detector used to be a sensitive film in a cassette combination that was developed to provide the x-ray for interpretation by a radiologist. In most cases today, the film and cassette system has been replaced by solid-state electronic detectors that produce a digital image for interpretation on a computer screen. Replacing the massive libraries used for storage of plain film radiographs in the past, electronic picture archiving and communication systems (PACS) are in common use today. These electronic databases allow for the evaluation of radiographic images on digital, computer-aided platforms and have enhanced our ability to collect and analyze images for large populations of patients across long periods of time. The digital nature of radiographic images also lends itself to computer-aided analysis, which adds another degree of reproducibility and efficiency in the research setting in addition to opening the door to more sophisticated statistical modeling of disease patterns.

The usefulness of radiographs in the diagnosis of an osteoarthritic joint has been recognized since the early part of the last century. In daily clinical practice, radiographic assessment of a joint for the presence of OA is based on obtaining and evaluating two orthogonally oriented images centered on the area of interest using the appropriate amount of radiation. Special projections may be acquired to increase the sensitivity of the examination for early radiographic manifestations of OA.

Radiographs allow differentiation of four different types of densities in human tissues: air, fat, water (soft tissue parts), and bone. In addition to the tissue densities mentioned above, metal objects, such as joint replacements, have a unique identifiable density that is distinct from human tissue densities. The two-dimensional human anatomy forms are identifiable on radiographs when the interfacing tissues have different radiographic densities. The forms of adjacent tissues that have the same radiographic density cannot be distinguished as a result, which is the main inherent limitation of this imaging modality. The diagnosis of the disease using radiography is based on the analysis of deviations from the normal state of these tissue densities.

High-quality radiographic images obtained on modern systems allow the evaluation of the fine internal structure of some tissues. This is especially true of bone, the structure of which is well suited for the evaluation with radiographs. The outer shell of bone, the cortex, is seen as a dense white line at the periphery of a bone, while the inner cavity of bone, the medullary cavity, is seen as a meshwork of fine thin white lines – the trabeculae. At a joint surface, the marginal white line represents the plate of bone that supports articular cartilage. This is termed the subchondral bone plate. The cartilage at the opposing surface of a joint cannot be distinguished normally because the radiographic density of the cartilage layers is identical (like other soft tissue or water). Hence, radiographs can only indirectly represent the apparent thickness of the two opposing layers of cartilage in a joint. This distance between the opposing bone ends in a joint – the distance between the subchondral bone plate white lines – is termed the joint space width (JSW). Assessment of the JSW is one of the cardinal parameters in the radiographic diagnosis and monitoring of OA.

The most common joints involved with OA are the interphalangeal and metacarpophalangeal joints in the hands, first carpometacarpal and trapezioscaphoid joints of the wrist, acromioclavicular and sternoclavicular joints, hip, knee, and the first tarsometatarsal and metatarsophalangeal joints of the foot. OA of the elbow, shoulder, and ankle joints is much less common and usually related to prior trauma, joint instability, or other joint disorders.

The radiographic appearance of OA, whether due to an identifiable or idiopathic cause, is sufficiently characteristic to allow differentiation from other diseases of the joints (see Fig. 7.1). The general radiographic features of OA are well known, consisting of joint space narrowing (JSN), osteophytes, subchondral sclerosis, and subchondral cysts. Joint malalignment, joint debris, effusions, and juxta-articular soft tissue swelling are additional nonspecific radiographic features that can be seen in OA or other disorders. The joint space is defined as the area between the opposing subchondral bone plates. This space contains the two cartilage layers articulating in a joint. In some joints, such as the acromioclavicular (AC) and the knee, this space also contains other tissue such as an articulating disk (AC joint) or menisci (knee)

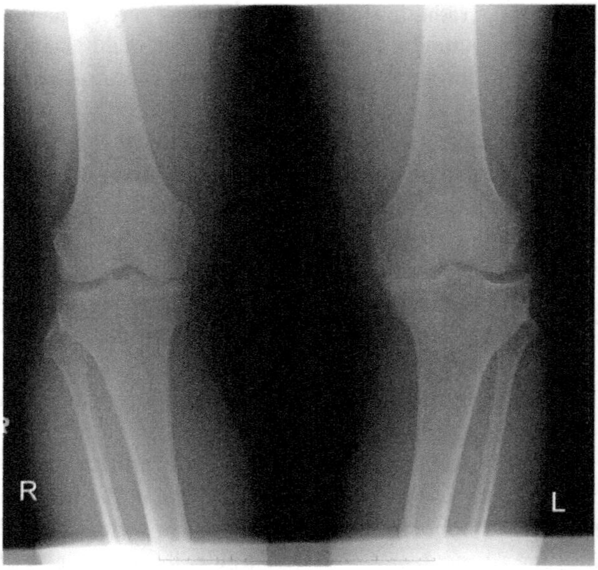

Fig. 7.1 Frontal radiograph of the knees demonstrating bilateral knee OA. There are features of severe OA in the left knee with bone on bone joint space loss in the medial compartment, large osteophytes, subchondral sclerosis, and a large cyst in the subspinous tibial plateau. Mild findings indicating early OA are seen in the right knee with spurring of the tibial spines and mild medial joint space narrowing. There is also varus malalignment of the knees, worse on the *left*

that contribute to the JSW. These structures are of similar radiographic density to adjacent cartilage and hence cannot be seen separately. In the setting of OA, the joint space narrows in a characteristic irregular fashion as opposed to uniform joint space narrowing seen in inflammatory arthropathies such as rheumatoid arthritis.

Osteophytes are spur-like bone outgrowths that typically develop at the margins of a joint, generally forming from a cartilaginous precursor that ossifies over time. They are thought to represent an adaptive response of the joint tissues to redistribution of pressure in OA joints. The presence of osteophytes is considered another cardinal feature for the radiographic diagnosis of OA and differentiates this disease from other joint diseases such as rheumatoid arthritis. The size and volume of osteophytes can be measured from radiographs and may help to stage the severity of the disease, as is discussed below.

Subchondral cysts (also termed pseudocysts or geodes) are well-defined areas of radiolucency that occur under the cartilage-bearing bone plate in OA or other disorders. They can be of variable size and may change over time. The cysts represent collections of joint fluid that are thought to form when overlying damaged cartilage and subchondral bone are penetrated by pressurized fluid or when the bone under the subchondral plate dies as a result of a bone contusion [1]. They are not true cyst pathologically as they do not contain a synovial lining.

Subchondral sclerosis is seen as areas of increased density and widening of the white line of the subchondral bone plate that represents new bone formation. Joint effusions associated with OA are generally small. Joint malalignment can develop as a result of progressive OA and is seen as abnormal position of the articular surfaces across the joint. Intra-articular bodies can be seen radiographically as bone or calcified fragments of various sizes. Joint ankylosis is an uncommon late complication of OA, represented by bone growth fusing a severely degenerated joint.

In addition to confirming the diagnosis, radiography can be used to stage the severity of OA in a joint. The oldest and most well-known radiographic staging system for OA is based on the work of Kellgren and Lawrence from 1957 [2] and 1963 [3]. The grading system was adopted by the World Health Organization as part of the definition of the disease. The atlas published by Kellgren and Lawrence contains descriptions of the radiographic findings for each grade of OA severity for several joints. The radiographic findings consist of osteophytes at the joint margin or at ligamentous attachments, joint space narrowing, sclerosis and cysts in the subchondral bone, as well as deformity of the bone ends for evidence of OA. The assignment of severity grade was based on an overall assessment of these features for a joint, referenced by the atlas of standards for each grade. Five grades of severity of OA were thus apportioned: none, doubtful, minimal, moderate, and severe. A written definition of each grade was subsequently provided in 1977 by Lawrence [4]. Grade zero was defined as the absence of the features of OA; Grade 1 as possible JSN and possible osteophyte lipping; Grade 2 as definite osteophyte, possible JSN, and slight sclerosis; Grade 3 as marked osteophyte, definite JSN, and some sclerosis; and Grade 4 as gross loss of joint space, large osteophytes, sclerosis, cysts, and marked deformity of bone ends.

The description of the grades provided by Lawrence focused on the presence or absence of particular radiographic features. As a result, the absolutely necessary presence of an osteophyte for the radiographic diagnosis of OA has become associated with the K-L system. Given the subtle differences in the source document descriptions, variations have arisen in the exact wording of the Kellgren-Lawrence (K-L) grades over time. This has led to different definitions of the radiographic presence of OA, which is usually taken to be a joint of at least Grade 2. Thus, some subsequent users of the K-L scale have defined the definite presence of OA as "definite osteophyte," while others as "definite osteophyte with possible joint space narrowing." As a result, studies that rely on a K-L Grade 2 definition for the detection of the presence of OA may include slightly different populations of subjects [5, 6]. In addition, increasing grade of OA in the K-L system has been taken to represent the natural progression of OA in a joint. These points have led to much controversy and disagreement in the literature regarding the radiographic classification of OA.

The K-L system has several limitations. The initial publications of Kellgren and Lawrence indicated a high reproducibility for a particular observer when using this grading system. At the same time, a poor reliability between different observers using this system was also documented in the original author's own work [4], where it was noted that one observer diagnosed the presence of definite OA in the hip four times more than another.

Additional drawbacks of this grading system became apparent in subsequent research. Studies using the K-L system for defining new onset of disease and progression of OA ran into difficulties as the K-L system was not designed to answer these questions. Large-scale longitudinal studies of OA, such as the Framingham Osteoarthritis Study [7], defined new onset of OA in the knee as K-L Grade 2 disease in a knee that was previously Grade 0 or 1. The Rotterdam Study [8], in comparison, defined new onset of disease as Grade 1 disease in a knee previously Grade 0. The onset and progression of OA is similarly heterogeneously defined in the literature.

To ameliorate the abovementioned shortcomings of the K-L system, several recommendations have been made. Defining the onset of OA as the definite presence of an osteophyte is one of the main limiting features of the K-L system. The exact point at which a possible osteophyte becomes a definite one is difficult to define leading to errors in the detection of osteophytes. Even using standardized x-ray acquisition leads to errors because of rotation of the knee. The suggested modification of the K-L grade 2 is that the combined presence of a definite osteophyte and definite JSN be required [9]. New-onset disease can then be defined as a K-L grade 2 knee, having both JSN and osteophyte, with at least one of these features being new. This approach is used by some of the largest longitudinal OA studies, namely, the MOST Study and the Osteoarthritis Initiative (OAI).

Using MRI assessment of cartilage damage, it was shown that cartilage damage is significantly more common in K-L Grade 2 disease with JSN than in Grade 2 disease without JSN [9]. A further limitation of radiographic detection of OA is that cartilage damage may be present in a joint that appears normal on radiographs, and the appearance of even Grade 1 disease may represent progression rather than new development of disease.

Using the K-L system for longitudinal follow-up to detect progression has given rise to additional variations in the use of the system in different studies [8, 10]. The annual risk of progression based on the K-L grades has been estimated at 5.6 % +/– 4.9 % and exhibits a negative linear relationship with follow-up time [11]. The original K-L Grade 3 results in difficulties in detecting progression of disease because this grade includes a wide breadth of JSN from mild to almost complete loss. Knees with progression of JSN over time might be classified as K-L Grade 3, hence showing no change in K-L grade.

A more accurate characterization of disease progression has been achieved by using JSN as the primary indicator, which can be assessed by semiquantitative scoring or with quantitation of JSN, rather than using the classic K-L grades [12]. The annual rate of progression of JSN has been estimated at 0.13 +/– 0.15 mm/year in one comprehensive literature review, and the rate of progression exhibits a negative linear relationship with follow-up time as seen with the risk of K-L grade progression [11]. The study noted that the variability of JSN rates in the literature is partly dependent on the radiographic approach and study design. An inherent limitation of radiographic interpretation of JSN is that joint space loss may be due to cartilage loss, meniscal loss, or both [13, 14]. Differentiation of the damage to these tissues may be important to better define the severity of the disease but is not possible radiographically.

Assessment of individual radiographic features of OA has been suggested as an alternative to the K-L score. The Osteoarthritis Research Society International (OARSI) atlas is a tool that provides standards for the grading of individual features of OA such as JSN and osteophytes [15]. The use of this tool can standardize the reading of radiographs in trials, but the inherent limitations of radiographic technique, such as variability in the appearance of JSN due to variations in beam angle or knee flexion, are not eliminated. When using the OARSI atlas to detect the presence of OA in the knee, up to twice as many cases of disease may be detected compared to using a modified K-L definition of disease [16, 17]. However, an argument against abandoning the K-L score is the large volume of historical data accumulated using this system, which would not inform a new system. In addition, OA pain is more strongly related to a global system score such as K-L than grading of individual features or a combined score of individual feature grades for the knee [18]. Other studies have shown that using the OARSI atlas for the grading of JSW is more reliable when the radiographic reading is centralized [19]. Due to the anatomic differences of various joints in the body, the specific progression of OA varies by joint. Various radiographic grading systems have been developed to reflect the specific feature of OA at many joints. The K-L score can be generically used for any joint and is often the gold standard comparison for joint-specific schemes.

Measuring JSN quantitatively is performed manually or using computer software. The standard metric used is minimal JSN. Quantitative JSN responsiveness depends on the degree of OA, severity, length of follow-up, and knee positioning used for the study [20, 21]. Good reliability has been shown in studies measuring JSN on knee radiographs with follow-up of at least 2 years using standardized knee positioning [22]. Radiographic JSW measurements using software analysis of the knee was shown to be comparable to MRI in detecting OA progression [21].

Radiography remains a useful and widely used method in clinical trials. Recent studies have shown the slowing of JSN progression in the medial compartment of the knee seen with doxycycline treatment, when the knees are in varus alignment [23]. In a study of patients with baseline knee pain, radiographic measurement of osteophyte area and minimum JSN was predictive of knee OA at 5-year follow-up [24]. In another study of knee OA, valgus knee alignment was shown to predispose to radiographic disease progression in knees with lateral knee OA [25]. Knees without any radiographic evidence of OA, having valgus alignment of as little as 3°, developed OA on follow-up in the lateral compartment.

Newly developed techniques have added to the capabilities of radiographically based methods in the evaluation and study of OA. The EOS system is based on a novel Nobel Prize-winning gaseous x-ray detector with multiwire proportional chamber. It can capture simultaneous spatially calibrated 2D images of the entire body under weight-bearing load, which can then be reconstructed in 3D. The system can acquire an entire skeletal survey at a fraction of the radiation typically required for such an evaluation, which makes it appealing especially for pediatric applications. The initial publications were focused on the evaluation of pediatric scoliosis with recent interest in lower extremity alignment in adult subjects with OA [26] and evaluation of patients with total joint replacements [27, 28].

Bone texture analysis and tomosynthesis are two older methods that have been revived for the study of OA. Bone texture analysis allows the evaluation of subchondral trabecular bone texture in 2D, which may be a predictor of progression of OA in the knee [29]. Tomosynthesis has been shown to be more sensitive in the detection of osteophytes and subchondral cysts in knee OA compared to radiography [30].

Magnetic Resonance Imaging (MRI)

MRI is an imaging technique exploiting the physical properties of subatomic particles, typically protons. When placed in a strong magnetic field, protons within biologic tissue can be induced to emit a radiofrequency signal that indicates their position, density, and chemical relationships. Radiofrequency pulses are delivered to the area of interest using radiofrequency coils that then also receive the signals emitted by the tissue under study. The timing of the pulse sequence determines which types of protons produce the most signal. This allows creation of images and identification of individual tissues (such as cartilage, menisci, bone marrow, synovium, ligaments, and capsule) which normally cannot be seen radiographically. A joint can be evaluated in its entirety using MRI, allowing assessment of individual tissue changes before structural changes occur, grading of the progression of OA at the individual tissue level, and detection of pre-radiographic disease.

Some of the limitations of MR imaging are its cost and availability. The strength of the magnet (commonly 1.5 or 3 T) and the type of coil used, which should be a dedicated coil for the joint imaged, are important inherent factors that influence the quality of the study. The specific parameters used to encode a particular type of sequence, the number of acquisition per sequence, the spatial resolution, as well as the combination of sequences used (the protocol) are variable between studies and reflect a compromise between image quality, time required for imaging, and patient comfort. Quality parameters such as signal homogeneity, patient positioning, image orientation, signal-to-noise ratio, and technical artifacts need to be optimized and consistently applied in both the clinical and research settings in order to maximize the potential of MR imaging. The overall quality of the study achieved can influence the sensitivity for the detection of the individual features of OA.

A consensus statement [31] by the OARSI-Outcome Measures in Rheumatoid Arthritis Clinical Trials (OMERACT) panel summarizes the requirements for an MRI protocol in the investigation of features of OA. In brief, the minimum number of sequences should be used such that the integrity of the whole-organ assessment of most articular features of OA is not compromised. In addition, fluid-sensitive fast spin echo sequences should be used in three orthogonal planes.

Because of the many different tissues that make up a synovial joint such as the knee, multiple sequences have to be used for a complete MRI evaluation. This allows the optimal evaluation of all tissues of interest. For example, assessment of focal cartilage defects and bone marrow lesions is most appropriate with a fluid-sensitive fast spin echo sequence with fat saturation [32]. A potential limitation of MRI is the occurrence of artifacts that can mimic pathology if the reader is unaware of them. These are signal changes that can arise from various sources such as a poorly performing sequence, foreign bodies such as metal in and around joints, or pathologic phenomena such as intra-articular gas that can form in the setting of OA and mimic pathology of the cartilage of meniscus. Certain sequences, such as gradient-recalled sequences which are well suited for the evaluation of cartilage, are particularly sensitive to such susceptibility artifacts [16]. Other sources of reader error are volume-averaging artifact which can occur, for example, at the periphery of joint margins simulating bone marrow lesions.

The use of MRI in OA has helped expand our understanding of the disease process. The traditional view that OA is a disease primarily of cartilage is currently felt to be true only of the final part in a series of events. The loss of cartilage and failure of the synovial organ are currently viewed as the final outcome of a range of different processes in OA. The radiologic-pathologic changes that occur in the early stages of OA can be seen on MRI. These include synovitis, effusions, joint debris, subchondral bone alterations, meniscal and other supporting structure damage, and osteophytes as well as a spectrum of cartilage alterations that culminate in full-thickness loss. Late changes that are classic of OA radiographically, such as subchondral sclerosis, cysts, and osteophytes, are also depicted on MRI.

An MRI definition of OA has been proposed under which the disease is definitely present in the knee if one of the two conditions is met [33].

1. A definite osteophyte and a full-thickness cartilage defect are present together.
2. A definite osteophyte or a full-thickness cartilage defect is present along with one of the following findings: a subchondral bone marrow lesion or cyst not associated with meniscal or ligamentous attachment; meniscal subluxation, maceration, or degenerative tear; partial-thickness cartilage loss; and bone attrition.

As was discussed in the previous section, radiographic markers of OA correlate with the degree of cartilage damage as detected on MRI. Osteophyte size increase was also shown to correlate with reduction of JSW radiographically, a surrogate marker for cartilage damage [34]. Experimentally, osteophyte growth has been shown to occur within days of inducing the disease [35], which suggests that cartilage damage may not be directly related to osteophyte formation in the early stages. To date, there are no reported longitudinal studies in humans that further evaluate this relationship. In a cross-sectional study of a large American population (the Framingham Osteoarthritis Cohort), the risk of severe cartilage damage on MRI was shown to correlate strongly with maximum osteophyte size [36] in the majority of the cohort. A small number of patients exhibited one of the two additional phenotypes, called atrophic and hypertrophic OA.

The atrophic OA phenotype has been defined based on MRI grading of cartilage and osteophytes using the WORMS grading system (see below) as severe cartilage damage and absence of osteophytes. The hypertrophic phenotype was defined as near intact tibiofemoral cartilage and large osteophytes. The prevalence of the phenotypes in the Framingham OA cohort was estimated at between 0.2 and 2.4 % [36]. The atrophic group of subjects was noted to have more structural damage such as meniscal and bone marrow lesions than the reference group. The lack of osteophytes in this phenotype may represent an imbalance in the rates of progression of cartilage damage and osteophyte formation with an increased rate of cartilage damage [37]. The subjects with a hypertrophic phenotype had a higher BMI and more bone marrow lesions than the reference group. This phenotype may be related to instability or malalignment due to ligament or other supporting structure damages [38]. The radiologic atrophic and hypertrophic phenotypes have been shown to correlate with different clinical patterns of OA in the knee [39].

MRI evaluation also allows the identification of the tissue source of pain in OA. The association of knee pain with MRI-detected bone marrow lesions [40], effusions, and synovitis [41] has been reported. MRI biomarkers of OA have been shown to be reliable and responsive [42] and to have predictive validity in knee OA [43]. MR imaging is currently recommended as an appropriate modality for the assessment of cartilage in clinical trials by the OARSI-FDA working group [44].

As in the case of radiographically based assessment of OA, MR-based grading of OA has been validated for several joint-specific scoring systems. These systems are semiquantitative in that they grade various features of OA – cartilage, menisci, ligaments, bone marrow lesions, synovitis, effusion, cystic lesions, and loose bodies in the case of the knee – according to a system-specific ordinal scale of severity. The individual scores can then be summed to give an overall grade of OA, similar to the OARSI atlas method of radiographic grading. This allows for a consistent approach to the evaluation of OA, allowing researchers to study the natural history of the disease, to correlate clinical symptoms to imaging findings, and to identify MRI-based risk factors of the disease.

Quantitative assessment of OA with MRI refers to the measurement of particular features such as cartilage thickness or volume as well as to the use of compositional methods such as T1 rho, T2 mapping, delayed gadolinium-enhanced MRI of cartilage, or other techniques that produce an objective measure of tissue signal intensity. These compositional measures allow for the detection of molecular changes in tissues that may be precursors to morphologic abnormalities seen in OA. As such, compositional assessment enables the detection of the earliest imaging evidence of OA.

Semiquantitative and quantitative assessment tools are primarily intended for the evaluation of osteoarthritic joints by trained musculoskeletal radiologists in a research environment and are currently not used for routine clinical joint evaluation. Semiquantitative assessment of a knee joint using one of the scoring systems by a trained specialist can take up to 45 min. Quantitative assessments require additional MRI time to obtain the sequences as well as additional time for segmentation of the tissue of interest. While segmentation can be performed manually or semiautomatically, it is labor intensive and requires special software and considerable operator input with segmentation method to produce reliable measurements.

Semiquantitative scoring systems have been developed for individual tissues involved in OA, such as the menisci, cartilage, ligaments, synovitis, and bone marrow allowing for a focused assessment. This can reduce the time required for scoring in studies limited in scope. Semiquantitative scoring systems are also available for joints other than the knee, including the hip, hand, spine, shoulder, and ankle, and are described below.

Knee

OA of the knee has received the most attention in the published literature. The knee is particularly well suited for study of OA by MRI in part due to the nature of its cartilage, which has the greatest thickness of all the joints in the body at the patella. Consequently, several MRI-based scoring systems have been developed for the semiquantitative grading of OA-related changes in the knee. There are five whole-joint scoring systems: WORMS, KOSS, BLOKS, MOAKS, and a system published by Meredith et al. [45].

The oldest and most widely used system is the Whole-Organ Magnetic Resonance Imaging Score (WORMS), first published in 2004 [46]. This system has been used in a large number of epidemiological studies including the Multicenter Osteoarthritis Study (MOST), the Framingham Knee Osteoarthritis Study, and the OA Initiative (OAI). The scoring in this system is based on a regional analysis of OA-related features rather than defining the exact number of lesions. The knee joint surface is split into 15 subregions. This division has the benefit of summarizing several features in a subregion, enabling interpretation and analysis. The system avoids the problems encountered when lesions are difficult to distinguish individually or when lesions split or merge over time [40]. In addition, WORMS is the only system that assesses subchondral bone attrition, defined as non-traumatic flattening or depression of the articular surface.

The Knee Osteoarthritis Scoring System (KOSS), published in 2005 [47], is the second most widely used score. KOSS assesses the same OA features as WORMS does and additionally scores meniscal subluxation. Scores in KOSS are assigned for individual OA-related features in a particular subregion rather than additively as in WORMS. The subregion definitions are different than in WORMS, and the grade of each individual feature is based on the size of the lesion.

The Boston Leeds Osteoarthritis Knee Score (BLOKS), published in 2008 [48], is relatively new. In this system, the knee is divided into weight-bearing and non-weight-bearing segments for the assessment of OA features, and a lesion-based approach is used for scoring bone marrow lesions. This enables longitudinal evaluation of individual lesions. The BLOKS assessment of individual lesions performed better than the WORMS approach for association with pain and cartilage loss [48].

The scoring system described by Meredith et al. [45] assesses individual cartilage lesions for signal change and size, summed over 17 subregions with a grade assigned for the overall severity of osteophytes, effusion, synovitis, and subchondral sclerosis. This is the only system that uses absolute size measurements for all features. This has the potential to bias results owing to natural patient size variations.

Most recently, the MRI Osteoarthritis Knee Score (MOAKS) was developed to address some of the limitations and concerns of the above described systems [49]. The same subregion definitions as WORMS are used in MOAKS with reduced redundancy of BML and cartilage scoring and refined scoring of bone marrow and cartilage lesions.

Scoring systems have also been developed for the individual features of OA. For cartilage assessment, at least five different scoring systems are available. These are mostly based on the surgical classification system of Outerbridge [50]. In the system proposed by Biswal et al. [51], cartilage lesions are graded similar to WORMS, on a 6-point scale with a further differentiation based on size less than or greater than 1 cm^2. Such a classification allowed the detection of progression of cartilage lesions in less than 2 years in the study population.

Signal alterations in Hoffa's fat pad on non-contrast MRI correlate with mild chronic synovitis histologically [52] in knees with OA. These signal changes can be scored semiquantitatively but are not specific since other etiologies such as nonspecific edema or chronic fibrosis can have similar appearances [53]. Accurate assessment of the extent of synovitis in the knee is currently best performed with contrast-enhanced MRI (CE-MRI) [54]. Several scoring systems based on CE-MRI assessment of synovitis are published [55–57], with the presence of synovitis correlating with histological evidence of synovial inflammation [58]. The synovitis score based on the CE-MRI scoring system of Baker et al. [56] was shown to correlate closely with severity of knee pain [56]. While the other scoring systems focus on the assessment of synovitis around the patella, the more comprehensive scoring system of Guermazi et al. [57] assesses additional sites such as the perimeniscal and peri-ACL and PCL recesses. A moderate to severe score in this system correlates significantly with the maximum Western Ontario and McMaster Osteoarthritis Index (WOMAC) pain score [57] as well as with meniscal damage and radiographic tibiofemoral OA [59]. As a result of the cross-sectional and longitudinal association of synovitis detected on CE-MRI and assessed semiquantitatively as demonstrated in these studies, this feature of OA can be used as an imaging marker of disease activity. This may prove useful in clinical trials assessing new disease-modifying OA drugs.

There are few scoring systems for MRI assessment of ligaments in knee OA. However, studies have shown that semiquantitative assessment of ligaments may have relevance in knee OA research. For example, an association between ligamentous injury and medial compartment knee OA or subjects with atraumatic knee pain without OA [60] was shown in one study, while another showed an association with crepitus of the knee [61]. A predisposition for lateral tibiofemoral joint damage in patients with OA and partial or complete tears of the anterior cruciate ligament (ACL) has been described [62].

Bone marrow lesions (BMLs) have been correlated with knee pain in a cross-sectional study as well as with progression of OA [40]. A scoring system based on lesion size was used for grading BMLs in this study. Another system using absolute size has shown response to BML changes over time [63]. Meniscal tear and extrusion also has an available grading system; the presence of tears and extrusion has been associated with the progression of symptomatic OA in the knee [64]. The presence of meniscal pathology [65] or elevated levels of total serum cholesterol [66] were found to be associated with incident or progressive BMLs.

Bone marrow lesions detected on MRI have gained much interest as an imaging marker of OA-related pain. Studies have shown that BMLs are associated with pain in patients with OA of the knee or at high risk of developing knee OA [40] and that an increase in the semiquantitative BML score over 15 months correlated with the development of OA-related knee pain [40], defined as aching, stiffness, or pain on most days. Other studies have shown that changes in knee pain in the setting of OA are reflected by changes in BML size [41], and others have indicated a direct relationship between pain as measured using the Western Ontario and McMaster Universities Arthritis Index (WOMAC) [48].

In addition to BMLs, semiquantitatively assessed synovitis on contrast-enhanced MRI is a well-established imaging marker of clinical disease activity in the knee. Other imaging markers that have been associated with the progression of OA in longitudinal studies include increased BMI (>30) [67], meniscal damage [68], malposition [13], and prevalent cartilage damage [69]. In the case of the patellofemoral joint, the presence of patella alta has been suggested as an additional risk factor for the progression of cartilage damage and BMLs [70].

Hip

A single MRI-based grading system of OA of the hip has been published, called the Hip Osteoarthritis MRI Scoring System (HOAMS) [71]. This system is based on a cross-sectional analysis, and its longitudinal responsiveness is unknown. HOAMS scores traditional OA parameters, consisting of cartilage, osteophytes, subchondral cysts, attrition, loose bodies, synovitis, and effusion. The evaluation of synovitis in this system uses contrast-enhanced MRI. In addition, hip joint-specific features, consisting of labrum, dysplasia, greater trochanteric tendonitis/bursitis, labral hypertrophy, paralabral cysts, and herniation pits, are scored. The severity of the traditional OA-related parameters listed above with the addition of BMLs and greater trochanteric tendonitis/bursitis using this scoring system was found to correlate well with the Kellgren-Lawrence severity of hip OA [71].

Hand

In the hand, the main published OA system is based on semiquantitative scoring of OA features of small distal joints, the PIP and DIP joints, of the second through the fifth fingers [72]. The Oslo Hand OA MRI (OHOA-MRI) Score, the score is applied to a contrast-enhanced evaluation that assesses synovitis and tenosynovitis in addition to JSN, osteophytes, BMLs, erosions, cysts, malalignment, and collateral ligament status. The original study published good inter and intra reader reliability. Compared to radiography, MRI-based assessment of osteoarthritic hands using this score detected twice the number of joints with osteophytes and erosions. Nevertheless, the frequency of MRI-detected features of OA was positively correlated with the radiographic severity of OA. Synovitis detected on MRI was found more frequently in low-grade radiographic disease (K-L 2) than in moderate disease (K-L 3). Several of the OHOA-MRI features – namely, BMLs, erosions, bone attrition, osteophytes, and moderate to severe synovitis – were independently associated with joint tenderness [73]. These studies suggest that MRI-based markers of OA may be useful targets in clinical trials of DMOAD development.

Spine

The spinal column contains a number of joints, all of which can become symptomatic as they degenerate. While MRI enables assessment of the numerous joints in the spine, there is no single grading system that accounts for changes in all of the different types of joints in the spine. Instead, MRI-based systems have been published that grade the features of OA in the intervertebral disks or facet joints only in the lumbar spine. The individual features that are assessed include signal and morphologic changes of the intervertebral disk, vertebral end plate changes, facet joint OA involvement, spinal canal, and neural foramen narrowing. The specific published grading systems are designed for the assessment of intervertebral disk degeneration [74], facet joint degeneration [75], and nerve root compromise [76]. The MRI protocols for these systems do not use contrast enhancement.

An intervertebral disk degeneration classification system was originally published by Pfirrmann et al. [74]. This was subsequently modified [77] as it was based on the evaluation of the spines in subjects with an average age of 40, resulting moderate to high grade for the majority of a cohort of older subjects with a mean age of 73 [77]. A cadaveric study using the Thomson scale for grading discovertebral joint degeneration [78] showed that both disk and facet joint degeneration progressed with age and that facet joint OA was most severe at the L4–L5 level.

Nerve root impingement due to intervertebral disk herniation has been assessed semiquantitatively on a four-level scale [76]. This MRI-based scale was shown to correlate well with surgical grading and to be reliable.

A semiquantitative system for grading facet joint degeneration [75] has been described and also grades disk degeneration and herniation, scoliosis, and anterolisthesis as well as facet joint BMLs. The study suggested that facet joint degeneration is mostly attributable to intervertebral disk degeneration and instability.

Shoulder

An MRI grading system has been published for the acromioclavicular joint (AC joint), which is a small joint at the tip of the shoulder between the distal end of the clavicle and the acromion [79]. This system grades the severity of OA in the AC joint on a scale of 1 to 3, depending on the presence and size of individual features. The features that are assessed are the presence of subchondral cysts, marginal osteophytes, bone sclerosis, joint soft tissue swelling, and impingement of the joint on the rotator cuff. Grading using this system on non-CE-MRI was shown to be more sensitive for the detection of AC joint OA than radiography.

Ankle

A single ankle-specific MRI-based grading system has been described [80], called the Ankle Osteoarthritis Scoring System (AOSS). This scale was reported in a small study showing good reproducibility compared to the Kellgren-Lawrence scale but was not correlated with arthroscopic findings. The score is based on a composite of parameters that were previously reported as clinically important: depth of cartilage damage (53), depth of subchondral bone defect (54), osteophyte size (55), size of bone marrow edema lesions (56), meniscoid impingement (57), effusion (58), loose bodies (59), synovitis (60), and soft tissue cysts (61).

Compositional MRI Techniques

MRI techniques have been developed that allow quantification of particular biochemical properties of different tissues of a joint such as cartilage, menisci, or ligaments. Techniques such as T2 mapping, T1 rho, CEST, and delayed gadolinium-enhanced MRI of cartilage (dGEMRIC) have allowed researchers to investigate early changes in the biochemical make up cartilage before the advent of any radiographic or gross morphologic changes. The T1 rho and dGEMRIC techniques are sensitive to loss of glycosaminoglycans (GAGs) in the cartilage, which has been associated with early damage in OA. Chemical exchange saturation transfer (CEST) can also be tuned to detect changes in GAG concentrations in the cartilage. In comparison, T2 mapping technique can be used to produce a color-coded representation of the average T2 values across a volume of tissue (see Fig. 7.2). Average T2 values are affected by changes in collagen orientation and hydration in the cartilage, seen as an increase of T2 values in areas of early OA [45, 55, 81].

While these techniques remain largely investigational and are not currently widely available, dGEMRIC, T2 mapping, and T1 rho techniques have been used in clinical studies of OA. Several studies have used dGEMRIC to assess cartilage in the knee to assess collagen hydrolysate in mild knee OA [82] or the effect of exercise on cartilage status [83]. The investigation of cartilage with average T2 maps has shown increasing values with increasing grade of cartilage defects (32, 33). Loading of the knee acutely has been shown to correlate with decreased T1 rho and T2 values in the medial knee compartment that was more marked in the presence of small

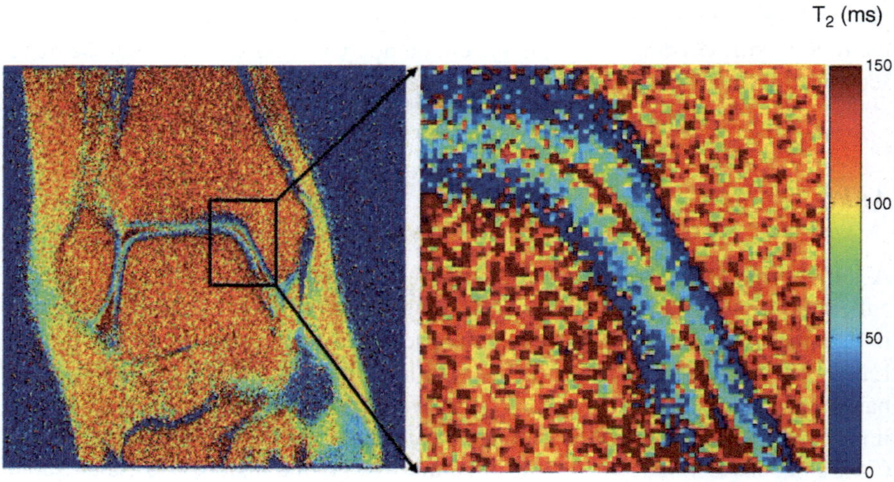

Fig. 7.2 Coronal plane T2 map of ankle cartilage obtained on 1.5 T MRI. The insert on the *right* shows in detail the normal T2 value gradients of the medial ankle cartilage. Low values (*blue*) are seen at the deepest layers and progressively increasing values (*red*) in the more superficial cartilage layers of both the talus and tibial surface. Color bar on the right represents average T2 values in milliseconds (ms)

focal cartilage defects [84]. Changes in T2, T1 rho, dGEMRIC, or CEST contrast values can therefore be used to detect and monitor OA severity and progression at the biochemical level before the onset of radiographic features, albeit still mostly used as experimental techniques.

Quantitative Techniques

Measurement of physical dimensions such as thickness, area, and volume of tissues of interest has been well established and was enabled by 3D MRI techniques. Measures such as cartilage volume, total area of subchondral bone (tAB), denuded area of subchondral bone (dAB), and mean cartilage thickness over total area of subchondral bone have been defined in the assessment of cartilage with MRI [85]. An efficient description of cartilage morphology and its longitudinal changes in knees with OA can be obtained by measuring tAB and dAB [86]. These measures allow the detection and tracking of cartilage changes in knees independent of anatomic location, as the location of cartilage loss in knees can be variable [87] and for better categorization of patients. Cartilage thinning and total area of denuded subchondral bone have been associated with progression to knee joint replacement [88].

CT

Computed tomography (CT) is a technology that creates images by rotating an x-ray source and opposing detector while passing the body through the plane of rotation. Computer algorithms then reconstruct images of the scanned volume in the desired plane, typically transverse to the body. The CT beam is attenuated in a similar way to conventional x-ray, but CT can display a wider range of density differences. This together with the tomographic scanning allows demonstration of much finer tissue details. The same features of OA seen with plain radiography are depicted with CT but in greater detail and in three dimensions. Semiquantitative analysis of OA using CT has been applied to facet joints in the lumbar spine [89], demonstrating increasing prevalence of facet OA, most commonly at L4 and L5 levels.

The ability of CT and MRI to acquire a volume of tissue allows visualization of the three-dimensional shape features that may not be visible on two-dimensional radiographs. Because the data acquired with CT, MRI, or radiography is digital, advanced statistical methods can be used for the analysis of morphologic features of bones, among others. This line of investigation has allowed for the description of bone shape changes in OA in three dimensions using CT or MRI images. In addition to osteophyte formation that can be seen radiographically, these techniques have shown flattening, widening, and ridge formation in the femoral, tibial, and patellar bones in joints with OA [90]. Furthermore, bone morphologic features in joints at risk of OA have also shown a predictive correlation with incidence of OA in the knee [90] and hip [91–93]. These studies suggest that bone morphologic features may be in part responsible for the development of OA. Detection of these features may therefore provide additional imaging biomarkers of OA.

Nuclear Medicine

Nuclear medicine imaging is based on the detection of decay photons originating from intravenously injected radioisotope tracers. The tracers are designed to identify particular features of metabolism. In OA, the radioisotopes redistribute to areas of increased bone turnover manifested by osteophyte formation, subchondral sclerosis, and bone marrow edema as well as synovitis [94]. Bone scintigraphy using technetium 99 m-hydroxymethane diphosphonate and positron emission scintigraphy (PET) using 2-^{18}F-fluoro-2-deoxy-D-glucose (18-FDG) or ^{18}F-fluoride (18-F^-) can be used to survey the entire body for bone or joint sources of pain in patients with complex pain symptoms [95]. PET scanning using 18-F^- showed increased bone metabolism in the proximal femur in patients with symptomatic hip OA suggesting that detection of early OA may be possible [96]. Nuclear medicine imaging suffers from a lack of resolution and imparts a significant radiation dose to the subject. Recently, efforts have been made to increase the resolution by combining the metabolic imaging capabilities of nuclear medicine with the resolution of CT [97] and MRI [98]. Further development of these technologies may provide powerful hybrid systems for the evaluation of OA in the future.

Ultrasound

Ultrasound uses high-frequency sound waves to interrogate tissues of interest around a joint. The advantage of ultrasound is its real-time, multiplanar capabilities at a relatively low cost. However, ultrasound is not capable of evaluating subchondral bone or intra-articular structures in adults due to the physical properties of sound. In addition, it is operator dependent. Nevertheless, many features of OA can be assessed and have shown clinical usefulness. In particular, ultrasound is useful in the assessment of synovial hypertrophy, vascularity, and joint effusion [99]. Evaluation of cartilage has been performed with ultrasound, demonstrating that early cartilage surface fibrillation can be detected to an accuracy of 20 μm [100]. In the evaluation of hand OA, a grading system has been published using semiquantitative scoring of synovial hypertrophy and vascularity [101] that showed moderately good reliability. JSN and osteophytes detected on ultrasound have been associated with pain in the hands [102]. In a large study of patients with painful knee OA, ultrasound-detected synovitis was associated with radiographically detected knee OA and clinical findings of an inflammatory flare [103].

Conclusions

Imaging evaluation of OA can be performed with many different modalities, each imaging modality providing an objective method of assessing the various features of OA. While radiography remains the primary modality of assessing and following the progression of OA in trials and routine clinical practice, developments in MRI techniques have propelled this imaging modality to the position of highest importance in furthering OA research. Compositional MRI techniques and new statistical methods are promising new avenues into the pathogenesis of OA and as imaging markers potentiating detection of early OA or joints at risk of developing the disease. Other imaging modalities such as ultrasound, CT, and nuclear medicine may provide valuable methods of evaluating OA in particular situations (see Table 7.1). The objective and noninvasive nature of diagnostic modalities makes them central to the management of OA and a key element in the development of DMOADs.

Table 7.1 Summary of benefits and limitations of different imaging techniques

Imaging modality	Benefits	Limitations
Radiography	Low cost	Limited responsiveness
	Global OA severity assessment	Early disease detection
	Scoring system	
Computed tomography	3D joint assessment	Radiation exposure
	Bone tissue assessment	Moderate cost
		Limited soft tissue evaluation
Magnetic resonance imaging	3D joint assessment	High cost
	Biochemical tissue evaluation	Complexity
	Scoring system	
Nuclear medicine imaging	Whole body assessment	Limited anatomic detail
	Metabolic assessment	Radiation exposure
Ultrasound	Low cost	Operator dependent
	Synovitis assessment	Limited joint penetration
	Scoring system	

References

1. Resnick D, Niwayama G, Coutts RD. Subchondral cysts (geodes) in arthritic disorders: pathologic and radiographic appearance of the hip joint. AJR Am J Roentgenol. 1977;128(5):799–806.
2. Kellgren JH, Lawrence JS. Radiological assessment of osteo-arthrosis. Ann Rheum Dis. 1957;16(4):494–502.
3. Kellgren JH, Jeffrey MR, Ball J. The epidemiology of chronic rheumatism: atlas of standard radiographs. Oxford: Blackwell Scientific; 1963.
4. Lawrence JS. Rheumatism in populations. London: W.M. Heinemann Medical Books; 1977.
5. Schiphof D, Boers M, Bierma-Zeinstra SM. Differences in descriptions of Kellgren and Lawrence grades of knee osteoarthritis. Ann Rheum Dis. 2008;67(7):1034–6.
6. Schiphof D, et al. Impact of different descriptions of the Kellgren and Lawrence classification criteria on the diagnosis of knee osteoarthritis. Ann Rheum Dis. 2011;70(8):1422–7.
7. Felson DT, et al. The incidence and natural history of knee osteoarthritis in the elderly. The Framingham Osteoarthritis Study. Arthritis Rheum. 1995;38(10):1500–5.
8. Reijman M, et al. Body mass index associated with onset and progression of osteoarthritis of the knee but not of the hip: the Rotterdam Study. Ann Rheum Dis. 2007;66(2):158–62.
9. Felson DT, et al. Defining radiographic incidence and progression of knee osteoarthritis: suggested modifications of the Kellgren and Lawrence scale. Ann Rheum Dis. 2011;70(11):1884–6.
10. Brouwer GM, et al. Association between valgus and varus alignment and the development and progression of radiographic osteoarthritis of the knee. Arthritis Rheum. 2007;56(4):1204–11.
11. Emrani PS, et al. Joint space narrowing and Kellgren-Lawrence progression in knee osteoarthritis: an analytic literature synthesis. Osteoarthritis Cartilage. 2008;16(8):873–82.
12. Felson DT, et al. A new approach yields high rates of radiographic progression in knee osteoarthritis. J Rheumatol. 2008;35(10):2047–54.
13. Hunter DJ, et al. The association of meniscal pathologic changes with cartilage loss in symptomatic knee osteoarthritis. Arthritis Rheum. 2006;54(3):795–801.
14. Gale DR, et al. Meniscal subluxation: association with osteoarthritis and joint space narrowing. Osteoarthritis Cartilage. 1999;7(6):526–32.
15. Altman RD, Gold GE. Atlas of individual radiographic features in osteoarthritis, revised. Osteoarthritis Cartilage. 2007;15 Suppl A:A1–56.
16. Hayashi D, Jarraya M, Guermazi A, et al. Frequency and fluctuation of susceptibility artifacts in the tibiofemoral joint space in painful knees on 3T MRI and association with meniscal tears, radiographic joint space narrowing and calcifications. Arthritis Rheum. 2012;64 Suppl 10:1030.
17. Culvenor AG, et al. Defining the presence of radiographic knee osteoarthritis: a comparison between the Kellgren and Lawrence system and OARSI atlas criteria. Knee Surg Sports Traumatol Arthrosc. 2014. [Epub ahead of print] doi:10.1007/s00167-014-3205-0.
18. Felson DT, et al. Defining radiographic osteoarthritis for the whole knee. Osteoarthritis Cartilage. 1997;5(4):241–50.
19. Guermazi A, et al. Different thresholds for detecting osteophytes and joint space narrowing exist between the site investigators and the centralized reader in a multicenter knee osteoarthritis study–data from the Osteoarthritis Initiative. Skeletal Radiol. 2012;41(2):179–86.
20. Nevitt MC, et al. Longitudinal performance evaluation and validation of fixed-flexion radiography of the knee for detection of joint space loss. Arthritis Rheum. 2007;56(5):1512–20.
21. Duryea J, et al. Comparison of radiographic joint space width with magnetic resonance imaging cartilage morphometry: analysis of longitudinal data from the Osteoarthritis Initiative. Arthritis Care Res (Hoboken). 2010;62(7):932–7.
22. Reichmann WM, et al. Responsiveness to change and reliability of measurement of radiographic joint space width in osteoarthritis of the knee: a systematic review. Osteoarthritis Cartilage. 2011;19(5):550–6.

23. Mazzuca SA, et al. Varus malalignment negates the structure-modifying benefits of doxycycline in obese women with knee osteoarthritis. Osteoarthritis Cartilage. 2010;18(8):1008–11.
24. Kinds MB, et al. Evaluation of separate quantitative radiographic features adds to the prediction of incident radiographic osteoarthritis in individuals with recent onset of knee pain: 5-year follow-up in the CHECK cohort. Osteoarthritis Cartilage. 2012;20(6):548–56.
25. Felson DT, et al. Valgus malalignment is a risk factor for lateral knee osteoarthritis incidence and progression: findings from the Multicenter Osteoarthritis Study and the Osteoarthritis Initiative. Arthritis Rheum. 2013;65(2):355–62.
26. Than P, et al. Geometrical values of the normal and arthritic hip and knee detected with the EOS imaging system. Int Orthop. 2012;36(6):1291–7.
27. Lazennec JY, et al. The EOS imaging system for understanding a patellofemoral disorder following THR. Orthop Traumatol Surg Res. 2011;97(1):98–101.
28. Lazennec JY, et al. Pelvis and total hip arthroplasty acetabular component orientations in sitting and standing positions: measurements reproductibility with EOS imaging system versus conventional radiographies. Orthop Traumatol Surg Res. 2011;97(4):373–80.
29. Woloszynski T, et al. Prediction of progression of radiographic knee osteoarthritis using tibial trabecular bone texture. Arthritis Rheum. 2012;64(3):688–95.
30. Hayashi D, et al. Detection of osteophytes and subchondral cysts in the knee with use of tomosynthesis. Radiology. 2012;263(1):206–15.
31. Peterfy CG, et al. MRI protocols for whole-organ assessment of the knee in osteoarthritis. Osteoarthritis Cartilage. 2006;14 Suppl A:A95–111.
32. Hayashi D, Guermazi A, Roemer FW. MRI of osteoarthritis: the challenges of definition and quantification. Semin Musculoskelet Radiol. 2012;16(5):419–30.
33. Hunter DJ, et al. Definition of osteoarthritis on MRI: results of a Delphi exercise. Osteoarthritis Cartilage. 2011;19(8):963–9.
34. Buckland-Wright JC, et al. Quantitative microfocal radiographic assessment of osteoarthritis of the knee from weight bearing tunnel and semiflexed standing views. J Rheumatol. 1994;21(9):1734–41.
35. Gilbertson EM. Development of periarticular osteophytes in experimentally induced osteoarthritis in the dog. A study using microradiographic, microangiographic, and fluorescent bone-labelling techniques. Ann Rheum Dis. 1975;34(1):12–25.
36. Roemer FW, et al. Prevalence of magnetic resonance imaging-defined atrophic and hypertrophic phenotypes of knee osteoarthritis in a population-based cohort. Arthritis Rheum. 2012;64(2):429–37.
37. Roemer FW, et al. Tibiofemoral joint osteoarthritis: risk factors for MR-depicted fast cartilage loss over a 30-month period in the multicenter osteoarthritis study. Radiology. 2009;252(3):772–80.
38. Pottenger LA, Phillips FM, Draganich LF. The effect of marginal osteophytes on reduction of varus-valgus instability in osteoarthritic knees. Arthritis Rheum. 1990;33(6):853–8.
39. Castaneda S, et al. Osteoarthritis: a progressive disease with changing phenotypes. Rheumatology (Oxford). 2014;53(1):1–3.
40. Felson DT, et al. The association of bone marrow lesions with pain in knee osteoarthritis. Ann Intern Med. 2001;134(7):541–9.
41. Zhang Y, et al. Fluctuation of knee pain and changes in bone marrow lesions, effusions, and synovitis on magnetic resonance imaging. Arthritis Rheum. 2011;63(3):691–9.
42. Hunter DJ, et al. Responsiveness and reliability of MRI in knee osteoarthritis: a meta-analysis of published evidence. Osteoarthritis Cartilage. 2011;19(5):589–605.
43. Hunter DJ, et al. Systematic review of the concurrent and predictive validity of MRI biomarkers in OA. Osteoarthritis Cartilage. 2011;19(5):557–88.
44. Conaghan PG, et al. Summary and recommendations of the OARSI FDA osteoarthritis Assessment of Structural Change Working Group. Osteoarthritis Cartilage. 2011;19(5):606–10.
45. Meredith DS, et al. Empirical evaluation of the inter-relationship of articular elements involved in the pathoanatomy of knee osteoarthritis using magnetic resonance imaging. BMC Musculoskelet Disord. 2009;10:133.

46. Peterfy CG, et al. Whole-Organ Magnetic Resonance Imaging Score (WORMS) of the knee in osteoarthritis. Osteoarthritis Cartilage. 2004;12(3):177–90.
47. Kornaat PR, et al. MRI assessment of knee osteoarthritis: Knee Osteoarthritis Scoring System (KOSS)–inter-observer and intra-observer reproducibility of a compartment-based scoring system. Skeletal Radiol. 2005;34(2):95–102.
48. Hunter DJ, et al. The reliability of a new scoring system for knee osteoarthritis MRI and the validity of bone marrow lesion assessment: BLOKS (Boston Leeds Osteoarthritis Knee Score). Ann Rheum Dis. 2008;67(2):206–11.
49. Hunter DJ, et al. Evolution of semi-quantitative whole joint assessment of knee OA: MOAKS (MRI Osteoarthritis Knee Score). Osteoarthritis Cartilage. 2011;19(8):990–1002.
50. Outerbridge RE. The etiology of chondromalacia patellae. J Bone Joint Surg Br. 1961; 43-B:752–7.
51. Biswal S, et al. Risk factors for progressive cartilage loss in the knee: a longitudinal magnetic resonance imaging study in forty-three patients. Arthritis Rheum. 2002;46(11):2884–92.
52. Fernandez-Madrid F, et al. Synovial thickening detected by MR imaging in osteoarthritis of the knee confirmed by biopsy as synovitis. Magn Reson Imaging. 1995;13(2):177–83.
53. Saddik D, McNally EG, Richardson M. MRI of Hoffa's fat pad. Skeletal Radiol. 2004;33(8):433–44.
54. Hayashi D, et al. Imaging of synovitis in osteoarthritis: current status and outlook. Semin Arthritis Rheum. 2011;41(2):116–30.
55. Rhodes LA, et al. The validation of simple scoring methods for evaluating compartment-specific synovitis detected by MRI in knee osteoarthritis. Rheumatology (Oxford). 2005;44(12):1569–73.
56. Baker K, et al. Relation of synovitis to knee pain using contrast-enhanced MRIs. Ann Rheum Dis. 2010;69(10):1779–83.
57. Guermazi A, et al. Assessment of synovitis with contrast-enhanced MRI using a whole-joint semiquantitative scoring system in people with, or at high risk of, knee osteoarthritis: the MOST study. Ann Rheum Dis. 2011;70(5):805–11.
58. Loeuille D, et al. Magnetic resonance imaging in osteoarthritis: which method best reflects synovial membrane inflammation? Correlations with clinical, macroscopic and microscopic features. Osteoarthritis Cartilage. 2009;17(9):1186–92.
59. Guermazi A, et al. Whole-knee synovitis semiquantitatively assessed on T1-weighted contrast-enhanced MRI is associated with radiographic tibiofemoral osteoarthritis and severe meniscal damage: the MOST Study [abstract 402]. Osteoarthritis Cartilage. 2009;17 Suppl 1:S211–2.
60. Bergin D, et al. Atraumatic medial collateral ligament oedema in medial compartment knee osteoarthritis. Skeletal Radiol. 2002;31(1):14–8.
61. Crema MD, et al. The association of magnetic resonance imaging (MRI)-detected structural pathology of the knee with crepitus in a population-based cohort with knee pain: the MoDEKO study. Osteoarthritis Cartilage. 2011;19(12):1429–32.
62. Stein V, et al. Pattern of joint damage in persons with knee osteoarthritis and concomitant ACL tears. Rheumatol Int. 2012;32(5):1197–208.
63. Brem MH, et al. Longitudinal evaluation of the occurrence of MRI-detectable bone marrow edema in osteoarthritis of the knee. Acta Radiol. 2008;49(9):1031–7.
64. Berthiaume MJ, et al. Meniscal tear and extrusion are strongly associated with progression of symptomatic knee osteoarthritis as assessed by quantitative magnetic resonance imaging. Ann Rheum Dis. 2005;64(4):556–63.
65. Englund M, et al. Meniscal pathology on MRI increases the risk for both incident and enlarging subchondral bone marrow lesions of the knee: the MOST Study. Ann Rheum Dis. 2010;69(10):1796–802.
66. Davies-Tuck ML, et al. Total cholesterol and triglycerides are associated with the development of new bone marrow lesions in asymptomatic middle-aged women - a prospective cohort study. Arthritis Res Ther. 2009;11(6):R181.
67. Laberge MA, et al. Obesity increases the prevalence and severity of focal knee abnormalities diagnosed using 3T MRI in middle-aged subjects–data from the Osteoarthritis Initiative. Skeletal Radiol. 2012;41(6):633–41.

68. Sharma L, et al. Relationship of meniscal damage, meniscal extrusion, malalignment, and joint laxity to subsequent cartilage loss in osteoarthritic knees. Arthritis Rheum. 2008;58(6):1716–26.
69. Ding C, et al. Association of prevalent and incident knee cartilage defects with loss of tibial and patellar cartilage: a longitudinal study. Arthritis Rheum. 2005;52(12):3918–27.
70. Stefanik JJ, et al. Association between patella alta and the prevalence and worsening of structural features of patellofemoral joint osteoarthritis: the multicenter osteoarthritis study. Arthritis Care Res (Hoboken). 2010;62(9):1258–65.
71. Roemer FW, et al. Hip Osteoarthritis MRI Scoring System (HOAMS): reliability and associations with radiographic and clinical findings. Osteoarthritis Cartilage. 2011;19(8):946–62.
72. Haugen IK, et al. Hand osteoarthritis and MRI: development and first validation step of the proposed Oslo Hand Osteoarthritis MRI score. Ann Rheum Dis. 2011;70(6):1033–8.
73. Haugen IK, et al. Associations between MRI-defined synovitis, bone marrow lesions and structural features and measures of pain and physical function in hand osteoarthritis. Ann Rheum Dis. 2012;71(6):899–904.
74. Pfirrmann CW, et al. Magnetic resonance classification of lumbar intervertebral disc degeneration. Spine (Phila Pa 1976). 2001;26(17):1873–8.
75. Friedrich KM, et al. The prevalence of lumbar facet joint edema in patients with low back pain. Skeletal Radiol. 2007;36(8):755–60.
76. Pfirrmann CW, et al. MR image-based grading of lumbar nerve root compromise due to disk herniation: reliability study with surgical correlation. Radiology. 2004;230(2):583–8.
77. Griffith JF, et al. Modified Pfirrmann grading system for lumbar intervertebral disc degeneration. Spine (Phila Pa 1976). 2007;32(24):E708–12.
78. Thompson JP, et al. Preliminary evaluation of a scheme for grading the gross morphology of the human intervertebral disc. Spine (Phila Pa 1976). 1990;15(5):411–5.
79. de Abreu MR, et al. Acromioclavicular joint osteoarthritis: comparison of findings derived from MR imaging and conventional radiography. Clin Imaging. 2005;29(4):273–7.
80. Schmal H, et al. Synovial cytokine expression in ankle osteoarthritis depends on age and stage. Knee Surg Sports Traumatol Arthrosc. 2015;23(5):1359–67. Epub 2013 Oct 19.
81. Roemer FW, et al. Presence of MRI-detected joint effusion and synovitis increases the risk of cartilage loss in knees without osteoarthritis at 30-month follow-up: the MOST study. Ann Rheum Dis. 2011;70(10):1804–9.
82. Roos EM, Dahlberg L. Positive effect of moderate exercise on glycosaminoglycan content in knee cartilage: a four-month randomized, controlled trial in patients at risk of osteoarthritis. Arthritis Rheum. 2005;52:3507–14.
83. McAlindon TE, et al. Change in knee osteoarthritis cartilage detected by delayed gadolinium enhanced magnetic resonance imaging following treatment with collagen hydrolysate: a pilot randomized controlled trial. Osteoarthritis Cartilage. 2011;19(4):399–405.
84. Souza RB, et al. The effects of acute loading on T1rho and T2 relaxation times of tibiofemoral articular cartilage. Osteoarthritis Cartilage. 2010;18(12):1557–63.
85. Eckstein F, et al. Proposal for a nomenclature for magnetic resonance imaging based measures of articular cartilage in osteoarthritis. Osteoarthritis Cartilage. 2006;14(10):974–83.
86. Buck RJ, et al. An efficient subset of morphological measures for articular cartilage in the healthy and diseased human knee. Magn Reson Med. 2010;63(3):680–90.
87. Guermazi A, et al. Osteoarthritis: a review of strengths and weaknesses of different imaging options. Rheum Dis Clin North Am. 2013;39(3):567–91.
88. Eckstein F, et al. Quantitative MRI measures of cartilage predict knee replacement: a case-control study from the Osteoarthritis Initiative. Ann Rheum Dis. 2013;72(5):707–14.
89. Kalichman L, et al. Facet joint osteoarthritis and low back pain in the community-based population. Spine (Phila Pa 1976). 2008;33(23):2560–5.
90. Neogi T, Bowes MA, Niu J, et al. MRI-based three-dimensional bone shape of the knee predicts onset of knee osteoarthritis: data from the osteoarthritis initiative. Arthritis Rheum. 2013;65(8):2048–58.

91. Gregory JS, et al. Early identification of radiographic osteoarthritis of the hip using an active shape model to quantify changes in bone morphometric features: can hip shape tell us anything about the progression of osteoarthritis? Arthritis Rheum. 2007;56(11):3634–43.
92. Lynch JA, et al. The association of proximal femoral shape and incident radiographic hip OA in elderly women. Osteoarthritis Cartilage. 2009;17(10):1313–8.
93. Baker-LePain JC, Lane NE. Relationship between joint shape and the development of osteoarthritis. Curr Opin Rheumatol. 2010;22(5):538–43.
94. Etchebehere EC, et al. Orthopedic pathology of the lower extremities: scintigraphic evaluation in the thigh, knee, and leg. Semin Nucl Med. 1998;28(1):41–61.
95. Omoumi P, et al. CT arthrography, MR arthrography, PET, and scintigraphy in osteoarthritis. Radiol Clin North Am. 2009;47(4):595–615.
96. Temmerman OP, et al. In vivo measurements of blood flow and bone metabolism in osteoarthritis. Rheumatol Int. 2013;33(4):959–63.
97. Moon YL, Lee SH, Park SY, et al. Evolution of shoulder disorders by 2-[F-18]-fluoro-2-deoxy-D-glucose positron emission tomography and computed tomography. Clin Orthop Surg. 2010;2:167–72.
98. Magee D, et al. Combining variational and model-based techniques to register PET and MR images in hand osteoarthritis. Phys Med Biol. 2010;55(16):4755–69.
99. Keen HI, Conaghan PG. Ultrasonography in osteoarthritis. Radiol Clin North Am. 2009;47(4):581–94.
100. Chiang EH, et al. Ultrasonic characterization of in vitro osteoarthritic articular cartilage with validation by confocal microscopy. Ultrasound Med Biol. 1997;23(2):205–13.
101. Keen HI, et al. The development of a preliminary ultrasonographic scoring system for features of hand osteoarthritis. Ann Rheum Dis. 2008;67(5):651–5.
102. Kortekaas MC, et al. Osteophytes and joint space narrowing are independently associated with pain in finger joints in hand osteoarthritis. Ann Rheum Dis. 2011;70(10):1835–7.
103. Conaghan PG, et al. Clinical and ultrasonographic predictors of joint replacement for knee osteoarthritis: results from a large, 3-year, prospective EULAR study. Ann Rheum Dis. 2010;69(4):644–7.

Chapter 8
Osteoarthritis: Joint Conservation Strategies

Rachel Schachar and Darrell Ogilvie-Harris

Key Points

- Patients with symptomatic osteoarthritis (OA) of the knee should participate in self-management programs, strengthening, low-impact aerobic exercises, and neuromuscular education.
- Patients with body mass index of equal to or greater than 25 should be encouraged by their physician to lose weight.
- Aerobic activity of at least 150 min per week of moderate intensity or 75 min per week of vigorous intensity performed in episodes of at least 10 min spread over 7 days and muscle-strengthening activities of moderate or high intensity should be included on 2 or more days per week.
- The evidence is inconclusive regarding the value of braces and orthotics for OA; cane or walking stick use was appropriate for knee-only OA.
- Therapeutic ultrasound, acupuncture, and electrotherapeutic therapies are subject to disagreement regarding their use, but there are no clear recommendations for benefit.
- From the evidence available, the AAOS clinical practice guideline cannot recommend performing knee arthroscopy and lavage or debridement procedures in patients with a primary diagnosis of symptomatic OA of the knee.

R. Schachar, MD, MSc
Division of Orthopedic Surgery, University of Toronto
(University of Toronto Orthopaedic Sports Medicine),
Toronto, ON, Canada

D. Ogilvie-Harris, MD (✉)
Division of Orthopedic Surgery, University Health Network,
UHN and Womens College Hospital, University of Toronto Orthopedic
Sports Medicine Program, Toronto, ON, Canada
e-mail: Darrell.Ogilive-Harris@uhn.ca

M. Kapoor, N.N. Mahomed (eds.), *Osteoarthritis: Pathogenesis, Diagnosis, Available Treatments, Drug Safety, Regenerative and Precision Medicine*,
DOI 10.1007/978-3-319-19560-5_8

- Patients with evidence of unstable meniscal tears had significantly improved pain and restored knee function when compared to treatment by physical therapy alone, but AAOS clinical practice guidelines published in 2013 were unable to recommend for or against arthroscopic partial meniscectomy in patients with OA.
- The AAOS clinical practice guidelines provide a limited recommendation for the use of a valgus-producing proximal tibial osteotomy in patients with symptomatic medial compartment OA of the knee.

Introduction

OA is the most common form of arthritis and is identified as one of the leading causes of pain and disability worldwide [1]. Approximately 70 % of the population greater than age 65 demonstrates radiographic evidence of OA [2]. With increased understanding of how the musculoskeletal system works, the standard of care for people suffering from arthritis has changed [3]. Not only is the goal for patients to regain movement, but for this movement to be pain-free and for quality of life to be maintained or improved.

Since the introduction of minimally invasive arthroscopy, attempts have been made to treat this disease [2]. There exists evidence that articular cartilage has some potential to regenerate, and current efforts in research are working toward cartilage restoration. This has so far proven to be difficult, as no technique currently exists that achieves a completely normal articular surface. For this reason, joint conservation strategies remain an important aspect in the management of OA.

There are a number of risk factors associated with OA, including age, gender, genetics, occupation, previous periarticular injury, and obesity [4]. Excessive intense high-impact exercise has also been identified as a risk factor for the development of OA [5]. Joint pain, specifically in the hip and knee, associated with OA can eventually lead to inactivity and loss of mobility, which in turn results in deconditioning, weight gain, loss of independence, and a decreased quality of life [6].

While conservative treatment for OA is limited, management goals are the same – joint preservation. Injury prevention, pain management and treatment of sustained injuries, and minimally invasive non-arthroplasty surgical interventions can achieve some of these goals (Fig. 8.1).

Exercise

The primary goal of OA treatment is to alleviate symptoms and prevent progression [4]. While there is no cure for knee OA treatment, options exist to improve quality of life and slow progression of joint deterioration, which can be expected to yield both immediate and long-term benefits (Fig. 8.2). The American Academy of Orthopedic Surgeons (AAOS) clinical practice guidelines published in 2013 recommends that patients with symptomatic OA of the knee participate

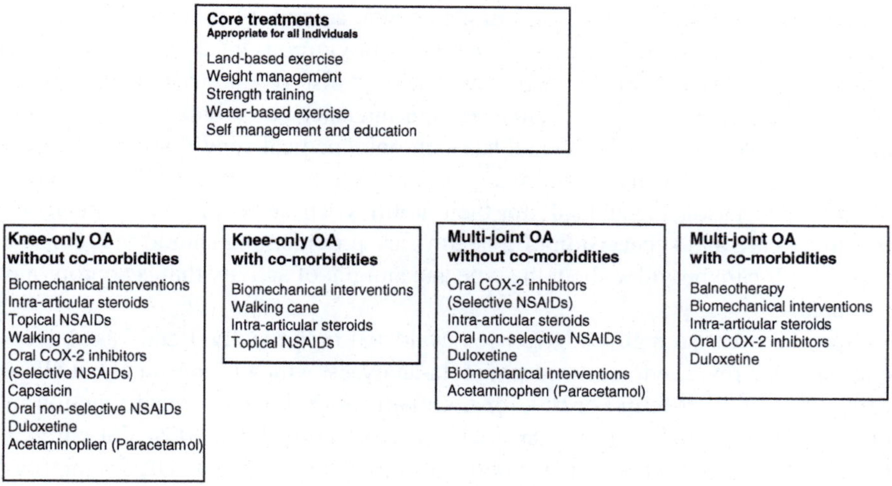

Fig. 8.1 OARSI guidelines for the nonsurgical management of knee OA (McAlindon et al. [10])

Fig. 8.2 Sports in OA (Vad [3])

Safe	Moderate	Harmful
Arthritis specific exercises	Golf	Jogging, running
Aquatherapy	Cross-country skiing	Step machine
Swimming	Softball	Football
Brisk walking	Elliptical trainer	Soccer
Cycling	Gardening (with stool)	Basketball
Low-impact aerobics	Tennis	Hockey
	Yoga, pilates	Rock climbing

in self-management programs, strengthening, low-impact aerobic exercises, and neuromuscular education and engage in physical activity consistent with national guidelines [7]. These guidelines were put forward as a "strong" recommendation for practitioners to follow.

The issue of weight loss is significant. This is a more difficult subject to broach with patients but is equally if not more important and is strongly recommended in the AAOS guidelines [7]. The evidence suggests that patients with symptomatic OA of the knee and a body mass index of equal to or greater than 25 should be encouraged by their physician to lose weight. This recommendation comes with the caveat to be sensitive to the patient and their preferences.

The 2008 Physical Activity Guidelines for Americans published by the Surgeon General provides key physical activity guidelines for the youth, adults, and older adults with the intended audience being policymakers and health professionals. In general, the recommendations encourage aerobic activity of at least 150 min per week of moderate intensity or 75 min per week of vigorous intensity performed in episodes of at least 10 min spread over 7 days. It also recommends that muscle-strengthening activities of moderate or high intensity be included on 2 or more days per week. When an individual has a chronic medical condition, the Surgeon General recommends that an individual still participate in regular physical activity at a level reasonable and safe for their abilities. These people should be under the direct care and supervision of a health-care provider and should first consult their health-care provider about the type and amount of activity that is appropriate for them.

Specific exercise regimes have been evaluated individually. Land-based exercise has been reviewed in four recent meta-analyses, which found small but clinically relevant short-term benefits for both pain control and physical function in knee OA. Interestingly, in two separate meta-analyses, the sport of t'ai chi was found to have strong favorable benefits for individuals with knee OA for improving pain and physical function. Overall the duration and type of land-based exercise programs varied – all included a combination of strength training, active range of motion exercise, and aerobic activity. The Osteoarthritis Research Society International (OARSI) felt that the quality of evidence was good and deemed land-based exercise to be an "appropriate" recommendation in the management of OA [8–10]. Along those same lines, water-based exercise, while not as extensively studied, was found to have small to moderate short-term benefits for function and quality of life in persons with OA of the hip and knee and was determined to be an appropriate recommendation for managing OA. However, a 2007 systematic review of water-based exercise for OA found only minor benefits for pain modification [11].

Strength training has also been demonstrated to be an appropriate recommendation for OA management – the programs primarily involve resistance-based lower extremity and quadriceps strengthening exercises. A 2011 meta-analysis and systematic review showed the strength training groups to have a moderate effect for reducing pain and improving physical function when compared to controls [12].

Biomechanical Interventions

Knee Bracing and Foot Orthoses

Patients consistently ask if a brace would be beneficial or provide relief (Fig. 8.3). Unfortunately, the evidence is somewhat mixed and inconclusive. In their 2013 clinical practice guidelines, the AAOS was unable to make recommendations for or against valgus-directed force brace (i.e., medial compartment unloader braces) for patients with symptomatic OA of the knee [7]. This recommendation of "inconclusive" was addressed by one level II systematic review and two randomized controlled trials (RCTs) that looked at the use of braces for patients presenting with

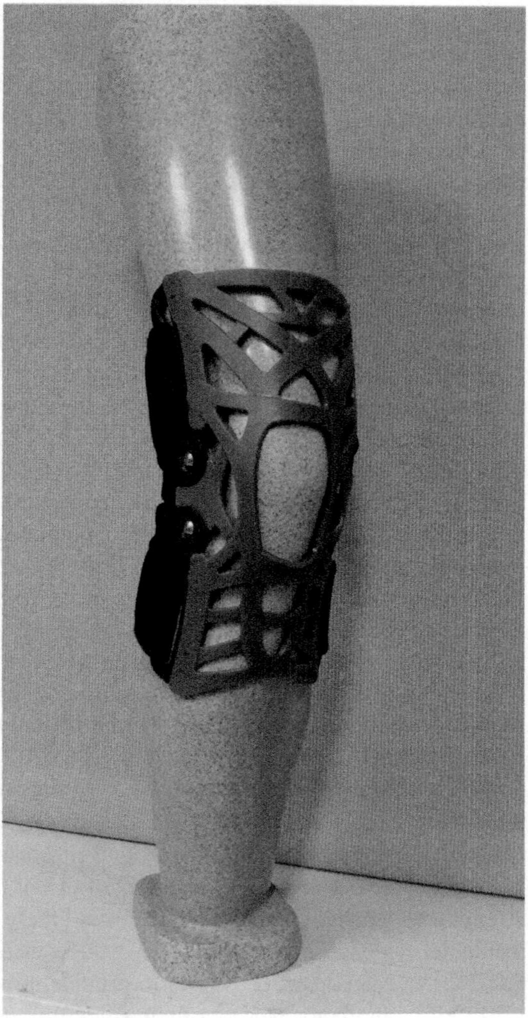

Fig. 8.3 OA unloader brace

isolated medial compartment OA of the knee. An inconclusive recommendation was also put forth for the use of braces with varus-directed force [7].

First of all, it is important to understand that OA of the entire knee is different from that of single compartment OA, which is often caused by a mechanical problem [13]. Patients with medial-sided compartment tend to have genu varum or varus knee alignment where the mechanical axis of the leg and body forces pass more through the medial compartment. The opposite is true of the lateral compartment OA. This joint malalignment places the knee at risk for progression of degenerative changes, worsening of pain, and impaired physical function [14]. In general, the purpose of a knee brace is to off-load the affected joint compartment, decrease pain, and improve function. In addition to the AAOS clinical practice guidelines, a Cochrane review on the topic concluded that there is very limited evidence for the effectiveness of brace treatment for OA, primarily due to lack of studies which addressed the issue [13]. The two knee brace studies reviewed did show improvement in both pain and function scores in the brace and neoprene sleeve group at 6 months and 1 year compared with the control groups [13].

A multicenter RCT following this set out to further investigate the use of bracing for knee [15]. This study effectively randomized 117 patients with unicompartment OA of the knee to receive a brace ($N=60$) or conservative treatment with no brace ($N=57$). The primary outcome measure was pain severity and knee function score, with secondary outcomes including walking distance and quality of life. Overall, their results also showed very little additional benefit for unicompartmental knee OA treated with an unloader brace versus conservative treatment alone [15]. It was felt that the main reason for this was that many patients do not adhere to the brace treatment long term. This was either because the positive effects were too small or because the adverse effects were too large. Fifteen out of the 60 patients in the brace group gave "no effect" as their reason for stopping. Other reasons for discontinuation included skin irritation, poor fit, and minimal symptoms. In favor for brace treatment, Kirkley et al. showed that if a patient is carefully selected, there could be potential benefit to brace treatment. They looked at patients with varus malalignment and found that knee pain was reduced with a neoprene sleeve relative to no treatment [16]. It is important to consider the patient population as well. A brace to reduce load can be viewed as a reasonable treatment option for younger patients with unicompartmental OA with varus alignment, given there are few conservative treatment alternatives that have proven effective and knee arthroplasty for younger patients with OA is not recommended [15].

Foot orthoses have also been used as an intervention for patients with symptomatic isolated unicompartmental OA of the knee, specifically lateral wedge insoles for medial compartment OA. The second edition of the AAOS evidence-based clinical practice guideline for the treatment of OA of the knee states that, with moderate strength, they cannot recommend the use of these insoles. As with knee bracing, the available evidence regarding lateral wedge insoles is conflicting. One published RCT shows lateral wedge insoles to provide no symptomatic or structural benefits [17], while another advocates their suitability as a possible alternative to valgus knee bracing in the setting of isolated medial knee OA [18]. Variable-stiffness walking shoes are another type of footwear which are felt to be more comfortable than lateral wedge insoles. These shoes have a stiffer lateral midsole, shown to reduce the external knee abduction moment and were shown in one recent RCT to reduce pain and improve function after a period of 6 months [19]. Unfortunately, this study did not show this benefit to be statistically significant when compared to constant-stiffness footwear.

The use of a cane or walking stick has also been viewed as a reasonable conservative treatment option for patients with knee pain and specifically due to knee OA. In medial knee OA, there is a strong association between excessive medial joint loading and disease progression [20]. As a result, and for generations, canes or walking aids have been recommended by health-care professionals in an attempt to off-load the painful knee. It has been estimated that 40–70 % of patients with OA use some type of walking aid [21, 22]. The use of assistive walking devices by older adults tends to primarily be for the management of knee pain or balance problems [23]. However, there is a paucity of evidence with respect to the impact of cane use in the treatment of OA. A single-blind RCT, conducted by Jones et al. 2012, concluded that a cane for gait assistance in patients with knee OA could be used to diminish pain and improve function and some aspects of quality of life compared with those not using a walking aid [24]. It was found that initially, during the first month, patients in the cane group had a substantial increase in energy expenditure, but this was no longer a factor by the end of the second month. Another interesting finding was that compared to the control group (no cane), patients using a cane consumed fewer nonsteroidal anti-inflammatory drugs or NSAIDs. This was statistically significant when measured at the end of the second month [24]. This study, despite a short follow-up period of only 2 months and the only RCT looking at cane use in this population, was well done and provides results that can be extrapolated to a similar patient population with knee OA. It was noted by the OARSI that this study lacked evidence for cane use for individuals with multiple affect joints and that caution should be used when trying to reduce knee pain at the expense of increasing load through other affected joints (i.e., hands) [10].

The Health, Aging and Body Composition (Health ABC) Study is a community-based, multicenter cohort study, which included 3075 men and women ages 70–79 recruited at the University of Pittsburgh that began in 1997 with the primary objective of examining the incidence of physical disability in relation to body composition and weight-based health conditions in healthy older adults [23]. A recently published prospective cohort study of a subset of 874 patients, from the Health ABC study group, with prevalent knee pain was assessed to identify factors that predicted incident use of walking aids and to assess whether their use was associated with changes in knee OA [23]. Main outcome measures included mean Western Ontario and McMaster Universities Osteoarthritis Index (WOMAC) pain scores and the frequency of joint space narrowing (JSN) on knee radiographs taken over a 3-year time period [23]. Unfortunately, only 10 % of the patient subset with radiographs and WOMAC data used walking aids, which could account for lack of difference between groups in both domains. However, while their longitudinal analysis looking at the association of walking aid use, with changes in JSN on radiographs, showed no relationship between use or nonuse of a walking aid and joint space changes, there was no evidence of progressive worsening in the walking aid group which was felt to be encouraging [23].

The ability to draw conclusions about these treatment modalities is limited by heterogeneity and poor quality of available evidence. From the available evidence, the OARS concluded that cane or walking stick use was appropriate for knee-only OA, but their recommendation was uncertain for multi-joint OA and suggested that further research be done in this area. The use of biomechanical interventions as directed by an appropriate specialist was advised [10]. Overall, these treatment options have greater benefit than risk if surgical intervention is not yet an option.

Physical Modalities

Joint pain associated with OA often leads to inactivity and loss of mobility, which in turn results in deconditioning, weight gain, loss of independence, and a decreased quality of life [6]. While a patient with knee OA may eventually need to employ pharmacotherapy and injection-based treatment or undergo a total knee arthroplasty, an intervention will have excellent outcomes for pain relief and improved quality of life. Due to associated risks of surgery or potential adverse effects of other invasive treatments, many patients may choose to pursue physical management options first [1].

A recent systematic review rigorously critically appraised 17 guidelines, which provided recommendations for physical management of OA [1]. Forty different therapeutic interventions were identified across all guidelines reviewed, and recommendations were graded from "strongly recommended" to "unsupported." From the identified treatment modalities, those felt to be most often used by patients and prescribed by health practitioners for management of OA are discussed further [1].

Ultrasound

Therapeutic ultrasound (US), the application of sound waves in tissue, is one of the many physical therapy modalities that are often employed when treating patients with pain and loss of function due to OA. While there is limited support from two systematic reviews compiled in 2010 that suggest a possible benefit of US in the treatment of knee OA, overall the evidence for the recommended use of therapeutic US for OA of the knee is poor [10]. The OARSI guidelines state that the quality of the analyzed evidence was low and therefore they were unable to make recommendation for its use. In the most recent Cochrane Collaboration Review, four additional trials were included for analysis, which included a total of 341 patients with knee OA [25]. The authors concluded that in comparison to the earlier version of the review (2001), the results suggest that therapeutic US may be beneficial for patients with knee OA. However, it was emphasized that there exists uncertainty about the magnitude of the effects on pain relief and function [25]. A recent systematic review and network meta-analysis (a means of evaluating the relative effectiveness of several interventions and synthesizing evidence across a network of RCTs) comparing continuous versus pulsed US for the management of knee OA indicated that pulsed US is more effective in both pain relief and functional improvement when compared to a control group [26]. It was noted by the authors that continuous US could only be considered as a pain relief treatment.

In a recent publication, a therapeutic US verses sham US randomized double-blind controlled clinical study, US was not found to have any additional benefit to conventional physical therapy programs alone in patients with knee OA [27].

Acupuncture

The efficacy of acupuncture for peripheral joint OA has been tested in numerous clinical trials. Trials that used a wait list or usual care control groups have generally found some clinically relevant benefit, but those using a sham acupuncture have been less positive [28]. A recent pooled analysis of 16 RCTs found statistically significant benefit of acupuncture in sham-controlled trials, though this did not reach the investigators' threshold for clinical significance. The most recent JAAOS clinical practice guidelines provided a strong recommendation against the use of acupuncture in patients with symptomatic knee OA [7]. Based on the best available evidence, the OARSI was "uncertain" about recommending acupuncture for the treatment of OA [10]. A harms analysis was not performed; it is outlined by the JAAOS guidelines that "strong" recommendations should be followed by health practitioners unless presented with a more convincing reason for an alternative approach [7].

Electrotherapeutics

Transcutaneous electrical nerve stimulation (TENS) [11] is often used as an adjunct by physical therapists when treating patients with joint pain associated with OA. The literature in this area is somewhat conflicting with respect to the results. The OARSI guidelines concluded that TENS was not appropriate for multiple-joint OA and were uncertain about the use for knee OA only [10]. This was based on a single systematic review that found inclusive results concerning the effect of TENS for pain relief in knee OA and a double-blind multicenter RCT, which showed no statistically significant difference between the TENS group and the sham TENS group for pain control [10]. Another randomized sham-controlled clinical trial looking at the additional effects of TENS for knee OA, when combined with a group education and exercise program, found that while all outcome measures improved over time (including the WOMAC pain scores, stiffness, quadriceps strength, exercise adherence, and exercise self-efficacy), there were no differences between the groups [29]. This may be explained by the fact that self-education and focused exercise programs seem to have the greatest impact for conservative management of knee OA. Finally, more recently a single-blinded RCT showed that the use of TENS significantly improved the quadriceps strength in patients with early-stage knee OA when compared with standard therapy [30]. Patients showed a significant reduction at 3-month follow-up in their pain visual analog scale.

While there are promising results from some RCTs, there is overall disagreement in the literature for the use of TENS for patients suffering from knee OA. This is supported by the JAAOS evidence-based clinical practice guidelines, which state that they are unable to recommend for or against the use of physical agents including electrotherapeutic therapies [7]. The strength of this recommendation, as outlined above, is inconclusive.

Thermotherapy

OA is a complex degenerative disease process that results in pain and stiffness and is often associated with joint swelling. Thermotherapy, also known as hot or cold therapy, involves applying heat or cold to the affected joints for the relief of pain symptoms [31]. This can be done through the use of hot or cold packs, damp towels, or wax baths. Heat applied to the body works to improve local circulation and muscle relaxation, whereas cold packs placed on the body tend to constrict blood vessels and block nerve impulses to the area resulting in decreased pain and swelling [31]. In the 2003 Cochrane Review, three RCTs were found to be appropriate for review. The authors' conclusions were that ice massage and cold packs decreased swelling resulting in a statistically beneficial effect on joint range of motion, knee strength, and patient function but not on pain control. Hot packs had no effect on joint swelling.

Non-arthroplasty Surgical Interventions

Arthroscopy

Arthroscopic lavage, arthroscopic abrasion, and debridement have had a basic role in the treatment of knee OA in the past [2]. More recently, its use in the treatment of knee OA has been called into question. It has been found that approximately 50–75 % of patients who undergo knee arthroscopy and debridement initially benefit from decreased pain and stiffness [32]. Unfortunately, 15 % of those patients progress to needing a total knee replacement within 1 year following surgery.

In 2002, Moseley et al. published a landmark study in which patients were randomized to receive arthroscopic lavage, debridement, or placebo surgery. Patients in the placebo group received skin incisions and underwent a simulated debridement without insertion of the arthroscope [33]. The 180 patients in the three treatment arms, most with moderate to severe knee OA, were then followed for a period of 2 years. During the follow-up period, no benefits were seen between the surgical groups and the sham surgery group. This study has been criticized on many levels but most importantly regarding the homogeneity of the study population, specifically that greater than 85 % of the patients were male making generalizability of the study results difficult. A more recent RCT by Kirkley et al. (2008), where patients were randomized to surgical lavage and arthroscopic debridement together with physical and medical therapy or to treatment with physical and medical therapy alone then followed for 2 years, found similar results [34]. The primary outcome measures were the WOMAC, the SF-36 short form physical component summary, and a pain and function scale. At the 2-year follow-up, there was no difference between the groups in either domain [32, 34]. One important point to note is that patients found, by clinical examination or MRI, to have large bucket handle meniscal tears were excluded from the study. Regardless, this study was very well executed with sound results. Their conclusions were that arthroscopic surgery does not provide any additional benefit to optimized physical and medical therapy for the treatment of knee OA [34]. Other studies have suggested that the need for arthroplasty may be delayed by arthroscopic surgery.

From the evidence available the AAOS clinical practice guideline cannot recommend performing knee arthroscopy and lavage or debridement procedures in patients with a primary diagnosis of symptomatic OA of the knee. This was put forward as a strong recommendation.

Partial Meniscectomy

The menisci are important with respect to knee function. They play a role in load sharing, shock absorption, reduction in joint contact stresses, passive stabilization, increasing congruity and contact area, limitation of extremes of flexion and extension, as well as proprioception [35]. These important functions are achieved by the transmission of load over the tibial plateau. Radiographic findings consistent with OA of the knee, including JSN, osteophyte formation, and squaring of the femoral condyles after total meniscectomy, suggest that the meniscus is an important structure in joint protection [35].

Biomechanical studies have demonstrated that the medial and lateral menisci transmit at least 50–70 % or more of the load when the knee is in extension with forces increasing to 85 % with 90° of knee flexion [36]. These loads are well distributed when the menisci are intact [37].

Removal of the medial meniscus results in a 50–70 % reduction in femoral condyle contact area and in a 100 % increase in contact stress. Total lateral meniscectomy causes a 40–50 % decrease in contact area and increases contact stress in the lateral compartment to 200–300 % that of normal.

Based on AAOS clinical practice guidelines published in 2013, they were unable to recommend for or against arthroscopic partial meniscectomy in patients with OA of the knee with a torn meniscus (Fig. 8.4). However, the strength of this recommendation was inconclusive, and therefore practitioners should feel little constraint in following this recommendation but should exercise good clinical judgment. Newly published research, in support of arthroscopic partial meniscectomy, showed that patients with evidence of unstable meniscal tears had significantly improved pain and restored knee function (using visual analog scale and Lysholm knee score outcome measures, respectively), when compared to treatment by physical therapy alone [38]. This study looked at 70 patients between the ages of 18–27, 29 % of whom had evidence of mild OA.

High Tibial Osteotomy

High tibial osteotomy (HTO) [33] was a procedure initially popularized in the 1970s by Coventry and Insall [32]. The basic principle of the HTO is to redirect the mechanical axis from the degenerated area of the knee joint to the relatively

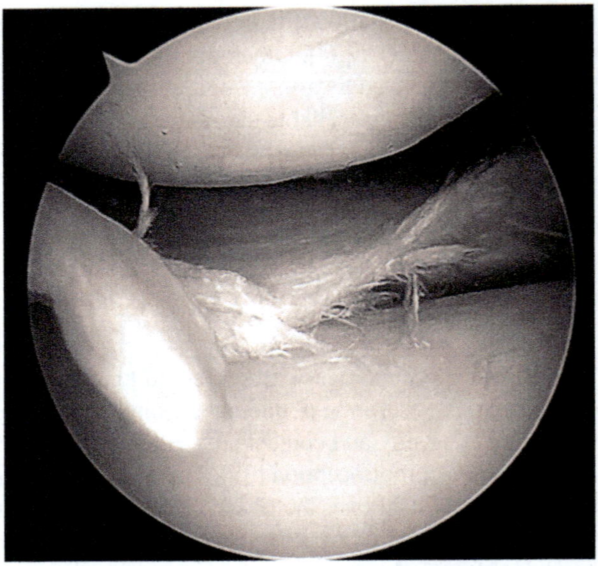

Fig. 8.4 OA knee with meniscal tear causing mechanical symptoms which may benefit from partial meniscectomy

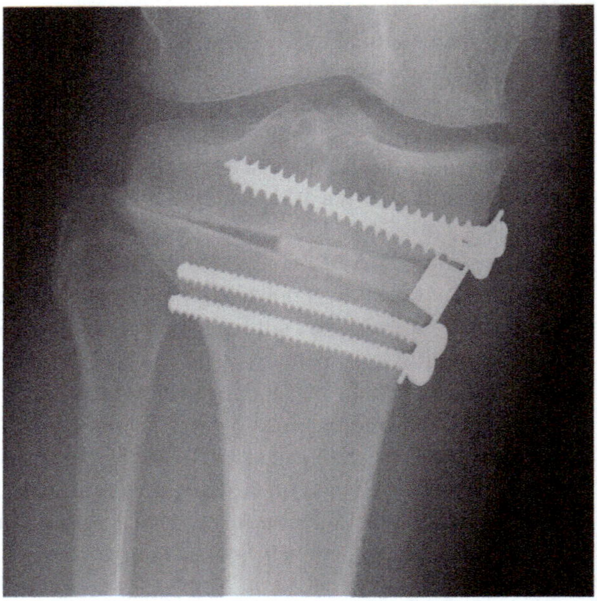

Fig. 8.5 High tibial osteotomy, opening medial wedge

well-preserved joint compartment (Fig. 8.5). Typically, this is done for the medial compartment OA of the knee resulting in the weight-bearing forces being shifted from the arthritic medial compartment over to the intact cartilage of the lateral side of the knee [32]. This procedure is typically indicated for highly active patients or laborers who have unicompartmental varus or valgus knee arthritis. Contraindications for this procedure include previous meniscectomy, significant degenerative changes in the compartment of the knee where the forces are to be transferred, inflammatory arthropathies, patients aged greater than 65, and symptomatic patellofemoral arthritis. There is good evidence for good-to-excellent functional outcomes with follow-up from 2 to 17 years [39–41].

The AAOS clinical practice guidelines provide a limited recommendation for the use of a valgus-producing proximal tibial osteotomy in patients with symptomatic medial compartment OA of the knee [7].

Conclusions

The evidence is clear that patients with symptomatic OA of the knee should participate in self-management programs, strengthening, low-impact aerobic exercises, and neuromuscular education. In addition, weight control is of value. Patients with body mass index of equal to or greater than 25 should be encouraged by their physician to lose weight and aerobic activity of at least 150 min per week of moderate intensity or 75 min per week of vigorous intensity performed in episodes of at least 10 min spread over 7 days. Along with this, muscle-strengthening activities of moderate or high intensity should be included on 2 or more days per week.

The evidence is inconclusive regarding the value of braces and orthotics for OA; cane or walking stick use was appropriate for knee-only OA. The evidence regarding physical modalities of treatment is generally equivocal. Therapeutic ultrasound, acupuncture, and electrotherapeutic therapies are subject to disagreement regarding their use, but there are no clear recommendations for their benefit.

Arthroscopic interventions should be limited to clear mechanical issues such as an unstable meniscus in an OA knee. From the evidence available, the AAOS clinical practice guidelines cannot recommend performing knee arthroscopy and lavage or debridement procedures in patients with a primary diagnosis of symptomatic OA of the knee. Recently, it was shown that patients with evidence of unstable meniscal tears had significantly improved pain and restored knee function when compared to treatment by physical therapy alone, but AAOS clinical practice guidelines published in 2013 were unable to recommend for or against arthroscopic partial meniscectomy in patients with OA. The AAOS clinical practice guidelines provide a limited recommendation for the use of a valgus-producing proximal tibial osteotomy in patients with symptomatic medial compartment OA of the knee.

References

1. Larmer PJ, et al. Systematic review of guidelines for the physical management of osteoarthritis. Arch Phys Med Rehabil. 2014;95(2):375–89.
2. Gifka J, Ogilvie-Harris DJ, editors. Osteoarthritis: fundamentals and strategies for joint-preserving treatment. Berlin/New York: Springer; 2000.
3. Vad V. Arthritis RX: a cutting-edge program for a pain-free life. 1st ed. New York: Gotham Books; 2006.

4. Dhawan P, Timothy Deakon R, Clarfield M. Solving Osteoarthritis Pain Control: Current Status of Hyaluronic Acid Knee Injections. 2014:1–6. https://themedicalxchange.com/en/article/2014/jul/14/solving-osteoarthritis-pain-control-current-stat-2/
5. Tveit M, et al. Former male elite athletes have a higher prevalence of osteoarthritis and arthroplasty in the hip and knee than expected. Am J Sports Med. 2012;40(3):527–33.
6. Loew L, et al. Ottawa panel evidence-based clinical practice guidelines for aerobic walking programs in the management of osteoarthritis. Arch Phys Med Rehabil. 2012;93(7):1269–85.
7. Jevsevar D. Treatment of osteoarthritis of the knee: evidence-based guideline, 2nd edition. J Am Acad Orthop Surg. 2013;21(9):571–6.
8. Zhang W, et al. OARSI recommendations for the management of hip and knee osteoarthritis, part I: critical appraisal of existing treatment guidelines and systematic review of current research evidence. Osteoarthritis Cartilage. 2007;15(9):981–1000.
9. Zhang W, et al. OARSI recommendations for the management of hip and knee osteoarthritis, Part II: OARSI evidence-based, expert consensus guidelines. Osteoarthritis Cartilage. 2008;16(2):137–62.
10. McAlindon TE, et al. OARSI guidelines for the non-surgical management of knee osteoarthritis. Osteoarthritis Cartilage. 2014;22(3):363–88.
11. Bartels EM, et al. Aquatic exercise for the treatment of knee and hip osteoarthritis. Cochrane Database Syst Rev. 2007;(4):CD005523.
12. Jansen MJ, et al. Strength training alone, exercise therapy alone, and exercise therapy with passive manual mobilisation each reduce pain and disability in people with knee osteoarthritis: a systematic review. J Physiother. 2011;57(1):11–20.
13. Brouwer RW, et al. Braces and orthoses for treating osteoarthritis of the knee. Cochrane Database Syst Rev. 2005;(1):CD004020.
14. Sharma L, Dunlop DD, Cahue S, Song J, Hayes KW. Quadriceps strength and osteoarthritis progression in malaligned and lax knees. Ann Intern Med. 2003;138(8):613–9.
15. Brouwer RW, et al. Brace treatment for osteoarthritis of the knee: a prospective randomized multi-centre trial. Osteoarthritis Cartilage. 2006;14(8):777–83.
16. Kirkley A, Webster-Bogaert S, Litchfield R, Amendola A, MacDonald S, McCalden R, Fowler P. The effect of bracing on varus gonarthrosis. J Bone Joint Surg Am. 1999;81(4):539–48.
17. Bennell KL, Bowles KA, Payne C, Cicuttini F, Williamson E, Forbes A, Hanna F, Davies-Tuck M, Harris A, Hinman RS. Lateral wedge insoles for medial knee osteoarthritis: 12 month randomised controlled trial. BMJ. 2011;18:342–50.
18. van Raaij TM, et al. Medial knee osteoarthritis treated by insoles or braces: a randomized trial. Clin Orthop Relat Res. 2010;468(7):1926–32.
19. Erhart JC, Mündermann A, Elspas B, Giori NJ, Andriacchi TP. Changes in knee adduction moment, pain, and functionality with a variable-stiffness walking shoe after 6 months. J Orthop Res. 2010;27(7):873–9.
20. Miyazaki T, Wada M, Kawahara H, Sato M, Baba H, Shimada S. Dynamic load at baseline can predict radiographic disease progression in medial compartment knee osteoarthritis. Ann Rheum Dis. 2002;61:617–22.
21. Van der Esch M, Heijmans M, Dekker J. Factors contributing to possession and use of walking aids among persons with rheumatoid arthritis and osteoarthritis. Arthritis Rheum. 2003;49:838–42.
22. Shrier I, et al. Conservative non-pharmacological treatment options are not frequently used in the management of hip osteoarthritis. J Sci Med Sport. 2006;9(1–2):81–6.
23. Carbone LD, et al. Assistive walking device use and knee osteoarthritis: results from the Health, Aging and Body Composition Study (Health ABC Study). Arch Phys Med Rehabil. 2013;94(2):332–9.
24. Jones A, et al. Impact of cane use on pain, function, general health and energy expenditure during gait in patients with knee osteoarthritis: a randomised controlled trial. Ann Rheum Dis. 2012;71(2):172–9.

25. Rutjes AW, et al. Therapeutic ultrasound for osteoarthritis of the knee or hip. Cochrane Database Syst Rev. 2010;(1):CD003132.
26. Zeng C, et al. Effectiveness of continuous and pulsed ultrasound for the management of knee osteoarthritis: a systematic review and network meta-analysis. Osteoarthritis Cartilage. 2014;22(8):1090–9.
27. Ulus Y, Tander B, Akyol Y, Durmus D, Buyukankncak O, Gul U, Canturk F, Bilgici A, Kuru O. Therapeutic ultrasound versus sham ultrasound for the management of patients with knee osteoarthritis: a randomized double-blind controlled clinical study. Int J Rheum Dis. 2012;15:197–206.
28. Manheimer E, et al. Acupuncture for peripheral joint osteoarthritis. Cochrane Database Syst Rev. 2010;(1):CD001977.
29. Palmer S, et al. Transcutaneous electrical nerve stimulation as an adjunct to education and exercise for knee osteoarthritis: a randomized controlled trial. Arthritis Care Res (Hoboken). 2014;66(3):387–94.
30. Cherian JJ, Kapadia BH, Bhave, A, McElroy MJ, Cherian C, Harwin SF, Mont MA. Use of Transcutaneous Electrical Nerve Stimulation Device in Early Osteoarthritis of the Knee. J Knee Surg. 2014.
31. Brosseau L, et al. Thermotherapy for treatment of osteoarthritis. Cochrane Database Syst Rev. 2003;(4):CD004522.
32. Feeley BT, Gallo RA, Sherman S, Williams R. Management of osteoarthritis of the knee in the active patient. J Am Acad Orthop Surg. 2010;18:406–16.
33. Moseley JB, O'Malley K, Petersen NJ, Menke TJ, Brody BA, Kuyendall DH, Hollingsworth JC, Ashton CM, Wray NP. Controlled trial of arthroscopic surgery for osteoarthritis of the knee. N Engl J Med. 2002;347(2):81–8.
34. Kirkley A, Birmingham TB, Litchfield R, Giffin R, Willits K, Wong C, Feagan B, Donner A, Griffin S, D'Ascanio L, Pope J, Fowler P. A randomized trial of arthroscopic surgery for osteoarthritis of the knee. N Engl J Med. 2008;359(11):1097–107.
35. Greis PE, Bardana DD, Holmstrom MC, Burks RT. Meniscal injury: I. Basic science and evaluation. J Am Acad Orthop Surg. 2002;10:168–76.
36. Ahmed AM, Burke DL. In-vitro measurement of static pressure distribution in synovial joints–Part I: Tibial surface of the knee. J Biomech Eng. 1983;105(3):216–25.
37. Radin EL, de Lamotte F, Maquet P. Role of the menisci in the distribution of stress in the knee. Clin Orthop Relat Res. 1984;185:290–4.
38. El Ghazaly SA, et al. Arthroscopic partial meniscectomy is superior to physical rehabilitation in the management of symptomatic unstable meniscal tears. Int Orthop. 2015;39(4):769–75.
39. Kuraishi J, Akizuki S, Takizawa T, Yamazaki I, Matsunaga D. Arthroscopic lateral meniscectomy in knees with lateral compartment osteoarthritis: a case series study. Arthroscopy. 2006;22(8):878–83.
40. Niemeyer P, Schmal H, Hauschild O, von Heyden J, Südkamp NP, Köstler W. Open-wedge osteotomy using an internal plate fixator in patients with medial-compartment gonarthritis and varus malalignment: 3-year results with regard to preoperative arthroscopic and radiographic findings. Arthroscopy. 2010;26(12):1607–16.
41. Omori G, Koga Y, Miyao M, Takemae T, Sato T, Yamagiwa H. High tibial osteotomy using two threaded pins and figure-of-eight wiring fixation for medial knee osteoarthritis: 14 to 24 years follow-up results. J Orthop Sci. 2008;13(1):39–45.

Chapter 9
Osteoarthritis Biomarkers

Ying-Hua Li, Christopher Kim, and Rajiv Gandhi

Key Points

- Biomarkers in OA can be categorized using the BIPEDS classification system: burden of disease, investigative, prognostic, efficacy of intervention, diagnostic, and safety.
- Urine CTX-II and serum COMP have the best performance and promise of all commercially available OA biomarkers.
- Identification and validation of panels of biomarkers correlated with imaging modalities may provide improved diagnosis, prediction, and understanding of the pathogenesis of OA.
- Catabolic factors reflecting the degradation of cartilage joint tissue remain the most promising OA biomarkers and are awaiting validation in clinical trials.
- Omics-based technology platforms, including DNA microarray, transcriptomics, proteomics, and metabolomics, are being increasingly applied in OA research and have identified significant amount of new potential OA biomarkers.
- Aberrantly expressed miRNAs contribute to the pathogenesis of OA and could serve as potential therapeutic targets to treat OA, as well as diagnostic biomarkers.
- Circulating miRNAs have emerged as a new class of minimally or noninvasive OA biomarkers due to their highly stability and ease of detection.

Y.-H. Li, PhD
Division of Genetics & Development, Toronto Western Research Institute,
Toronto Western Hospital, University Health Network, Toronto, ON, Canada

C. Kim, MD, MSc • R. Gandhi, MD, MSc (✉)
Division of Orthopedic Surgery, Toronto Western Hospital,
University Health Network, Toronto, ON M5T 2S8, Canada
e-mail: Rajiv.Gandhi@uhn.ca

M. Kapoor, N.N. Mahomed (eds.), *Osteoarthritis: Pathogenesis, Diagnosis, Available Treatments, Drug Safety, Regenerative and Precision Medicine*,
DOI 10.1007/978-3-319-19560-5_9

Introduction

The hallmark of osteoarthritis (OA) is progressive degradation of cartilage, leading to whole joint destruction and clinical symptoms of pain and loss of function [1]. The accepted gold standard diagnosis of OA is currently based on radiographic criteria, typically a Kellgren-Lawrence (K-L) grade ≥ 2 with pain and impairment of mobility [2]. However, radiographic measures have limitations with diagnosing and assessing the progression of OA, as radiographs indicate changes in bone and indirectly assess the progression of cartilage loss. Also, radiographic changes characteristic of OA appear after significant joint deterioration, and the change may occur relatively slowly with poor correlation with patient joint function [3]. Given these limitations, there has been considerable interest in the identification and development of biomarkers to quantify joint remodeling and disease progression.

The National Institutes of Health (NIH) defines a biomarker as a characteristic that is objectively measured and evaluated as an indicator of normal biologic processes, pathogenic processes, or pharmacologic responses to a therapeutic intervention [4]. The term biomarker encompasses proteins, protein fragments, metabolites, carbohydrate biomarkers, genomic RNA and DNA biomarkers, cellular biomarkers, and imaging biomarkers [5]. In a systematic review of the literature in OA biomarkers, van Spil et al, identified 84 relevant publications covering 26 different biomarkers published up to 2010 [6].

The goal of biomarkers in OA is to measure and predict disease progression and outcome. Therefore, identifying OA biomarkers that can capture the full spectrum of the pathogenesis of OA is needed.

Classification of Osteoarthritis Biomarkers

In 2006, the NIH funded OA Biomarkers Network proposed a classification scheme for OA biomarkers represented by the acronym BIPED to connote the five categories of markers: Burden of Disease, Investigative, Prognostic, Efficacy of Intervention and Diagnostic [3]. Through the recent Osteoarthritis Research Society International (OARSI)/US Food and Drug Administration (FDA) initiative, the BIPED classification system added a sixth category, Safety of Interventions, to become BIPEDS [7]. The same OA biomarkers working group proposed to divide biomarkers in two major groups: wet biomarkers and dry biomarkers. The soluble or wet biomarkers are measured in blood, serum, plasma, urine, or synovial fluid and represent a modulation of endogenous substances in these fluids, whereas dry biomarkers consist of visual analog scales, performed tasks, or imaging [8].

Based upon the BIPEDS classification, Bauer et al. and Kraus et al. proposed the following clinical use of biological markers in OA [3, 7]. (a) *Diagnostic markers:* as indicated by Bauer et al., diagnostic markers are defined by the ability to classify individuals as either diseased or non-diseased with good positive and negative likelihood ratios and area under the curve in the receiving operator curve [3]. (b) *Burden of disease markers:* these markers assess the severity or extent of disease, typically at a single point in time, among individuals with OA [3]. (c) *Prognostic markers:* prognostic markers predict the future onset of OA among those without OA at baseline or the progression of OA among those with existing disease. These biomarkers may be used to determine risk in those without OA, clinical outcomes in individuals with OA, or the efficacy of potential new disease-modifying osteoarthritis drugs (DMOADs) [3]. (d) *Efficacy of intervention markers:* these biomarkers provide information about the efficacy of treatment among those with OA or those at high risk of developing OA. These biomarkers can be used in randomized controlled trials (RCTs) to evaluate short- and long-term changes associated with DMOADs [3]. (e) *Investigative markers:* as stated by Bauer et al., an investigative marker is one on which there is insufficient information to allow inclusion into one of the existing categories [3]. (f) *Safety of intervention markers:* finally, safety biomarkers provide information about exposure to new potential drugs, radiation, and contrast agents. These biomarkers are expected to be of increasing significance as new biomarkers are identified and studied [7].

Circulatory and Inflammatory Biomarkers

Increasingly, indicators of inflammation have gained credibility as OA biomarkers because they have been shown to predict outcomes in OA.

Adipokines (adiponectin and leptin) are emerging as modulators of joint disease by promoting and perpetuating the inflammatory response. Several studies have revealed associations between adipokines and joint disease. Perruccio and colleagues have shown a dose response association between overall painful joint burden and plasma levels of adipokines in individuals with hip and knee OA [9]. As well, plasma adiponectin levels have been reported to be significantly higher in individuals with OA compared to healthy controls [10]. In a recent study, serum leptin was found to correlate with the severity of knee OA [11]. In another study, the investigators reported a negative association between serum leptin levels and knee cartilage volume [12]. Stannus and associates reported a positive association between serum leptin and radiographic hip joint space narrowing [13].

The presence of high-sensitivity C-reactive protein (CRP) and interleukin 6 (IL-6) has been shown to predict outcomes in OA. In a group of 54 patients with idiopathic OA undergoing total hip and knee arthroplasty, increased synovial inflammation correlated with elevated plasma CRP levels [14]. In a cross-sectional study of 105 women with knee OA who were followed for 2 years, increased levels of CRP were found, which predicted disease progression in these patients compared to 740 women without OA [15]. Increased serum levels of CRP predicted cartilage loss associated with knee OA and poorer functional outcomes post total knee arthroplasty as well [16, 17]. Similar results have been reported for IL-6. In a study of 172 randomly selected patients followed over 3 years, baseline levels of serum IL-6 could predict loss of both medial and lateral tibial cartilage volume, and changes in

IL-6 over 3 years were associated with changes in tibial cartilage volume [18]. In a study of 908 women who were followed prospectively for 15 years, Livshits and colleagues reported that prevalent radiographic OA was significantly associated with both increased circulating levels of CRP and IL-6, and incident radiographic OA was significantly predicted by IL-6 [19]. In another study of 161 patients with knee OA followed over 2 years, baseline levels of CRP and IL-6 predicted cartilage volume loss in the medial compartment of the knee [20]. The predictive value of baseline CRP and IL-6 levels on cartilage volume loss was possibly related to the fact that both are known inflammatory biomarkers. Synovitis, followed over 1 year arthroscopically in 422 patients, was a potential predictive factor of rapid progression of cartilage lesions in the medial tibiofemoral compartment [21].

These studies show the involvement of inflammatory biomarkers in OA pathogenesis and support the association between inflammation and joint disease (Table 9.1).

Catabolic Osteoarthritis Biomarkers

A hallmark feature of OA pathology is the higher rate of cartilage degradation than cartilage synthesis, leading to chronic cartilage loss. Cartilage, composed of chondrocytes and the extracellular matrix (ECM), is a connective tissue possessing unique biological and mechanical properties which supports its load-bearing function [22]. The dry weight of cartilage is mainly made of type II collagen and some type I, along with certain amount of proteoglycans and integral proteins. Fragments of these components generated during cartilage degeneration can be released into the bloodstream, synovial fluid, and urine and therefore be utilized as biomarkers [23].

Table 9.1 Circulatory and inflammatory OA biomarkers

Biomarker subtypes	Biomarkers	BIPEDS classification
Cytokine and protein biomarkers	CRP	P
	IL-6	P
	IL-1β	P
	IL-8	P
	TNF-α	P
	15-HETE	P
	PGE2	P
Obesity-related inflammatory biomarkers	Leptin	P
	Adiponectin	P
	Resistin	P
	Visfatin	P

Abbreviations: *P* prognostic, *CRP* C-reactive protein, *IL* interleukin, *TNF* tumor necrosis factor, *15-HETE* 15-hydroxyeicosatetraenoic acid, *PGE2* prostaglandin E2

C-Telopeptides of Type II Collagen

Since type II collagen is the major collagen type and most abundant protein in cartilage, C-terminal telopeptides of type II collagen (CTX-II), a catabolic product of type II collagen, has become the widely accepted biomarker for assessing collagen breakdown [24]. Urinary levels of CTX-II (uCTX-II) have been used as a marker for cartilage metabolism, disease severity, and monitoring drug response in OA patients [25–27]. Reijman et al. studied the association between the concentration of uCTX-II and the prevalence and progression of radiographic OA of the knee and hip. The 1,235 subjects were 55 years of age and older and were followed for 6.6 years on average. They found that subjects with a uCTX-II level in the highest quartile had a 4.2-fold increased risk of having radiographic knee or hip OA, compared with subjects with a uCTX-II level in the lowest quartile. Furthermore, subjects with an uCTX-II level in the highest quartile had a 6.0-fold increased risk for progression of radiographic knee OA at the knee and an 8.4-fold increased risk for progression of radiographic hip OA. In addition to its strong correlation with radiographic OA, another advantage of uCTX-II or serum CTX-II is that it is noninvasive. However, as collagen type II breakdown correlates with radiographic features of OA, the use of uCTX-II as a pre-radiographic diagnostic biomarker is limited. Additional biomarkers originated from collagen type II include cleavage of collagen type II triple helix (C2C), triple helix collagen type II cleavage (Coll2-1), nitrated form of Coll2-1 (Coll2-1NO2), collagen type II propeptides (PIINP, PIIANP, PIIBNP, PIICP, CPII), and collagen type I and II cleavage neoepitope (C1, C2). These additional collagenous biomarkers either provide complementary information on collagen type II catabolism or help to distinguish subtypes of OA [28]. For example, Coll2-1 and Coll2-1NO2 are more useful for studying oxidative stress-related collagen II degradation in OA [29, 30].

Cartilage Oligomeric Matrix Protein

Cartilage oligomeric matrix protein (COMP) is a structural glycoprotein binding to and stabilizing type I, II, and IX collagen fibers, fibronectin, and aggrecan [31]. COMP has been considered as an OA biomarker and has been tested in OA diagnosis, prognosis, and therapeutic intervention. Many large population studies have shown that serum COMP (sCOMP) levels correlated with cartilage degradation and disease severity. In the Johnston County OA Project involving 143 patients with radiographic knee OA and 148 healthy controls, a significant elevation of sCOMP levels were detected in the OA group compared to controls. Moreover, sCOMP levels were upregulated with knee OA K-L grade and the number of joints involved [32]. Sharif et al. suggested the use of sCOMP levels to predict OA progression. In this longitudinal study lasting 5 years, 115 patients with OA were grouped as non-progressors and progressors defined by either a reduction in the tibiofemoral joint space width by at least 2 mm or total knee arthroplasty at follow-up. They found that the chance to have radiographic OA progression was increased by 15 % with every 1 unit increase in sCOMP levels [33]. The existence of COMP fragments and their release into the culture medium were also confirmed recently which may provide complement to total COMP in use as biomarkers [34].

Hyaluronic Acid

Hyaluronic acid (HA) is a common component of most connective tissues, as well as a principal component of the synovial fluid. During the degenerative process, HA is secreted by the synovium and cartilage. Serum levels of HA were proposed to be a marker to predict the progression of knee OA [35]. OA patients had increased serum HA (sHA), and patients with higher initial sHA values displayed a more rapid progression of the disease [36, 37]. More recent studies also suggested that sHA can be available as a burden of disease marker for patients with radiographic or severe OA [38, 39]. The major problem associated with HA as an OA biomarker is its specificity and sensitivity, as HA is ubiquitously present in all connective tissues and tends to be affected by physical activities and food intake [40].

Despite the existence of multiple catabolic biomarkers in research, currently, there is no single biomarker validated for clinical use for OA. Given the unique advantages and disadvantages of these biomarkers, combined use of different biomarkers might be of benefit in the future (Table 9.2). Also, majority of the abovementioned biomarkers are systemic, for example, from serum or urine, and their concentrations are subject to systemic conditions or illnesses. Therefore, obtaining local biomarkers from synovial fluid may provide more specificity and sensitivity. Moreover, local biomarkers would ensure the ability to detect OA in a particular joint.

Table 9.2 Catabolic OA biomarkers

Biomarkers	Catabolic process	Tissue of origin	BIPEDS classification
uCTX-II	Type II collagen degradation	Cartilage, bone	BPED
sCOMP	Cartilage matrix degradation	Cartilage, bone, meniscus, synovium, tendon	BPD
sHA	Cartilage degradation	Cartilage, synovium, ubiquitous in all ECM	BPED
s/uColl2-1	Triple helix type II collagen degradation	Cartilage	BPD
s/uColl2-1NO2	Triple helix type II collagen (nitrated) degradation	Cartilage	BPD
s/uC2C	Type II collagen degradation	Cartilage	BED
s/uC1, C2	Collage type I and type II degradation	Cartilage, bone, synovium, meniscus	D

Abbreviations: *B* burden of disease, *P* prognostic, *E* efficacy of intervention, *D* diagnostic, *u* urine, *s* serum

Note: Adapted from Mobasheri and Henrotin [97].

Post-Genomic Osteoarthritis Biomarkers

Following completion of the Human Genome Project, the generation of massive genomic information has rapidly transformed the field of biomedical research into the post-genomic era [41]. Post-genomics, or so-called system biology, studies the expression and functions of the entire set of genes and proteins present in a whole genome by using high-throughput methodologies including microarray, transcriptomics, proteomics, and metabolomics. With thousands of genes and proteins being analyzed simultaneously, these omics-based technology platforms have significantly contributed to the discovery of the new crop of biomarkers over the past decade [42]. The post-genomic strategies have been applied in various fields, including OA.

Transcriptomic Osteoarthritis Biomarkers

Transcriptome refers to all the ribonucleic acids (RNAs) that are transcribed from the genome containing messenger RNAs (mRNAs), ribosomal RNAs (rRNAs), transfer RNAs (tRNAs), and noncoding RNAs. Transcriptomic analysis has been performed through gene microarrays or RNA sequencing (RNA-Seq) to quantify the abundance of all transcripts in a particular biological specimen [43].

Gene microarrays have been widely used in gene expression studies and have proven to be a powerful tool to identify candidate RNA biomarkers for various pathological conditions including OA. Geyer et al. performed a transcriptomic analysis of affected versus intact articular cartilage from the same joint using high-density synthetic oligonucleotide hybridization arrays (HG-U133 Plus 2.0 GeneChips), and 411 transcripts out of 54,675 probes appeared to be differentially expressed. Of these, 6 genes were upregulated in the affected cartilage of all patients, including insulin-like growth factor-binding protein 3 (IGFBP-3), Wnt-1-inducible signaling protein 1 (WISP-1), aquaporin 1 (AQP-1), delta/notch-like EGF-repeat containing transmembrane (DNER), decay-accelerating factor (DAF), and complement factor I [44]. The Research Arthritis and Articular Cartilage (RAAK) study which involved a larger patient cohort was carried out to determine the genome-wide gene expression in 33 pairs of matched OA affected and intact cartilage from the same joint of patients. About 1,717 genes were found to be differentially expressed, and 18 were present with a change of twofold or higher in OA affected cartilage compared with preserved cartilage.

Comparing gene expression at damaged focal areas of cartilage to those preserved areas provides information of dynamic changes of genes and pathways involved in OA progression [45]. However, macroscopic assessment of damaged or preserved cartilage is relatively subjective and less accurate, which may partially explain the low consistency of the differentially expressed genes between studies with similar design using comparable tissues. Xu et al. identified 998 differentially expressed genes between femoral neck fractures and cartilage from hip OA patient using the Illumina Human HT-12 V3 microarrays. These target genes were enriched within 71 canonical pathways and showed excellent correlation with previous studies using similar tissues but revealed discord between hip and knee OA, indicating different mechanisms may be present for knee and hip OA pathophysiology [46].

The RNA-Seq transcriptome platform, as a relatively new technology still at the development stage and due to high costs, has just started to be applied in OA research. In a study, RNA sequence libraries were prepared from normal cartilage of the metacarpophalangeal joints from 4 young (4 years old) and 4 old (>15 years old) horses, and sequencing was undertaken using the Illumina HiSeq platform. Levels of 396 transcripts, including noncoding RNAs, were significantly different in old compared to young cartilage. The majority of cartilage genes relating to ECM, proteases, matrix synthetic enzymes, cytokines, and growth factors, as well as Wnt signaling, were reduced in old cartilage relative to young cartilage. As aging is an important risk factor of OA, altered expressions of transcripts identified in old cartilage could provide valuable information to understand the pathogenesis of OA [47].

Blood samples have also been subject to transcriptomic analysis in OA. A complementary DNA (cDNA) microarray was used to screen for differentially expressed genes in 85 subjects with mild OA and 76 controls. Six genes were significantly downregulated in mild OA: heat shock 90 kDa protein 1, alpha; inhibitor of kappa light polypeptide gene enhancer in B cells, kinase complex-associated protein; interleukin 13 receptor, alpha 1; laminin, gamma 1; platelet factor 4 (also known as chemokine (C-X-C motif) ligand 4); and tumor necrosis factor, alpha-induced protein 6. A nine-gene signature (abovementioned six genes plus early growth response 1; alpha glucosidase II alpha subunit; and v-maf musculoaponeurotic fibrosarcoma oncogene homologue B) was identified as a diagnostic biomarker to discriminate mild OA from controls, with a higher diagnostic capacity than any of the individual nine genes [48]. Another transcriptomic screen of peripheral blood leukocytes from patients with symptomatic knee OA and controls identified 173 abnormally expressed genes. Cluster analysis revealed 2 distinct OA subgroups: those with or without the interleukin 1-beta (IL-1β) signature, defined as ≥2 fold IL-1β overexpression. Patients with IL-1β signature had more pain, decreased function, and higher risk of radiographic progression of OA [49]. This study suggested a novel method to classify OA based on IL-1β expression and moreover that the transcriptomic profile of peripheral blood leukocytes had the potential as a prognostic biomarker for OA patients.

Transcriptome analysis has generated valuable information on the molecular changes across the whole genome, which will improve our understanding of the complexity of OA phenotypes. With the popularization of the powerful RNA-Seq platform, the discovery of multiple panels of new OA biomarkers is warranted.

Proteomics Biomarkers

By studying the presence and functions of an entire set of proteins in a particular biological sample, proteomics is being increasingly applied in cartilage research and OA pathology [50]. It also elucidates information regarding protein structure and interactions, thereby providing mechanistic insight into disease pathogenesis and a new powerful tool for biomarker exploration. In OA research, proteomic studies have been applied to cartilage tissue, chondrocytes, synovial fluid, serum, urine, and culture supernatant, and have identified significant panels of novel candidate biomarkers [51].

Wu et al. measured the protein compositions in cartilage from OA and healthy donors and found 59 differently expressed proteins by liquid chromatography–mass spectrometry. In particular, HtrA1, a serine protease, was upregulated at high levels in OA cartilage [52]. Another study by Guo et al. performed proteomics on cartilage extractions from individuals with and without OA and identified 16 differentially expressed proteins which belonged to the following five function groups including glycolysis and energy production (ADH, ADK, ENOA, KPYM, and FR), signaling (ANNX-I, PEBP, and TUB), redox (PRDX3 and SODM), and cartilage matrix (COLL-I and COLL-VI) [53]. Proteomic profiling of chondrocytes also revealed that 19 proteins were increased and 9 decreased significantly in OA cells compared to normal. Among these, three stress response proteins (HSP90beta, GRP78, and GRP94) were upregulated and three glycolysis-related proteins (enolase, glyceraldehyde 3-phosphate dehydrogenase, and fructose biphosphate aldolase) were downregulated [54]. This study indicated an impaired glycolytic metabolism and an increased stress response in OA chondrocytes, both of which have been reported previously to be implicated in cartilage degradation [55, 56].

With the goal of searching for new OA biomarkers, intensive proteomic profiling studies have focused on bodily fluids from OA and non-OA individuals. Fernandez-Puente et al. measured protein levels in serum from 50 moderate OA patients, 50 severe OA patients, and 50 non-symptomatic controls using isobaric tags for relative and absolute quantitation (iTRAQ) and matrix-assisted laser desorption/ionization (MALDI)-TOF/TOF mass spectrometry. They identified 349 total proteins in serum, and of these, 6 were modulated only in moderate OA, 13 only in severe OA, and 7 in both groups. In addition to COMP, most of these differentially expressed proteins were novel candidate biomarkers for OA including a few complement components, lipoproteins, von Willebrand factor, tetranectin, and lumican [57]. Han et al. analyzed synovial fluid samples from 36 OA patients and 24 rheumatoid arthritis (RA) patients. Three protein peaks were identified and able to differentiate between OA and RA patients at a sensitivity of 89.4 % and a specificity of 91.2 % by artificial neural networks analysis. One peak was identified as S100A12 which was also reported to be upregulated in human OA elsewhere [58]. Ritter et al. performed a proteomic analysis of knee synovial fluid from 20 OA patients and 10 controls. Sixty-six proteins were differentially present in both OA and control synovial fluid. Analysis showed that these proteins were associated with the acute-phase response pathway, the complement pathway, and the coagulation pathway [59]. The complement pathway has been identified in numerous studies to play a critical role in the pathogenesis of OA and a potential biomarker [60].

While a considerable amount of candidate protein markers have been identified from proteomic studies, the studies are not sufficiently consistent. For example, there was less than 25 % reliability of the synovial fluid protein list between Ritter et al. and Kamphorst et al. studies [59, 61]. However, proteomics has emerged as a powerful approach to identify proteins in pathological conditions and to discover new potential biomarkers.

Metabolomic Biomarkers

Metabolomics, defined as large-scale profiling of small molecular metabolites present in a cell, tissue, body fluids, or any biological system, has opened new avenues for biomarker identification [62]. Metabolites include various low-molecular end products of diverse cellular processes, such as lipids, amino acids, peptides, vitamins, organic acids, carbohydrates, and nuclear acids. The levels of metabolites are considered to be the ultimate response of biological systems to genetic, environmental, and lifestyle factors under normal or diseased states. Current commonly used methods for studying metabolomics are nuclear magnetic resonance and mass spectrometry, along with gas chromatography, liquid chromatography, or capillary electrophoresis for sample separations.

Zhai and coworkers utilized targeted metabolite profiling to investigate the association of metabolite ratios in serum with the development of knee OA. They found 14 ratios that were significantly associated with knee OA at discovery stage in their cohort. By replicating this study in the Chingford cohort, two of these 14 ratios (valine/histidine and xleucine/histidine) were successfully confirmed to correlate with radiographic severity of OA. Mechanically, as these branched-chain amino acids (BCAAs) including valine and xleucine could not be synthesized by the body, an increase in BCAAs metabolites implied the breakdown of collagen [63]. This was the first study using serum-based metabolomics and demonstrated that the BCAAs to histidine ratio have potential clinical use as an OA biomarker.

Jiang et al. reported a mass spectrometry-based metabolic study to identify the global metabolic defects in the serum of four major types of arthritis including RA ($n=27$), OA ($n=27$), ankylosing spondylitis ($n=27$), and gout ($n=33$) compared with healthy control subjects ($n=60$). They identified a global metabolic profile in all arthritic patients, suggesting these four types of arthritis share common metabolic defects possibly resulting from joint inflammation. Meanwhile, a unique metabolic signature, potential biomarker for diagnosis, was discovered for each type of arthritis. This report demonstrated the applicability of metabolomic profiling as a novel diagnostic tool for arthritis including OA, along with current clinical detection methods [64]. Another group conducted a global metabolite profiling of conditioned medium of synovial tissue cultures from patients with severe OA or non-OA patients undergoing ligament or meniscal repair. They identified 13 compounds significantly elevated in the end stage OA group [65]. Given the difficulty in translating synovium culture method into clinical practice, they also performed metabolomics on ankle synovial fluid of patients with and without ankle OA. One hundred and six metabolites were significantly elevated in the OA sample, representing abnormalities in almost all pathways involving metabolism including amino acid, carbohydrate, mitochondrial oxidation, lipid, peptide, vitamin, nucleotide synthesis, and redox homeostasis [66].

Taken together, these studies have linked abnormal metabolic changes to the pathogenesis of OA, and metabolomics have proven to be a new robust tool for biomarker discovery in OA. This is in accordance with the emerging new subtype of OA, metabolic syndrome OA, which has recently been recognized because of the increased incidence of OA in patients with metabolic syndrome such as dyslipidemia, hypertension, obesity, and type 2 diabetes. Therefore, biomarkers identified by metabolomics will also help discriminate between different OA subtypes.

MicroRNAs Biomarkers in Osteoarthritis

MicroRNA and Its Biogenesis

MicroRNAs (miRNAs) belong to the family of small noncoding RNAs, about 19–23 nucleotides long when eventually processed as functioning mature miRNA. Though not coding for proteins, miRNAs play important roles in regulating gene expression at the posttranscriptional level through complementary base-pairing within 3' untranslated region (3'UTR) of target mRNA [67]. According to miRNA databases, the targeting strategy between miRNAs and mRNAs is not simply a one to one relationship, rather, one mRNA can be synergistically targeted by multiple miRNAs or a single miRNA can target multiple genes [68, 69]. There are more than 2,000 annotated miRNAs from the human genome and the number is still increasing. It is estimated that human miRNAs regulate as much as 60 % of genes and play pivotal roles in various physiological processes such as cell proliferation, differentiation, genomic stability, metabolism, apoptosis, and aging. Not surprisingly, deregulation of miRNA has been associated with many pathological conditions including OA [70].

There are three forms of miRNAs which are long primary miRNAs (pri-miRNA), hairpin precursor miRNAs (pre-miRNA), and short mature miRNAs. In the nucleus, the miRNA gene is transcribed into large pri-miRNA which is subsequently cleaved by Drosha, an RNase III enzyme, to make pre-miRNA. Pre-miRNA is a 70–125 nucleotide long hairpin structure with 2 nucleotides overhanging at the 3' end. It is then exported by RanGTP and exportin5 proteins into the cytoplasm where it is processed by a second RNase III enzyme Dicer, to form the short mature miRNA. At this point, it is incorporated into an RNA-induced silencing complex to induce target mRNA degradation and protein translation depression [71].

MicroRNA Biomarkers in Joint Tissues

The critical role of miRNA regulation during skeletal development has been highlighted by a study with Dicer-null mice where chondrocytes from these mice displayed reduced proliferation and accelerated differentiation into cell hypertrophy [72].

MiR-140 is the most studied miRNA involved in OA. It was first reported as cartilage-specific miRNA in mouse and directly targeted HDAC4 [73]. Microarray profiling by Miyaki et al. discovered that miR-140 was upregulated during chondrogenesis but downregulated in OA chondrocytes compared to normal [74].

A further study demonstrated that IL-1β treatment of normal chondrocytes suppressed miR-140 expression, while overexpression of miR-140 downregulated IL-1β-induced ADAMTS5 expression and rescued the IL-1β-dependent repression of AGGRECAN gene expression. An additional study in vivo in mice by the same group showed that MiR-140-null mice developed age-related OA-like phenotypes, including proteoglycan loss and articular cartilage fibrillation. The crucial role of miR-140 in OA cartilage protection was further demonstrated by resistance to antigen-induced arthritis through miR-140 overexpression [75]. Meanwhile, another group identified matrix metalloproteinases-13 (MMP-13) and insulin-like growth factor-binding protein 5 as two more targets for miR-140 [76]. NFAT3 and SMAD3 seemed to activate and repress miR-140 expression respectively, providing novel strategies for treating OA [77].

Similar as miR-140, miR-27b has been shown to be downregulated in IL-1β-stimulated OA chondrocytes. MiR-27b directly targeted MMP-13, indicating that decreased miR-27b might be responsible for the overexpression of MMP-13 in response to IL-1β [78].

Yamasaki et al. reported expression of miR-146a in early-stage OA cartilage compared to normal. Interestingly, miR-146a levels were decreased in later stage OA when Mankin scores were increased [79]. MiR-146a is inducible by IL-1β stimulation in normal human chondrocytes, by lipopolysaccharide in THP-1 cells and by mechanical pressure injury [79–82]. MiRNA-146a has also been linked to pain by modulating inflammatory cytokines such as tumor necrosis factor-alpha (TNF-α), COX-2, iNOS, IL-6, IL-8, RANTS, and ion channel TRPV1. Therefore, miRNA-146a may serve as target for therapeutic intervention to alleviate OA-related pain [83, 84].

Using human miRNA qPCR array, a few studies have examined the expression of hundreds of miRNAs in chondrocytes, cartilage, or bone tissue. Iliopoulos et al. measured the expression of 352 miRNAs in OA versus normal cartilage. They found that 16 miRNAs were deregulated in OA cartilage and were able to distinguish OA chondrocytes from normal chondrocytes. Among these, nine miRNAs were upregulated and seven downregulated. Interestingly, levels of five miRNA (miR-22, miR-103, miR-25, miR-337, and miR-29a) statistically correlated with body mass index (BMI), suggesting the potential role of these miRNA in lipid metabolism and OA pathology [85]. In another study, Jones and associates identified that some miRNAs were differentially expressed in late-stage human OA, 17 in cartilage, and 30 in bone. Further functional analysis revealed that miR-9, miR-98, and miR-146 might play a role in inflammatory regulation mediating IL-1β-induced TNF-α production and MMP-13 secretion [81]. Another study conducted a profiling of 723 miRNAs in cultured chondrocytes and discovered 1 upregulated (has-miR-483-5p) and 6 downregulated (hsa-miR-149, hsa-miR-582-3p, hsa-miR-1227, hsa-miR-634, hsa-miR-576-5p, hsa-miR-641) miRNAs in OA chondrocytes versus controls [86].

Given the essential regulatory roles of miRNAs in mRNA stability and protein translation, identification of differentially expressed miRNAs in OA joint tissue will deepen our understanding of the mechanism underlying cartilage degradation and OA pathology. Moreover, aberrantly expressed miRNAs involved in the pathogenesis of OA could serve as potential therapeutic targets to treat OA, as well as diagnostic biomarkers.

Promising Circulating MicroRNA Biomarkers

Majority of miRNAs exist and function intracellularly; however, non-tissue and cell-free circulating miRNAs are also present in extracellular compartments in all tested body fluids such as serum, plasma, synovial fluid, urine, cerebrospinal fluid, and saliva [87]. Unlike mRNA and other nuclear acids, miRNAs in human plasma and serum are highly stable and protected from ribonuclease digestion [88]. In addition to its stability, other distinct advantages associated with using miRNAs as biomarkers include high sensitivity, easy accessibility, and detection. Therefore, attention has been drawn to the development of circulating miRNAs as clinical biomarkers in OA [89–90].

In 2010, Murata et al. first investigated the presence of miR-16, miR-132, miR-146a, miR-155, and miR-223 in plasma and synovial fluid, as well as their high stability under multiple freezing–thawing cycles [91]. They found that both synovial fluid and serum miRNAs were quite stable for storage at −20 °C and were still stable after as many as eight freeze–thawing cycles from −20 to 4 °C. The concentrations of the five miRNAs in synovial fluid were found to be much lower than those in plasma in both OA and RA patients. In addition, there was no correlation between plasma and synovial fluid miRNAs. Finally, the authors reported that the levels of miR-132 in plasma of both OA and RA were significantly reduced compared to normal [64].

Subsequently, a 3 miRNAs signature consisting of miR-454, miR-885-5p, and let-7e was identified in serum which could predict the risk of developing severe knee or hip OA [92]. This study followed 816 individuals over a 15-year period and assessed the occurrence of severe knee or hip OA using total knee or hip arthroplasty, with at least one joint as a definitive outcome. At follow-up, 67 individuals had developed severe knee or hip OA. In the initial screening, Taqman qPCR array analyses of 377 miRNAs were performed in 13 individuals with severe OA versus 13 controls matched for sex, menopausal status, age, and BMI. Screening results revealed that 12 miRNAs were differentially expressed, which were subsequently validated in the entire cohort by Taqman qPCR. Validation showed that miR-454, miR-885-5p, and let-7e were strongly associated with the development of severe OA. Let-7e appeared to be the most promising biomarker to predict severe OA. Another study identified 12 differentially expressed miRNAs in the plasma of 54 patients with primary OA at early and intermediate stages (stages 2 and 3, respectively), indicating the value of these miRNAs as disease progression markers. Analysis showed that these miRNAs could regulate mRNAs that are crucial in chondrocyte maintenance and differentiation, including SMAD1, IL-1β, COL3A, VEGFA, and FGFR1 [93].

The origin and functions of circulating miRNAs remain largely unknown. It is widely believed that these miRNAs might be released directly from blood cells into

Table 9.3 Potential OA miRNA biomarkers in body fluids. Shown are potential miRNAs biomarkers identified in body fluids from OA patients compared to controls with statistical significance ($p<0.05$)

Types of fluid	Differentially expressed miRNAs ($p \leq 0.05$)/FC	Research population	References
Plasma and synovial fluid	miR-132 down/NA	30 OA, 30 normal	Murata et al. [91]
Serum	Let- 7e down/0.75 miR-454 down/0.77	67 severe OA, 749 non-OA	Beyer et al. [92]
Plasma	miR-93 up/3.18 miR-126 up/3.96 miR-146a up/2.96 miR-184 up/2.47 miR-186 up/4.44 miR-195 up/3.53 miR-345 up/3.51 miR-885-5p up/3.51	27 OA, 27 normal	Borgonio Cuadra et al. [93]

Abbreviations: *FC* fold changes compared to controls, *down* downregulated, *up* upregulated

the bloodstream or from circulating cells from damaged tissue at disease states [94]. Murata et al. also reported that the expression patterns of four miRNAs (miR-16, miR-132, miR-146a, and miR-223) in synovial fluid are similar to those in synovial tissue from OA patients, suggesting that synovial tissue might release miRNAs directly into the surrounding extracellular environment through an unknown mechanism [91]. Currently, it is not clear if the secretion of miRNA from synovial tissue is certain miRNA selective or is merely a universal mechanism for all miRNAs. Further studies are also required to clarify the correlation of circulating miRNAs in synovial fluid to OA disease activity as well as to explore the feasibility of use circulating miRNAs as biomarkers in clinical practice (Table 9.3).

Conclusions

Despite much active research into various OA biomarkers, there is no single biomarker that is sufficiently well validated and recognized to diagnose OA or aid the progression of individuals with or without OA [95]. In a systematic review applying the BIPED classification, van Spil and associates indicated that uCTX-II and serum COMP seemed to have the best performance and promise of all commercially available OA biomarkers [6]. However, the authors commented on the current limitations of OA biomarker studies including an overall lack of consistent evidence, differences between the clinical trial populations versus population-based cohort studies, and differences in sample collection and possible publication bias [6]. Presently, no OA biomarker is consistent to function as an OA outcome measure in clinical trials as a secondary or supportive endpoint [96]. As a result, the European Society for Clinical and Economic Aspects of Osteoporosis and Osteoarthritis (ESCEO) convened a meeting in October of 2012 to discuss the direction of future research in OA biomarkers. The ESCEO group outlined 3 areas of future research including mechanisms of disease and development of new biomarkers, assays and technological development, and prognosis and risk. Briefly, ESCEO discussed research into the underlying mechanism of disease to validate existing biomarkers and identify new candidates, improve assays and standardize protocols that can accurately and reproducibly measure OA biomarkers in serum or urine, and identify biomarkers for early stages of OA so treatments can be started to slow down the progression of OA [95]. Furthermore, future research advancements and refinements in genetic, proteomic, and metabolomics approaches, as well as identification and validation of panels of biomarkers that may be correlated with imaging modalities, may provide improved diagnosis, prediction, and understanding of the pathogenesis of OA [97]. Today, there remains a need for more active research in the area of OA biomarkers.

References

1. Bijlsma JW, Berenbaum F, Lafeber FP. Osteoarthritis: an update with relevance for clinical practice. Lancet. 2011;377:2115–26.
2. Altman R, Asch E, Bloch D, Bole G, Borenstein D, Brandt K, et al. Development of criteria for the classification and reporting of knee osteoarthritis. Arthritis Rheum. 1986;29(8):1039–49.
3. Bauer DC, Hunter DJ, Abramson SB, et al. Classification of osteoarthritis biomarkers: a proposed approach. Osteoarthritis Cartilage. 2006;14:723–7.
4. Atkinson AJ, Colburn WA, DeGruttola VG, Biomarkers Definitions Working Group, et al. Biomarkers and surrogate endpoints: preferred definitions and conceptual framework. Clin Pharmacol Ther. 2001;69:89–95.
5. De Gruttola VG, Clax P, DeMets DL, Downing GJ, Ellenberg SS, Friedman L, et al. Considerations in the evaluation of surrogate endpoints in clinical trials. Summary of a National Institutes of Health workshop. Control Clin Trials. 2001;22(5):485–502.
6. van Spil WE, Degroot J, Lems WF, et al. Serum and urinary biochemical markers for knee and hip-osteoarthritis: a systematic review applying the consensus BIPED criteria. Osteoarthritis Cartilage. 2010;18:605–12.
7. Kraus VB, Nevitt M, Sandell LJ. Summary of the OA biomarkers workshop 2009–biochemical biomarkers: biology, validation, and clinical studies. Osteoarthritis Cartilage. 2010;18(6):742–5.
8. Kraus VB, Burnett B, Coindreau J, Cottrell S, Eyre D, Gendreau M, et al. Application of biomarkers in the development of drugs intended for the treatment of osteoarthritis. OARSI FDA Osteoarthritis Biomarkers Working Group. Osteoarthritis Cartilage. 2011;19(5):515–42.
9. Perruccio AV, Mahomed NN, Chandran V, Gandhi R. Plasma adipokine levels and their association with overall burden of painful joints among individuals with hip and knee osteoarthritis. J Rheumatol. 2014;41(2):334–7.
10. Laurberg TB, Frystyk J, Ellingsen T, Hansen IT, Jorgensen A, Tarp U, et al. Plasma adiponectin in patients with active, early, and chronic rheumatoid arthritis who are steroid- and disease-modifying antirheumatic drug-naive compared with patients with osteoarthritis and controls. J Rheumatol. 2009;36:1885–91.
11. Staikos C, Ververidis A, Drosos G, Manolopoulos VG, Verettas DA, Tavridou A. The association of adipokine levels in plasma and synovial fluid with the severity of knee osteoarthritis. Rheumatology. 2013;52:1077–83.

12. Ding C, Parameswaran V, Cicuttini F, Burgess J, Zhai G, Quinn S, et al. Association between leptin, body composition, sex and knee cartilage morphology in older adults: the Tasmanian older adult cohort (TASOAC) study. Ann Rheum Dis. 2008;67:1256–61.
13. Stannus OP, Jones G, Quinn SJ, Cicuttini FM, Dore D, Ding C. The association between leptin, interleukin-6, and hip radiographic osteoarthritis in older people: a cross-sectional study. Arthritis Res Ther. 2010;12:R95.
14. Pearle AD, Scanzello CR, George S, Mandl LA, DiCarlo EF, Peterson M, et al. Elevated high-sensitivity C-reactive protein levels are associated with local inflammatory findings in patients with osteoarthritis. Osteoarthritis Cartilage. 2007;15:516–23.
15. Spector TD, Hart DJ, Nandra D, et al. Low-level increases in serum C-reactive protein are present in early osteoarthritis of the knee and predict progressive disease. Arthritis Rheum. 1997;40:723–7.
16. Sharif M, Shepstone L, Elson CJ, et al. Increased serum C reactive protein may reflect events that precede radiographic progression in osteoarthritis of the knee. Ann Rheum Dis. 2000;59:71–4.
17. Smith JW, Martins TB, Gopez E, et al. Significance of C-reactive protein in osteoarthritis and total knee arthroplasty outcomes. Ther Adv Musculoskelet Dis. 2012;4:315–25.
18. Stannus O, Jones G, Cicuttini F, et al. Circulating levels of IL-6 and TNF-alpha are associated with knee radiographic osteoarthritis and knee cartilage loss in older adults. Osteoarthritis Cartilage. 2010;18:1441–7.
19. Livshits G, Zhai G, Hart DJ, Kato BS, Wang H, Williams FMK, et al. Interleukin-6 is a significant predictor of radiographic knee osteoarthritis: the Chingford Study. Arthritis Rheum. 2009;60:2037–45.
20. Pelletier JP, Raynauld JP, Caron J, Mineau F, Abram F, Dorais M, et al. Decrease in serum level of matrix metalloproteinases is predictive of the disease-modifying effect of osteoarthritis drugs assessed by quantitative MRI in patients with knee osteoarthritis. Ann Rheum Dis. 2010;69(12):2095–101.
21. Ayral X, Pickering EH, Woodworth TG, et al. Synovitis: a potential predictive factor of structural progression of medial tibiofemoral knee osteoarthritis – results of a 1 year longitudinal arthroscopic study in 422 patients. Osteoarthritis Cartilage. 2005;13:361–7.
22. Goldring SR, Goldring MB. Clinical aspects, pathology and pathophysiology of osteoarthritis. J Musculoskelet Neuronal Interact. 2006;6(4):376–8.
23. Garvican ER, et al. Biomarkers of cartilage turnover. Part 1: Markers of collagen degradation and synthesis. Vet J. 2010;185(1):36–42.
24. Jayabalan P, Sowa GA. The development of biomarkers for degenerative musculoskeletal conditions. Discov Med. 2014;17(92):59–66.
25. Christgau S, et al. Collagen type II C-telopeptide fragments as an index of cartilage degradation. Bone. 2001;29(3):209–15.
26. Reijman M, et al. A new marker for osteoarthritis: cross-sectional and longitudinal approach. Arthritis Rheum. 2004;50(8):2471–8.
27. Gineyts E, et al. Effects of ibuprofen on molecular markers of cartilage and synovium turnover in patients with knee osteoarthritis. Ann Rheum Dis. 2004;63(7):857–61.
28. Ameye LG, et al. The chemical biomarkers C2C, Coll2-1, and Coll2-1NO2 provide complementary information on type II collagen catabolism in healthy and osteoarthritic mice. Arthritis Rheum. 2007;56(10):3336–46.
29. Henrotin Y, et al. Collagen catabolism through Coll2-1 and Coll2-`O and myeloperoxidase activity in marathon runners. Springerplus. 2013;2(1):92.
30. Deberg M, et al. New serum biochemical markers (Coll 2–1 and Coll 2–1 NO2) for studying oxidative-related type II collagen network degradation in patients with osteoarthritis and rheumatoid arthritis. Osteoarthritis Cartilage. 2005;13(3):258–65.
31. Tseng S, Reddi AH, Di Cesare PE. Cartilage oligomeric matrix protein (COMP): a biomarker of arthritis. Biomark Insights. 2009;4:33–44.
32. Clark AG, et al. Serum cartilage oligomeric matrix protein reflects osteoarthritis presence and severity: the Johnston County Osteoarthritis Project. Arthritis Rheum. 1999;42(11):2356–64.

33. Sharif M, et al. Suggestion of nonlinear or phasic progression of knee osteoarthritis based on measurements of serum cartilage oligomeric matrix protein levels over five years. Arthritis Rheum. 2004;50(8):2479–88.
34. Ahrman E, et al. Novel cartilage oligomeric matrix protein (COMP) neoepitopes identified in synovial fluids from patients with joint diseases using affinity chromatography and mass spectrometry. J Biol Chem. 2014;289(30):20908–16.
35. Sharif M, et al. Serum hyaluronic acid level as a predictor of disease progression in osteoarthritis of the knee. Arthritis Rheum. 1995;38(6):760–7.
36. Bierma-Zeinstra SM, Koes BW. Risk factors and prognostic factors of hip and knee osteoarthritis. Nat Clin Pract Rheumatol. 2007;3(2):78–85.
37. Pavelka K, et al. Hyaluronic acid levels may have predictive value for the progression of knee osteoarthritis. Osteoarthritis Cartilage. 2004;12(4):277–83.
38. Kaneko H, et al. Reference intervals of serum hyaluronic acid corresponding to the radiographic severity of knee osteoarthritis in women. BMC Musculoskelet Disord. 2013;14:34.
39. Elliott AL, et al. Serum hyaluronan levels and radiographic knee and hip osteoarthritis in African Americans and Caucasians in the Johnston County Osteoarthritis Project. Arthritis Rheum. 2005;52(1):105–11.
40. Chua Jr SD, et al. Effect of an exercise and dietary intervention on serum biomarkers in overweight and obese adults with osteoarthritis of the knee. Osteoarthritis Cartilage. 2008;16(9):1047–53.
41. Peltonen L, McKusick VA. Genomics and medicine. Dissecting human disease in the postgenomic era. Science. 2001;291(5507):1224–9.
42. Gharbi M, Deberg M, Henrotin Y. Application for proteomic techniques in studying osteoarthritis: a review. Front Physiol. 2011;2:90.
43. Pedrotty DM, Morley MP, Cappola TP. Transcriptomic biomarkers of cardiovascular disease. Prog Cardiovasc Dis. 2012;55(1):64–9.
44. Geyer M, et al. Differential transcriptome analysis of intraarticular lesional vs intact cartilage reveals new candidate genes in osteoarthritis pathophysiology. Osteoarthritis Cartilage. 2009;17(3):328–35.
45. Ramos YF, et al. Genes involved in the osteoarthritis process identified through genome wide expression analysis in articular cartilage; the RAAK study. PLoS One. 2014;9(7):e103056.
46. Xu Y, et al. Identification of the pathogenic pathways in osteoarthritic hip cartilage: commonality and discord between hip and knee OA. Osteoarthritis Cartilage. 2012;20(9):1029–38.
47. Peffers M, Liu X, Clegg P. Transcriptomic signatures in cartilage ageing. Arthritis Res Ther. 2013;15(4):R98.
48. Marshall KW, et al. Blood-based biomarkers for detecting mild osteoarthritis in the human knee. Osteoarthritis Cartilage. 2005;13(10):861–71.
49. Attur M, et al. Increased interleukin-1beta gene expression in peripheral blood leukocytes is associated with increased pain and predicts risk for progression of symptomatic knee osteoarthritis. Arthritis Rheum. 2011;63(7):1908–17.
50. Williams A, et al. Applications of proteomics in cartilage biology and osteoarthritis research. Front Biosci (Landmark Ed). 2011;16:2622–44.
51. Hsueh MF, Onnerfjord P, Kraus VB. Biomarkers and proteomic analysis of osteoarthritis. Matrix Biol. 2014;39C:56–66.
52. Wu J, et al. Comparative proteomic characterization of articular cartilage tissue from normal donors and patients with osteoarthritis. Arthritis Rheum. 2007;56(11):3675–84.
53. Guo D, et al. Proteomic analysis of human articular cartilage: identification of differentially expressed proteins in knee osteoarthritis. Joint Bone Spine. 2008;75(4):439–44.
54. Ruiz-Romero C, et al. Proteomic analysis of human osteoarthritic chondrocytes reveals protein changes in stress and glycolysis. Proteomics. 2008;8(3):495–507.
55. Kubo T, et al. Stress-induced proteins in chondrocytes from patients with osteoarthritis. Arthritis Rheum. 1985;28(10):1140–5.

56. Tillmann K. Pathological aspects of osteoarthritis related to surgery. Inflammation. 1984;8(Suppl):S57–74.
57. Fernandez-Puente P, et al. Identification of a panel of novel serum osteoarthritis biomarkers. J Proteome Res. 2011;10(11):5095–101.
58. Han MY, et al. Identification of osteoarthritis biomarkers by proteomic analysis of synovial fluid. J Int Med Res. 2012;40(6):2243–50.
59. Ritter SY, et al. Proteomic analysis of synovial fluid from the osteoarthritic knee: comparison with transcriptome analyses of joint tissues. Arthritis Rheum. 2013;65(4):981–92.
60. Wang Q, et al. Identification of a central role for complement in osteoarthritis. Nat Med. 2011;17(12):1674–9.
61. Kamphorst JJ, et al. Profiling of endogenous peptides in human synovial fluid by NanoLC-MS: method validation and peptide identification. J Proteome Res. 2007;6(11):4388–96.
62. Blanco FJ, Ruiz-Romero C. Osteoarthritis: metabolomic characterization of metabolic phenotypes in OA. Nat Rev Rheumatol. 2012;8(3):130–2.
63. Zhai G, et al. Serum branched-chain amino acid to histidine ratio: a novel metabolomic biomarker of knee osteoarthritis. Ann Rheum Dis. 2010;69(6):1227–31.
64. Jiang M, et al. Serum metabolic signatures of four types of human arthritis. J Proteome Res. 2013;12(8):3769–79.
65. Adams Jr SB, et al. Global metabolic profiling of human osteoarthritic synovium. Osteoarthritis Cartilage. 2012;20(1):64–7.
66. Adams Jr SB, Setton LA, Nettles DL. The role of metabolomics in osteoarthritis research. J Am Acad Orthop Surg. 2013;21(1):63–4.
67. Bartel DP. MicroRNAs: genomics, biogenesis, mechanism, and function. Cell. 2004;116(2):281–97.
68. Li Y, et al. Mirsynergy: detecting synergistic miRNA regulatory modules by overlapping neighbourhood expansion. Bioinformatics. 2014;30(18):2627–35.
69. Kozomara A, Griffiths-Jones S. MiRBase: annotating high confidence microRNAs using deep sequencing data. Nucleic Acids Res. 2014;42(Database issue):D68–73.
70. Wu C, et al. MicroRNAs play a role in chondrogenesis and osteoarthritis. Int J Mol Med. 2014;34(1):13–23.
71. Nair VS, et al. Design and analysis for studying microRNAs in human disease: a primer on -Omic Technologies. Am J Epidemiol. 2014;180(2):140–52.
72. Kobayashi T, et al. Dicer-dependent pathways regulate chondrocyte proliferation and differentiation. Proc Natl Acad Sci U S A. 2008;105(6):1949–54.
73. Tuddenham L, et al. The cartilage specific microRNA-140 targets histone deacetylase 4 in mouse cells. FEBS Lett. 2006;580(17):4214–7.
74. Miyaki S, et al. MicroRNA-140 is expressed in differentiated human articular chondrocytes and modulates interleukin-1 responses. Arthritis Rheum. 2009;60(9):2723–30.
75. Miyaki S, et al. MicroRNA-140 plays dual roles in both cartilage development and homeostasis. Genes Dev. 2010;24(11):1173–85.
76. Tardif G, et al. Regulation of the IGFBP-5 and MMP-13 genes by the microRNAs miR-140 and miR-27a in human osteoarthritic chondrocytes. BMC Musculoskelet Disord. 2009;10:148.
77. Tardif G, et al. NFAT3 and TGF-beta/SMAD3 regulate the expression of miR-140 in osteoarthritis. Arthritis Res Ther. 2013;15(6):R197.
78. Akhtar N, et al. MicroRNA-27b regulates the expression of matrix metalloproteinase 13 in human osteoarthritis chondrocytes. Arthritis Rheum. 2010;62(5):1361–71.
79. Yamasaki K, et al. Expression of MicroRNA-146a in osteoarthritis cartilage. Arthritis Rheum. 2009;60(4):1035–41.
80. Nakasa T, et al. Expression of microRNA-146 in rheumatoid arthritis synovial tissue. Arthritis Rheum. 2008;58(5):1284–92.
81. Jones SW, et al. The identification of differentially expressed microRNA in osteoarthritic tissue that modulate the production of TNF-alpha and MMP13. Osteoarthritis Cartilage. 2009;17(4):464–72.

82. Jin L, et al. Role of miR-146a in human chondrocyte apoptosis in response to mechanical pressure injury in vitro. Int J Mol Med. 2014;34(2):451–63.
83. Li X, et al. MicroRNA-146a is linked to pain-related pathophysiology of osteoarthritis. Gene. 2011;480(1–2):34–41.
84. Li X, et al. Altered spinal microRNA-146a and the microRNA-183 cluster contribute to osteoarthritic pain in knee joints. J Bone Miner Res. 2013;28(12):2512–22.
85. Iliopoulos D, et al. Integrative microRNA and proteomic approaches identify novel osteoarthritis genes and their collaborative metabolic and inflammatory networks. PLoS One. 2008;3(11):e3740.
86. Diaz-Prado S, et al. Characterization of microRNA expression profiles in normal and osteoarthritic human chondrocytes. BMC Musculoskelet Disord. 2012;13:144.
87. Weber JA, et al. The microRNA spectrum in 12 body fluids. Clin Chem. 2010;56(11):1733–41.
88. Mitchell PS, et al. Circulating microRNAs as stable blood-based markers for cancer detection. Proc Natl Acad Sci U S A. 2008;105(30):10513–8.
89. Kumar P, et al. Circulating miRNA biomarkers for Alzheimer's disease. PLoS One. 2013;8(7):e69807.
90. Ward J, et al. Circulating microRNA profiles in human patients with acetaminophen hepatotoxicity or ischemic hepatitis. Proc Natl Acad Sci U S A. 2014;111(33):12169–74.
91. Murata K, et al. Plasma and synovial fluid microRNAs as potential biomarkers of rheumatoid arthritis and osteoarthritis. Arthritis Res Ther. 2010;12(3):R86.
92. Beyer C, et al. Signature of circulating microRNAs in osteoarthritis. Ann Rheum Dis. 2015;74(3):e18.
93. Borgonio Cuadra VM, et al. Altered expression of circulating microRNA in plasma of patients with primary osteoarthritis and in silico analysis of their pathways. PLoS One. 2014;9(6):e97690.
94. Redova M, Sana J, Slaby O. Circulating miRNAs as new blood-based biomarkers for solid cancers. Future Oncol. 2013;9(3):387–402.
95. Lotz M, Martel-Pelletier J, Christiansen C, Brandi ML, Bruyère O, Chapurlat R, Collette J, Cooper C, Giacovelli G, Kanis JA, Karsdal MA, Kraus V, Lems WF, Meulenbelt I, Pelletier JP, Raynauld JP, Reiter-Niesert S, Rizzoli R, Sandell LJ, Van Spil WE, Reginster JY. Republished: Value of biomarkers in osteoarthritis: current status and perspectives. Postgrad Med J. 2014;90(1061):171–8.
96. Kraus VB. Biomarkers in osteoarthritis. Curr Opin Rheumatol. 2005;17(5):641–6.
97. Mobasheri A, Henrotin Y. Biomarkers of osteoarthritis: a review of recent research progress on soluble biochemical markers, published patents and areas for future development. Recent Pat Biomarkers. 2011;1:25–43.

Chapter 10
Drug/Agent Treatments for Osteoarthritis: Present and Future

Camille Roubille, Jean-Pierre Pelletier, and Johanne Martel-Pelletier

Key Points

- Osteoarthritis (OA) management is currently based on a wide spectrum of therapeutic options to relieve pain, but other OA drugs with disease-modifying properties (DMOADs) are being developed.
- There are presently agents that are symptomatic slow-acting drugs for OA (SYSADOA), which not only reduce joint pain but could also slow the structural disease progression in the joint.
- Targeting cartilage changes (catabolism and anabolism), subchondral bone remodeling, and synovial inflammation are the three main thrusts of research in DMOAD development. Promising emerging therapies include platelet-rich plasma (PRP), bone remodeling modulators, and inflammatory inhibitors.
- OA should be considered a dynamic process and may be a systemic disease with several tissues and pathways to target for DMOAD development.
- With the advent of DMOADs, physicians should aim at treating the "patient" rather than the "disease." Combining therapeutics at both local and systemic levels to impact both symptoms and joint structural changes will likely be the future strategy instead of a sole drug, at least at the beginning of the treatment.
- Selectively targeting some phenotypes of OA patients evidenced by sensitive tools, such as magnetic resonance imaging (MRI), may allow the development of DMOADs based on personalized medicine.

C. Roubille, MD • J.-P. Pelletier, MD • J. Martel-Pelletier, PhD (✉)
Osteoarthritis Research Unit, University of Montreal Hospital Research Centre (CRCHUM), Montreal, QC, Canada
e-mail: jm@martelpelletier.ca

M. Kapoor, N.N. Mahomed (eds.), *Osteoarthritis: Pathogenesis, Diagnosis, Available Treatments, Drug Safety, Regenerative and Precision Medicine*,
DOI 10.1007/978-3-319-19560-5_10

Introduction

OA is the most common form of arthritis resulting in pain and reduced quality of life. While a structure-modifying treatment remains the highest unmet need in OA, several symptomatic treatments are already available on the market. A multimodal approach combining non-pharmacological and pharmacological treatment is at present the best option for OA management, yet the current options only relieve pain. While the overall goal in OA management is to slow the natural progression of structural damage, a global approach should be considered as OA is a dynamic process involving the main tissues of the joint. In brief, OA is a whole joint disease characterized by degradation and loss of articular cartilage, hypertrophic bone changes with osteophyte formation, subchondral bone remodeling, and inflammation of the synovial membrane. Advances in the understanding of the pathological process have contributed to underlining the interconnection between the three joint tissues as well as to defining certain phenotypes. Finding novel therapeutics that will modify the structural changes occurring in the joint tissues during the disease process is one of the most exciting challenges in the field of rheumatology, but the development of new OA treatment requires innovative and global approaches. Such new strategies would be cost-effective by reducing the need for pharmacological interventions and surgical management, while targeting specific pathways leading to OA.

Currently, symptomatic therapies include mostly analgesics such as acetaminophen, non-steroidal anti-inflammatory drugs (NSAIDs), duloxetine, and intra-articular injections of corticosteroids and of hyaluronate. With regard to the development of disease-modifying OA drugs or agents (DMOADs), targeting cartilage changes (catabolism and anabolism), subchondral bone remodeling, and synovial inflammation are the three main thrusts of research. The present review will focus on the conventional pharmacological treatments and on future therapies with DMOADs.

Currently Available Pharmacological Therapies

Because OA is a chronic disease, more common in people older than 60, safety remains critical. Guidelines for the medical management of OA focus on controlling pain and improving the function and quality of life while minimizing therapeutic toxicity [1–3]. For hand OA, the American College of Rheumatology (ACR) guidelines [4] recommend topical capsaicin, topical NSAIDs, oral NSAIDs including cyclooxygenase (COX)-2 inhibitors, and tramadol. They also advise not to use opioids or intra-articular treatments for that condition. For knee and hip OA, acetaminophen, oral NSAIDs, topical NSAIDs (except for hip OA), tramadol, and intra-articular steroid injections are recommended [4].

Rapid-Acting Symptomatic Agents

The rapid-acting symptomatic treatments for OA consist mainly of analgesics and NSAIDs.

Analgesics

Acetaminophen remains the first-line therapeutic agent for OA [2] because of its low cost, as well as its efficacy and safety profile. It is recommended that it should be the preferred long-term oral analgesic to be used [1]. It has been reported that acetaminophen is less effective at relieving OA than NSAIDs [5] but more effective than placebo. However, this was not confirmed when using the Western Ontario and McMaster Universities Osteoarthritis Index (WOMAC) and the Lequesne index [6]. The preferred use of analgesics in OA should take into account the clinical context in which such treatment is prescribed. Indeed, significant adverse effects of acetaminophen have been reported, including gastric ulcerations and bleeding, increased risk of mild loss of renal function with long-term consumption, and hypertension for doses up to 3 g per day [7–9]. Furthermore, even at therapeutic doses, acetaminophen could cause asymptomatic elevation of liver enzymes in healthy people [10]. It is recommended that acetaminophen should not be used in patients who have existing liver dysfunction or such risk factors. Based on the above information, it is recommended that the lowest effective dose of acetaminophen to obtain pain relief should be used.

Opioids

Opioids have become more widely prescribed (often in combination with acetaminophen), especially for OA patients who experience lack of efficacy, have contraindications or intolerance to NSAIDs [2], and cannot undergo total joint arthroplasty because of comorbidities contraindicating surgery and anesthesia [4]. It is common to start with a weak opioid such as codeine or tramadol, often in combination with acetaminophen and, if ineffective or not tolerated, to use a stronger opioid such as hydrocodone, oxycodone, morphine, or transdermal fentanyl. However, opioids show several, sometimes severe, adverse events, resulting from binding of opioids to δ, κ, and μ receptors that also cause analgesia, including sedation, vomiting, and respiratory depression. Coordination and judgment impairment can lead to falls, particularly in older adults who are more susceptible to opioid-related effects due to renal insufficiency and lower lean body mass. In elderly people, opioids may cause severe injuries from falls, such as hip fractures or even death. Fracture risk appears to be greater with opioids than with NSAIDs in older people and increases with higher opioid dosage, especially during the first 2 weeks after initiating short-term opioid therapy [11]. Moreover, it seems that opioids do not improve patients' functioning [12] or quality of life. The benefits of using opioids should be weighed as judiciously as possible.

Duloxetine

Another analgesic, duloxetine, may improve knee OA pain as well as function [13]. Duloxetine is a selective serotonin and norepinephrine reuptake inhibitor, but the direct analgesic effect is independent of improvement of depression or anxiety. Serotonin and norepinephrine have been involved in the mediation of endogenous descending inhibitory pain pathways and central sensitization. In chronic pain states, their inhibitory effect is reduced or lost, leading to pain facilitation. Thus, duloxetine, by inhibiting their reuptake, can increase their activity and reduce persistent and chronic pain in OA [14]. Duloxetine was found to improve knee OA pain as well as function, as evaluated by clinically relevant outcomes in two 13-week trials [13]. The main adverse events include nausea, constipation, and hyperhidrosis. Duloxetine is recommended [4] as an alternative treatment for patients with symptomatic knee OA who have failed to respond to both pharmacological and non-pharmacological options. Controlled trials to compare duloxetine with other interventions in OA and to evaluate its efficacy in combination with other therapies may be useful to enhance prospective treatment.

NSAIDs

Other rapid symptomatic treatments that aim to block or reduce joint inflammation are the NSAIDs and specific cyclooxygenase-2 (COX-2) inhibitors, also named coxibs. These are recommended for patients who are unresponsive to acetaminophen, preferentially during inflammatory flares [2]. The use of NSAIDs is limited by gastrointestinal, renal, and cardiovascular side effects, which increase with age due to comorbidities. Coxibs demonstrate fewer gastrointestinal complications than NSAIDs but pose a potential cardiovascular risk [15]. The absence of COX-2 in platelets may explain that thromboxane A2 (TXA2) generation is unaffected as it is mediated by COX-1, whereas prostacyclin production is inhibited. A coxib-induced imbalance based on an inhibition of COX-2-generated prostacyclin, without an opposing reduction in TXA2, has been one hypothesis to explain the coxib-related cardiovascular risk. This imbalance could create continued TXA2 production and increased risk of thrombosis. Another explanation could be that some coxibs have been found to increase blood pressure.

Topical Treatments

Adjuvant therapies are interesting means that could be used to decrease analgesic consumption. NSAIDs can be used orally or topically with similar efficacy. Topical NSAIDs have been reported to be as effective as oral NSAIDs [16, 17], with a lower risk of systemic exposure and gastrointestinal complications. Their principal reported side effect is local skin reactions. They are recommended as alternative or adjuvant therapy [2], and ACR guidelines recommend them for the initial management of knee OA and prefer them to oral NSAIDs for patients older than 75 [4].

Capsaicin, the active principle of hot chili peppers, can cause depletion of substance P from sensory nerve endings and reduce or abolish the transmission of painful stimuli. However, its effectiveness and safety in pain relief remain controversial [18]. A burning sensation is the most common side effect, particularly during the first week of application [18]. It is still unclear if long-term capsaicin treatment can cause persistent desensitization of the skin, which may not be totally reversible. Capsaicin is recommended by guidelines for the initial management of hand OA but not of knee OA [1, 4].

Lidocaine patches, which are approved for postherpetic neuralgia, were also reported to reduce neuropathic pain associated with moderate-to-severe OA of the knee, without any reported treatment-related adverse effects [19].

Intra-articular Treatments

Corticosteroids are potent anti-inflammatory drugs that inhibit, among other factors, phospholipase A2. Intra-articular corticosteroid injection is recommended for OA inflammatory flares, especially if accompanied by effusion [2]. Short-term pain reduction in knee OA occurs between 2 and 3 weeks but has no significant effect on function. The Cochrane Review [20] reported that after 4 weeks, there was no effect on pain, physical function, or stiffness. However, repeated injections of intra-articular corticosteroids every 3 months for 2 years showed efficacy for pain relief after 1 year but not after 2 years [20]. Long-term safety of repeated intra-articular steroid injections in symptomatic knee OA has been demonstrated with improvement of OA symptoms up to 2 years [21]. Comparisons between corticosteroids revealed that triamcinolone hexacetonide was superior to betamethasone [20].

Hyaluronic acid (HA) is a constitutive glycosaminoglycan (GAG) component of the extracellular matrix and of the synovial fluid. HA is involved in the maintenance of joint homeostasis and its concentration is reduced in OA patients. Intra-articular HA injection (viscosupplementation) is recommended for knee OA patients who have had an inadequate response to initial therapy [4], despite possible induced transient pain and swelling at the injection site [22]. Compared with intra-articular corticosteroids, viscosupplementation has a delayed but prolonged effect [22].

Slow-Acting Symptomatic Drugs

Disease-modifying agents that not only reduce joint pain but also could slow the progression of the disease are of interest to alleviate the manifestations of OA in the long-term. Among the symptomatic slow-acting drugs for OA (SYSADOA) are glucosamine and chondroitin sulfate. For the past 10 years, glucosamine and chondroitin sulfate have been widely prescribed and used by OA patients for symptom relief. They are safe and with possible structure-modifying effects [2].

Glucosamine is a substrate used in the formation of GAGs (important constituents of articular cartilage) and shows a protective structural effect. The protective effect of glucosamine on structural progression of knee OA was reported in two studies exploring the radiological progression of knee OA after a daily administration of glucosamine for 3 years [23–27]. Chondroitin, a sulfated GAG, improves joint swelling and delays progression in patients with knee OA evaluated by X-rays [27, 28] or by magnetic resonance imaging (MRI) [29]. In the latter study, chondroitin was shown to reduce cartilage loss and the progression of bone marrow lesions (BML) [29].

Diacerein, an inhibitor mainly of interleukin-1β (IL-1β) but also of some proteases, was shown to be effective in patients with knee [30] and hip OA [31]. Diacerein provides sustained pain relief for several weeks after discontinuation, suggesting a long carry-over effect, with an analgesic-sparing effect [30]. Moreover, the effect of diacerein was found to be additive to that of NSAIDs. Interestingly, it did not inhibit COX or prostaglandin E_2. Diarrhea is the most frequent adverse event, which likely occurs due to prostaglandin synthesis induced by rhein, the active metabolite of diacerein, leading to an increase in gut motility. It is safer than NSAIDs for the upper gastrointestinal system and is therefore an alternative option to NSAIDs for the treatment of OA as it has a good global safety profile.

Treatment with avocado-soybean unsaponifiables (ASU) was found to reduce pain in knee OA, with a carry-over effect that persisted after treatment discontinuation [32] and in hip OA to reduce the percentage of radiologically assessed progressors [33]. Inhibition of IL-1β and matrix metalloproteinases (MMPs), as well as a potential action on subchondral bone osteoblasts, have been proposed as potential mechanisms of action [33].

Perspectives: Disease-Modifying Osteoarthritis Drugs (DMOADs)

No DMOAD has yet been approved, but some promising emerging agents can be speculated to have DMOAD effects in the future. Several drugs are in development or currently being tested in clinical trials. These treatments fall under one of the following categories.

DMOADs Targeting Pathways of Cartilage Catabolism and Anabolism

Metalloproteinase (MMP) Inhibitors

MMP inhibitors aim to block MMPs and extracellular matrix degradation, but clinical trials were limited by various adverse events including musculoskeletal effects. One of them, doxycycline, a member of the tetracycline antibiotics group with calcium chelating effect, thus inhibiting some MMPs, demonstrated a minimal structural beneficial effect but no effect on pain [34].

Growth Factors: Bone Morphogenetic Protein-7 and Fibroblast Growth Factor-18

Two growth factors involved in OA cartilage repair are currently in clinical trials: bone morphogenetic protein-7 (BMP-7), also known as osteogenic protein-1 (OP-1), and fibroblast growth factor-18 (FGF-18).

In vivo, in animal models, BMP-7 demonstrated reparative effects on articular cartilage degradation [35]. In vitro, human chondrocytes also promoted cartilage formation in response to BMP-7 treatment [36]. One completed Phase I trial using a weekly intra-articular injection of BMP-7 found no dose-limiting toxicity. By the 12th week of treatment, there was a trend toward a greater symptomatic improvement compared to placebo in knee OA patients who received 0.1 and 0.3 mg of BMP-7 [37].

In a meniscal tear rat model of OA, bi-weekly intra-articular injections of FGF-18 for 3 weeks induced chondrogenesis and cartilage repair, with dose-dependent increases in cartilage thickness of the tibial plateau [38]. Two Phase I studies have been completed. A randomized, double-blind, placebo-controlled, proof-of-concept trial evaluated the DMOAD effects of intra-articular administration of FGF-18 at doses of 10, 30, and 100 μg [39]. Outcomes were central medial tibiofemoral compartment cartilage volume change assessed by qMRI, and loss of joint space width (JSW) measured by X-rays, as well as the WOMAC pain and function scores after 6 and 12 months. FGF-18 was associated with a dose-dependent reduction in cartilage volume loss, not in the medial compartment but in the lateral compartment. A reduction in the lateral JSW loss was also evidenced in the FGF-18 group compared to placebo. All groups had improved WOMAC pain scores, with significance achieved at 12 months in patients receiving a 100 μg dose of the growth factor compared to placebo. Tolerance of the active treatment was good and no safety issue was observed.

Platelet-Rich Plasma

The rationale for using platelet-rich plasma (PRP) is that platelets contain storage pools of growth factors, including transforming growth factor-β (TGF-β), platelet-derived growth factor (PDGF), and vascular endothelial growth factor (VEGF), as well as cytokines, chemokines, and other mediators [40], which are currently thought to accelerate the natural healing process and promote cartilage repair after local injection. Moreover, as TGF-β and PDGF can stimulate the proliferation of mesenchymal stem cells (MSCs), these factors may direct the local mesenchymal and epithelial cells to migrate, divide, and increase collagen and matrix synthesis [41]. Nevertheless, the exact mechanism of how PRP could improve cartilage healing in OA remains to be determined. It is suggested that PRP may have an indirect effect by reducing synovial inflammation and modulating cytokinic local environment or a direct effect by stimulating the chondral anabolism and slowing the catabolic activity [42]. Indeed, growth factors contained in PRP may increase expression of the chondrocyte phenotype and stimulate the differentiation of MSCs as well as reduce IL-1 synthesis. Moreover, platelet-released growth factors may regulate endogenous HA synthesis [41], which could contribute to its action.

First reports of PRP efficacy in musculoskeletal conditions concerned sports- and overuse-related injuries, such as tendinitis, acute rotator cuff tears, and knee cartilage lesions [43]. Nowadays, a growing literature portrays PRP as a simple, low-cost, minimally invasive, and promising therapy for knee OA because of its potential for articular cartilage repair. However, high-quality studies sufficiently powered to support such postulate are lacking [42]; indeed, the literature contains mostly anecdotal reports and case series or studies of small sample size or uncontrolled studies [44–47].

On the other hand, some studies compared PRP to HA for ethical reasons, while others used placebo. Explanation of the data is also complicated by a lack of standardization of study protocols, especially PRP preparation and subsequent variability in platelet concentrations, as well as platelet activation status. Some used fresh PRP, avoiding cold storage which is thought to potentially alter platelet function [42], while others preferred to freeze PRP and delay intra-articular injection to assess the sample quality [48]. Moreover, the role of white blood cell (WBC) filtering during PRP preparation remains uncertain as WBCs are not only a source of cytokines and enzymes but can also release proteases and reactive oxygen [48]. Additional issues are the number and frequency of injections for optimal results and for which OA patients this therapy would be the most effective [42]. Future clinical trials are needed to address these issues.

Three main clinical trials in knee OA, two comparing PRP to HA and one to placebo, have been published [42, 48, 49]. The first one [48] compared the PRP treatment (three weekly injections) at 2, 6, and 12 months to HA. PRPs were obtained through a double-spinning procedure providing a high concentration of platelets but also containing WBCs and were frozen before injection. Both groups improved and no statistical differences were found between HA and PRP patients. A trend favoring the PRP group was noted only in patients with low-grade articular degeneration (KL grade up to 2) at 6 and 12 months. The second one [49] compared plasma rich in growth factors (PRGF), a single spinning procedure providing WBC-free PRP with a low platelet concentration, with HA at a short-term follow-up of 24 weeks, both administered three times on a weekly basis. The primary outcome measure was a 50 % decrease in knee pain from baseline to week 24. Compared with

HA, the rate of response to PRGF was significant at 14.1 percentage points higher. However, no significant differences were found between PRGF and HA groups with regard to all secondary outcomes measured, including WOMAC. More recently, Patel et al. [42] evaluated patients with knee OA divided into three groups, one receiving a single injection of PRP (WBC filtered), one receiving two injections of PRP 3 weeks apart, and one receiving a single injection of saline as placebo control. WOMAC, visual analogue scale (VAS) pain score, and overall satisfaction were measured at 6 weeks, and at 3 and 6 months. Both groups treated with PRP compared to the placebo group had statistically significantly better results within 2–3 weeks lasting up to 6 months.

It is noteworthy that all these studies described improvement in pain scores but did not assess cartilage damage. However, given the rationale of using PRP in OA, partly based on the fact that growth factors may influence cartilage repair through their potential effects on stem cells, PRP may be a future DMOAD. For this reason, investigation of its structural effects in future trials is needed.

Blocking Nitric Oxide

Nitric oxide (NO) contributes to extracellular matrix damage in OA [50]. Inducible NO synthase (iNOS) is responsible for excessive and sustained NO production by chondrocytes. Selective inhibition of iNOS reduced the progression of experimental OA in an animal model [51]. However, a recent 2-year randomized controlled trial (RCT) (Phase II/III) of cindunistat, an oral iNOS inhibitor, showed no superiority over placebo for rate of change in joint space narrowing (JSN) and no effect on pain or function. Only a transient slowing of JSN was noted in KL grade 2 OA patients at 48 weeks, which was not sustained at 96 weeks of follow-up. No slowing of OA progression was evidenced in KL grade 3 OA patients [52].

DMOADs Targeting Subchondral Bone Remodeling

Subchondral bone is at the interface between articular cartilage and trabecular bone. Loss of integrity of the osteochondral junction in OA removes the barrier between intra-articular and subchondral compartments and is associated with the invasion of articular cartilage by vascular channels originating from the subchondral bone. A cross talk between subchondral bone and cartilage as well as an increased subchondral turnover was shown to play a key role in the development of OA, and interest in subchondral bone as a therapeutic target is growing [53, 54]. The potential DMOAD effect of anti-osteoporotic agents is currently being explored in OA [55].

After promising preclinical findings in OA animal models, particularly in early OA [56, 57], clinical trials with bisphosphonates in human OA have provided mixed results. In a cross-sectional study in postmenopausal women with knee OA, alendronate and estrogen therapy decreased the frequency of BMLs detected by qMRI, and alendronate use alone was associated with less severity of knee pain [58]. In a double-blind 1-year trial in patients with mild-to-moderate knee OA, risedronate decreased the WOMAC score, but the reduction in JSN was found to be non-significant compared to placebo [59]. In contrast, a 2-year clinical trial found no significant effect of risedronate on WOMAC score or radiographic progression [60]. On the other hand, in a qMRI study in knee OA patients, a significant reduction in pain and BMLs at 6 months after a single infusion of zoledronic acid compared to placebo was reported [61].

While most commonly used osteoporosis treatments including bisphosphonates act by inhibiting bone resorption, another class of agents, strontium ranelate (SrRan), not only decreases bone resorption but also increases bone formation and is currently portrayed as the first potential DMOAD. In vitro, SrRan was found to inhibit the resorptive properties of human subchondral bone osteoblasts by reducing the synthesis of some MMPs and modulating osteoprotegerin (OPG) and receptor activator of nuclear factor-κB ligand (RANKL) levels [62]. SrRan was also reported to stimulate cartilage matrix formation by human chondrocytes in vitro [63]. In vivo, in an experimental dog OA model, therapeutic dosages of SrRan significantly reduced the progression of OA structural changes and inhibited the expression of IL-1β and key proteases involved in cartilage degradation [64]. Together, these data suggest that SrRan could target the three major tissues involved in OA, namely, the cartilage, subchondral bone, and synovium. In clinical studies, SrRan was found to reduce the radiological progression of spinal OA and back pain in women with osteoporosis and OA after a 3-year treatment [65]. A 3-year double-blind, randomized trial demonstrated that treatment with SrRan was associated with a significant protective effect on joint structure and clinically relevant improvement of symptoms in patients with knee OA [66]. In brief, the groups treated with SrRan at both 1 g/day and 2 g/day had less JSN and fewer radiological progressors compared to placebo. In addition, patients treated with SrRan 2 g/day had a greater reduction in WOMAC total score, as well as pain and physical function subscores, than those receiving placebo. Treatment with SrRan 2 g/day over 3 years was also associated with a clinically meaningful improvement in pain starting at 6 months, as well as physical function and stiffness as assessed by the number of responders above thresholds of clinical relevance [67].

A subgroup of patients from that trial was included in a study exploring the effect of SrRan on cartilage volume loss and BMLs using qMRI [68]. Data showed that SrRan has a beneficial impact on both cartilage and subchondral bone. As in vitro and in vivo data [62–64] demonstrated that SrRan has combined anti-catabolic and pro-anabolic properties, although speculative, SrRan could have a direct impact on cartilage as well as a positive effect on the cross talk between subchondral bone and cartilage. The loss of osteochondral integrity may expose the cartilage to mediators released from subchondral channels stimulating chondrocytes, combined with a possible direct effect on the chondrocytes, and may partly account for the impact of SrRan on cartilage loss, in addition to its preponderant effect on BMLs.

The data on the DMOAD properties of SrRan open the door to other promising bone pathways to target OA. Hence, targeting the OPG/RANKL system, which is critical for bone turnover [54, 69, 70], appears interesting. RANKL, localized on osteoblasts, enhances osteoclastogenesis via interaction with the receptor RANK, localized on osteoclasts. OPG, produced by osteoblasts, is a secreted decoy receptor for RANKL that serves as a physiological inhibitor of RANKL-driven osteoclast activities. Data showed that OPG, RANK, and RANKL are also expressed and produced by human chondrocytes [71], and on human OA chondrocytes, the OPG/RANKL ratio was reduced whereas the RANK/RANKL ratio was increased [71]. An imbalance in the OPG/RANKL system, both in synovial fluid and serum, has been associated with OA severity [72]. The pro-resorptive effect of RANKL on the osteoclastogenesis process could therefore be targeted by the use of either OPG or an anti-RANKL antibody. A study carried out in an experimental mouse model of OA revealed, upon OPG administration, reduced cartilage degradation through an effect on the trabecular bone [73]. The potential of RANKL inhibition as a DMOAD is therefore interesting. Denosumab is a fully human IgG2 monoclonal antibody that binds human RANKL with a high affinity and which has been approved for use in postmenopausal osteoporosis [74] and in oncology. By analogy, in rheumatoid arthritis (RA), a Phase II trial evaluated the effects of denosumab in addition to methotrexate on structural damage. At 6 months, the increase in the MRI erosion score from baseline was lower in patients receiving 60 mg of denosumab and significance was reached with 180 mg of denosumab compared to placebo [75]. Denosumab has not yet been evaluated as a DMOAD.

Cathepsin K inhibitors may also be prospective DMOADs. In preclinical models, cathepsin K inhibition showed beneficial effects on protection of subchondral bone loss and against cartilage degradation and suggested reduced osteophyte formation [76].

The use of parathyroid hormone (PTH) as a DMOAD is also conceivable but has not yet been evaluated. Recombinant human PTH 1–34, teriparatide, is a bone anabolic therapy used for osteoporosis. In a mouse meniscal/ligamentous injury model of knee OA, intermittent teriparatide systemic injections decreased cartilage degeneration and induced matrix regeneration [77].

Calcitonin also appears an option. In a Phase IIa clinical trial in knee OA [78], oral calcitonin improved the Lequesne function score, whereas no difference was found in terms of pain relief compared to placebo. Moreover, the nasal form of calcitonin was found to improve WOMAC total and subscale scores (pain, stiffness, and function) [79]. This study was limited by the absence of a control group. A 2-year Phase III trial in knee OA patients resulted in the symptom-modifying efficacy of oral calcitonin with a significant improvement in WOMAC pain, function, and stiffness scores compared to placebo. With regard to structural effects, oral calcitonin did not impact JSW, which was the primary endpoint, but significantly increased cartilage volume compared to placebo, suggesting some structure-modifying efficacy [80]. Another Phase III trial was terminated early, probably due to an imbalance in prostate cancer events in male subjects. Of note, the European Medicines Agency's Committee for Medicinal Products for Human Use (CHMP) recommended in 2012 that calcitonin therapy should only be used for short-term periods because of an increased risk of cancer of 0.7–2.4 % with long-term use, especially with intranasal calcitonin [81]. This could limit the potential use of calcitonin as a DMOAD.

Vitamin D supplementation failed to reduce WOMAC pain or cartilage volume loss assessed by qMRI compared to placebo in a recent 2-year knee OA trial [82]. Another work evaluating whether vitamin D supplementation can slow knee cartilage loss assessed by qMRI in OA patients is ongoing [83].

Targeting Inflammatory Pathways

Several proinflammatory cytokines play a pivotal role in the pathogenesis of OA. In particular, IL-1β and TNF-α are key cytokines favoring the degeneration of articular cartilage matrix, which makes them prime targets for OA treatment [84]. IL-1β stimulates joint tissue to produce several proteases involved in cartilage degradation and reduces the production of matrix macromolecules such as aggrecan. It was recently reported that one IL-1 receptor antagonist (IL-1Ra) haplotype could be associated with increased OA progression [85]. Targeting IL-1β in OA seems a logical approach to slow the disease progression, either directly with recombinant human IL-1Ra, antibodies against the cytokine or its specific receptor, or through gene therapy. Intra-articular injection of recombinant human IL-1Ra was found to be protective against the development of induced OA in a dog model and associated with a reduction in the expression of some MMPs [86], providing evidence of a role of IL-1 in cartilage degradation. However, after a promising pilot clinical study [87] reporting that intra-articular injection of anakinra (a recombinant non-glycosylated version of the human IL-1Ra) was well tolerated in OA patients and improved pain as well as WOMAC total scores through 3 months, Chevalier et al. [88] performed a 12-week double-blind study assessing the efficacy of a single intra-articular injection of 50 mg or 150 mg of anakinra versus placebo in patients with moderate-to-severe knee OA evaluated 4 weeks later. Anakinra was found to be safe and well tolerated. Patients treated with anakinra showed no significant difference versus placebo in score change from baseline to week 4 in the WOMAC index. However, significant short-term pain relief was evidenced at day 4 with the 150 mg anakinra injection compared to placebo. In this study, several factors could have negatively impacted the evaluation of treatment response such as the inclusion of patients with low-level pain at baseline; the short half-life of the drug, suggesting that repeated injections are necessary to obtain a sustained symptomatic effect; and a strong placebo effect. Of note, the structural effect of such strategy has not been investigated, and the absence of symptomatic effect does not mean absence of structural effect. In contrast, 3 months of daily subcutaneous injections of anakinra in three patients with erosive hand OA showed improvement of pain and disability [89]. Additionally, a double-blind, placebo-controlled RCT using a systemic administration of a monoclonal antibody (AMG 108) directed against the functional type 1 receptor of IL-1 demonstrated no significant difference in the level of pain at 6 weeks when compared to the placebo [90]. However, a trend toward efficacy favoring AMG 108 was found in patients with high baseline WOMAC pain [91]. Additionally, although no difference in the incidence of serious infections related to the reduction of neutrophil count was seen compared to placebo, such biological therapy may expose patients to serious adverse events [91].

Briefly, most of the studies so far have failed to show a beneficial symptomatic effect of IL-1β inhibition in OA. Recently, a Phase II proof-of-concept study assessing the efficacy and safety of subcutaneous injections of gevokizumab, a potent anti-IL-1β antibody, compared to placebo, in the treatment of active erosive OA of the hand revealed no drug-related benefits after 6 months of treatment [92]. Another study on the safety and effect on pain of a single intra-articular administration of canakinumab, an anti-IL-1β monoclonal antibody, in patients with knee OA is completed but not yet published. Further studies evaluating the effect of anti-IL-1β, especially of repeated intra-articular injections, for instance, on a weekly basis, or of biologic agents with sustained half-life, are needed before burying the concept of IL-1 inhibition in OA management [93]. Moreover, as mentioned above, studies should evaluate the effect not only on pain but also on the joint structure, which is the target benefit that we are looking for.

Another approach is the intra-articular injection of an autologous anti-proinflammatory cytokine product named Orthokin, consisting of autologous conditioned serum obtained after incubation with glass beads to induce the synthesis of various anti-inflammatory cytokines such as IL-1Ra, IL-4, IL-10, and IL-13. Two clinical studies provided controversial results. The first reported study failed to show any difference between WOMAC, VAS, and Knee Injury and Osteoarthritis Outcome Score (KOOS) pain scores between Orthokin and saline over 12 months of follow-up [94]. The second demonstrated significantly better outcomes compared to saline and to HA [95]. Further studies will be needed before considering this technique in routine practice.

Targeting TNF-α in OA with infliximab and adalimumab has also been evaluated in a few trials providing conflicting results. Two antibodies against TNF-α (adalimumab, infliximab) were also shown to relieve symptoms of hand [96] and knee OA [97], but results are still controversial, as another study reported no significant symptomatic or DMOAD structural effect of adalimumab in hand OA [98].

In an open-label pilot trial in 10 patients with erosive OA of the hands, monthly intra-articular injections of infliximab reduced pain in all patients, without adverse reactions after 1 year of follow-up [96]. In contrast, another open-label study [99] in patients with erosive hand OA who received subcutaneous injections of adalimumab every 2 weeks for 12 weeks showed no improvement in the number of tender joints, grip strength, disability, pain, and global disease assessment. However, there was a statistically significant improvement in the number of swollen joints compared to baseline. A clinical trial [98] in patients with erosive hand OA treated with subcutaneous injections of adalimumab or placebo every 2 weeks for 12 months failed to demonstrate the control of structural damage on radiography as similar percentages of patients in both groups had either development of new erosions or progression of existing erosions. There were also no significant differences between groups with regard to pain and swelling on palpation, grip strength, morning stiffness, pain severity score, and function. However, palpable soft tissue swelling in interphalangeal finger joints at baseline was identified as the strongest predictor of erosive progression in these joints, and adalimumab was found to halt the erosive progression compared to placebo in these joints with destructive features on radiography and palpable effusion [98]. A Phase II study also showed the lack of efficacy of adalimumab in hand OA [100]. A recent open-label evaluation of adalimumab for 12 weeks in 20 patients with knee OA and clinical effusion reported that 70 % of the patients achieved an Osteoarthritis Research Society International/Outcome Measures in Rheumatology Clinical Trials (OARSI/OMERACT) response at week 12 [97]. In these studies, differences within results from erosive hand OA and knee OA could reflect different disease phenotypes.

To summarize, the current evidence does not support the use of anti-cytokine therapy in all OA patients. Further trials are needed, especially with respect to the selection of OA patients who may be speculated to benefit most from such therapy [101]. As for strategies targeting subchondral bone remodeling, selecting patients with early OA and synovitis may be necessary in future studies for targeted and personalized OA management. However, the method for selecting inflammatory OA patients, whether only clinically based with synovial effusion of a swollen and painful joint or MRI based with radiological synovitis, remains to be determined.

Another proinflammatory cytokine, IL-6, could be of therapeutic benefit to OA patients, but to our knowledge, no study has yet assessed IL-6 inhibition in OA.

Conclusion

OA drug management is based on a wide spectrum of therapeutic options to relieve pain and to try to delay progression. The focus is now on the development of DMOADs that could be associated with conventional therapy to provide a more effective treatment, which remains a huge unmet medical need worldwide given that OA prevalence is likely to increase with the aging population. An exciting and promising new era in DMOAD development may be within reach, provided that future clinical trials are sufficiently powered and systematically designed, use the right evaluation techniques, and target the appropriate and more homogeneous categories of OA patients.

References

1. Jordan KM, Arden NK, Doherty M, Bannwarth B, Bijlsma JW, Dieppe P, et al. EULAR Recommendations 2003: an evidence based approach to the management of knee osteoarthritis: Report of a Task Force of the Standing Committee for International Clinical Studies Including Therapeutic Trials (ESCISIT). Ann Rheum Dis. 2003;62:1145–55.

2. Zhang W, Moskowitz RW, Nuki G, Abramson S, Altman RD, Arden N, et al. OARSI recommendations for the management of hip and knee osteoarthritis, part II: OARSI evidence-based, expert consensus guidelines. Osteoarthritis Cartilage. 2008;16:137–62.
3. Zhang W, Nuki G, Moskowitz RW, Abramson SB, Altman RD, Arden NK, et al. OARSI recommendations for the management of hip and knee osteoarthritis: part III: changes in evidence following systematic cumulative update of research published through January 2009. Osteoarthritis Cartilage. 2010;18:476–99.
4. Hochberg MC, Altman RD, April KT, Benkhalti M, Guyatt G, McGowan J, et al. American College of Rheumatology 2012 recommendations for the use of nonpharmacologic and pharmacologic therapies in osteoarthritis of the hand, hip, and knee. Arthritis Care Res (Hoboken). 2012;64:455–74.
5. Zhang W, Jones A, Doherty M. Does paracetamol (acetaminophen) reduce the pain of osteoarthritis? A meta-analysis of randomised controlled trials. Ann Rheum Dis. 2004;63:901–7.
6. Towheed TE, Maxwell L, Judd MG, Catton M, Hochberg MC, Wells G. Acetaminophen for osteoarthritis. Cochrane Database Syst Rev. 2006;(1):CD004257.
7. Curhan GC, Knight EL, Rosner B, Hankinson SE, Stampfer MJ. Lifetime nonnarcotic analgesic use and decline in renal function in women. Arch Intern Med. 2004;164:1519–24.
8. Forman JP, Rimm EB, Curhan GC. Frequency of analgesic use and risk of hypertension among men. Arch Intern Med. 2007;167:394–9.
9. Rahme E, Barkun A, Nedjar H, Gaugris S, Watson D. Hospitalizations for upper and lower GI events associated with traditional NSAIDs and acetaminophen among the elderly in Quebec, Canada. Am J Gastroenterol. 2008;103:872–82.
10. Heard KJ, Green JL, Dart RC. Serum alanine aminotransferase elevation during 10 days of acetaminophen use in nondrinkers. Pharmacotherapy. 2010;30:818–22.
11. Miller M, Sturmer T, Azrael D, Levin R, Solomon DH. Opioid analgesics and the risk of fractures in older adults with arthritis. J Am Geriatr Soc. 2011;59:430–8.
12. Avouac J, Gossec L, Dougados M. Efficacy and safety of opioids for osteoarthritis: a meta-analysis of randomized controlled trials. Osteoarthritis Cartilage. 2007;15:957–65.
13. Hochberg MC, Wohlreich M, Gaynor P, Hanna S, Risser R. Clinically relevant outcomes based on analysis of pooled data from 2 trials of duloxetine in patients with knee osteoarthritis. J Rheumatol. 2012;39:352–8.
14. Skljarevski V, Zhang S, Iyengar S, D'Souza D, Alaka K, Chappell A, et al. Efficacy of duloxetine in patients with chronic pain conditions. Curr Drug Ther. 2011;6:296–303.
15. Trelle S, Reichenbach S, Wandel S, Hildebrand P, Tschannen B, Villiger PM, et al. Cardiovascular safety of non-steroidal anti-inflammatory drugs: network meta-analysis. BMJ. 2011;342:c7086.
16. Tugwell PS, Wells GA, Shainhouse JZ. Equivalence study of a topical diclofenac solution (pennsaid) compared with oral diclofenac in symptomatic treatment of osteoarthritis of the knee: a randomized controlled trial. J Rheumatol. 2004;31:2002–12.
17. Underwood M, Ashby D, Cross P, Hennessy E, Letley L, Martin J, et al. Advice to use topical or oral ibuprofen for chronic knee pain in older people: randomised controlled trial and patient preference study. BMJ. 2008;336:138–42.
18. McCleane G. The analgesic efficacy of topical capsaicin is enhanced by glyceryl trinitrate in painful osteoarthritis: a randomized, double blind, placebo controlled study. Eur J Pain. 2000;4:355–60.
19. Gammaitoni AR, Galer BS, Onawola R, Jensen MP, Argoff CE. Lidocaine patch 5% and its positive impact on pain qualities in osteoarthritis: results of a pilot 2-week, open-label study using the Neuropathic Pain Scale. Curr Med Res Opin. 2004;20 Suppl 2:S13–9.
20. Bellamy N, Campbell J, Robinson V, Gee T, Bourne R, Wells G. Intraarticular corticosteroid for treatment of osteoarthritis of the knee. Cochrane Database Syst Rev. 2006;(2):CD005328.
21. Raynauld JP, Buckland-Wright C, Ward R, Choquette D, Haraoui B, Martel-Pelletier J, et al. Safety and efficacy of long-term intraarticular steroid injections in osteoarthritis of the knee: a randomized, double-blind, placebo-controlled trial. Arthritis Rheum. 2003;48:370–7.

22. Bellamy N, Campbell J, Robinson V, Gee T, Bourne R, Wells G. Viscosupplementation for the treatment of osteoarthritis of the knee. Cochrane Database Syst Rev. 2005;(2):CD005321.
23. Reginster JY, Deroisy R, Rovati LC, Lee RL, Lejeune E, Bruyere O, et al. Long-term effects of glucosamine sulphate on osteoarthritis progression: a randomised, placebo-controlled clinical trial. Lancet. 2001;357:251–6.
24. Pavelka K, Gatterova J, Olejarova M, Machacek S, Giacovelli G, Rovati LC. Glucosamine sulfate use and delay of progression of knee osteoarthritis: a 3-year, randomized, placebo-controlled, double-blind study. Arch Intern Med. 2002;162:2113–23.
25. Bruyere O, Pavelka K, Rovati LC, Deroisy R, Olejarova M, Gatterova J, et al. Glucosamine sulfate reduces osteoarthritis progression in postmenopausal women with knee osteoarthritis: evidence from two 3-year studies. Menopause. 2004;11:138–43.
26. Poolsup N, Suthisisang C, Channark P, Kittikulsuth W. Glucosamine long-term treatment and the progression of knee osteoarthritis: systematic review of randomized controlled trials. Ann Pharmacother. 2005;39:1080–7.
27. Lee YH, Woo JH, Choi SJ, Ji JD, Song GG. Effect of glucosamine or chondroitin sulfate on the osteoarthritis progression: a meta-analysis. Rheumatol Int. 2010;30:357–63.
28. Hochberg MC, Zhan M, Langenberg P. The rate of decline of joint space width in patients with osteoarthritis of the knee: a systematic review and meta-analysis of randomized placebo-controlled trials of chondroitin sulfate. Curr Med Res Opin. 2008;24:3029–35.
29. Wildi LM, Raynauld JP, Martel-Pelletier J, Beaulieu A, Bessette L, Morin F, et al. Chondroitin sulphate reduces both cartilage volume loss and bone marrow lesions in knee osteoarthritis patients starting as early as 6 months after initiation of therapy: a randomised, double-blind, placebo-controlled pilot study using MRI. Ann Rheum Dis. 2011;70:982–9.
30. Pelletier JP, Yaron M, Haraoui B, Cohen P, Nahir MA, Choquette D, et al. Efficacy and safety of diacerein in osteoarthritis of the knee: a double-blind, placebo-controlled trial. The Diacerein Study Group. Arthritis Rheum. 2000;43:2339–48.
31. Dougados M, Nguyen M, Berdah L, Mazieres B, Vignon E, Lequesne M, et al. Evaluation of the structure-modifying effects of diacerein in hip osteoarthritis: ECHODIAH, a three-year, placebo-controlled trial. Evaluation of the Chondromodulating Effect of Diacerein in OA of the Hip. Arthritis Rheum. 2001;44:2539–47.
32. Maheu E, Mazieres B, Valat JP, Loyau G, Le Loet X, Bourgeois P, et al. Symptomatic efficacy of avocado/soybean unsaponifiables in the treatment of osteoarthritis of the knee and hip: a prospective, randomized, double-blind, placebo-controlled, multicenter clinical trial with a six-month treatment period and a two-month followup demonstrating a persistent effect. Arthritis Rheum. 1998;41:81–91.
33. Maheu E, Cadet C, Marty M, Moyse D, Kerloch I, Coste P, et al. Randomised, controlled trial of avocado-soybean unsaponifiable (Piascledine) effect on structure modification in hip osteoarthritis: the ERADIAS study. Ann Rheum Dis. 2014;73:376–84.
34. Nuesch E, Rutjes AW, Trelle S, Reichenbach S, Juni P. Doxycycline for osteoarthritis of the knee or hip. Cochrane Database Syst Rev. 2009;(4):CD007323.
35. Jelic M, Pecina M, Haspl M, Kos J, Taylor K, Maticic D, et al. Regeneration of articular cartilage chondral defects by osteogenic protein-1 (bone morphogenetic protein-7) in sheep. Growth Factors. 2001;19:101–13.
36. Gavenis K, Heussen N, Schmidt-Rohlfing B. Effects of low concentration BMP-7 on human osteoarthritic chondrocytes: comparison of different applications. J Biomater Appl. 2012;26:845–59.
37. Hunter DJ, Pike MC, Jonas BL, Kissin E, Krop J, McAlindon T. Phase 1 safety and tolerability study of BMP-7 in symptomatic knee osteoarthritis. BMC Musculoskelet Disord. 2010;11:232.
38. Moore EE, Bendele AM, Thompson DL, Littau A, Waggie KS, Reardon B, et al. Fibroblast growth factor-18 stimulates chondrogenesis and cartilage repair in a rat model of injury-induced osteoarthritis. Osteoarthritis Cartilage. 2005;13:623–31.
39. Lohmander LS, Hellot S, Dreher D, Krantz EF, Kruger DS, Guermazi A, et al. Intraarticular sprifermin (recombinant human fibroblast growth factor 18) in knee osteoarthritis: a randomized, double-blind, placebo-controlled trial. Arthritis Rheumatol. 2014;66:1820–31.

40. Anitua E, Andia I, Ardanza B, Nurden P, Nurden AT. Autologous platelets as a source of proteins for healing and tissue regeneration. Thromb Haemost. 2004;91:4–15.
41. Dhillon RS, Schwarz EM, Maloney MD. Platelet-rich plasma therapy – future or trend? Arthritis Res Ther. 2012;14:219.
42. Patel S, Dhillon MS, Aggarwal S, Marwaha N, Jain A. Treatment with platelet-rich plasma is more effective than placebo for knee osteoarthritis: a prospective, double-blind, randomized trial. Am J Sports Med. 2013;41:356–64.
43. Taylor DW, Petrera M, Hendry M, Theodoropoulos JS. A systematic review of the use of platelet-rich plasma in sports medicine as a new treatment for tendon and ligament injuries. Clin J Sport Med. 2011;21:344–52.
44. Kon E, Mandelbaum B, Buda R, Filardo G, Delcogliano M, Timoncini A, et al. Platelet-rich plasma intra-articular injection versus hyaluronic acid viscosupplementation as treatments for cartilage pathology: from early degeneration to osteoarthritis. Arthroscopy. 2011;27:1490–501.
45. Kon E, Buda R, Filardo G, Di Martino A, Timoncini A, Cenacchi A, et al. Platelet-rich plasma: intra-articular knee injections produced favorable results on degenerative cartilage lesions. Knee Surg Sports Traumatol Arthrosc. 2010;18:472–9.
46. Sampson S, Reed M, Silvers H, Meng M, Mandelbaum B. Injection of platelet-rich plasma in patients with primary and secondary knee osteoarthritis: a pilot study. Am J Phys Med Rehabil. 2010;89:961–9.
47. Sanchez M, Anitua E, Azofra J, Aguirre JJ, Andia I. Intra-articular injection of an autologous preparation rich in growth factors for the treatment of knee OA: a retrospective cohort study. Clin Exp Rheumatol. 2008;26:910–3.
48. Filardo G, Kon E, Di Martino A, Di Matteo B, Merli ML, Cenacchi A, et al. Platelet-rich plasma vs hyaluronic acid to treat knee degenerative pathology: study design and preliminary results of a randomized controlled trial. BMC Musculoskelet Disord. 2012;13:229.
49. Sanchez M, Fiz N, Azofra J, Usabiaga J, Aduriz Recalde E, Garcia Gutierrez A, et al. A randomized clinical trial evaluating plasma rich in growth factors (PRGF-Endoret) versus hyaluronic acid in the short-term treatment of symptomatic knee osteoarthritis. Arthroscopy. 2012;28:1070–8.
50. Martel-Pelletier J, Wildi LM, Pelletier JP. Future therapeutics for osteoarthritis. Bone. 2012;51:297–311.
51. Pelletier JP, Jovanovic D, Fernandes JC, Manning P, Connor JR, Currie MG, et al. Reduced progression of experimental osteoarthritis in vivo by selective inhibition of inducible nitric oxide synthase. Arthritis Rheum. 1998;41:1275–86.
52. Graverand MP, Clemmer RS, Redifer P, Brunell RM, Hayes CW, Brandt KD, et al. A 2-year randomised, double-blind, placebo-controlled, multicentre study of oral selective iNOS inhibitor, cindunistat (SD-6010), in patients with symptomatic osteoarthritis of the knee. Ann Rheum Dis. 2013;72:187–95.
53. Suri S, Walsh DA. Osteochondral alterations in osteoarthritis. Bone. 2012;51:204–11.
54. Kwan Tat S, Lajeunesse D, Pelletier JP, Martel-Pelletier J. Targeting subchondral bone for treating osteoarthritis: what is the evidence? Best Pract Res Clin Rheumatol. 2010;24:51–70.
55. Lajeunesse D, Pelletier JP, Martel-Pelletier J. Osteoporosis and osteoarthritis: bone is the common battle ground. Medicographia. 2010;32:391–8.
56. Pelletier JP, Troncy E, Bertaim T, Thibaud D, Goulet AC, Abram F, et al. Treatment with tiludronic acid helps reduce the development of experimental osteoarthritis lesions in dogs with anterior cruciate ligament transection followed by reconstructive surgery: a 1-year study with quantitative magnetic resonance imaging. J Rheumatol. 2011;38:118–28.
57. Moreau M, Rialland P, Pelletier JP, Martel-Pelletier J, Lajeunesse D, Boileau C, et al. Tiludronate treatment improves structural changes and symptoms of osteoarthritis in the canine anterior cruciate ligament model. Arthritis Res Ther. 2011;13:R98.
58. Carbone LD, Nevitt MC, Wildy K, Barrow KD, Harris F, Felson D, et al. The relationship of antiresorptive drug use to structural findings and symptoms of knee osteoarthritis. Arthritis Rheum. 2004;50:3516–25.

59. Spector TD, Conaghan PG, Buckland-Wright JC, Garnero P, Cline GA, Beary JF, et al. Effect of risedronate on joint structure and symptoms of knee osteoarthritis: results of the BRISK randomized, controlled trial [ISRCTN01928173]. Arthritis Res Ther. 2005;7:R625–33.
60. Bingham 3rd CO, Buckland-Wright JC, Garnero P, Cohen SB, Dougados M, Adami S, et al. Risedronate decreases biochemical markers of cartilage degradation but does not decrease symptoms or slow radiographic progression in patients with medial compartment osteoarthritis of the knee: results of the two-year multinational knee osteoarthritis structural arthritis study. Arthritis Rheum. 2006;54:3494–507.
61. Laslett LL, Dore DA, Quinn SJ, Boon P, Ryan E, Winzenberg TM, et al. Zoledronic acid reduces knee pain and bone marrow lesions over 1 year: a randomised controlled trial. Ann Rheum Dis. 2012;71:1322–8.
62. Tat SK, Pelletier JP, Mineau F, Caron J, Martel-Pelletier J. Strontium ranelate inhibits key factors affecting bone remodeling in human osteoarthritic subchondral bone osteoblasts. Bone. 2011;49:559–67.
63. Henrotin Y, Labasse A, Zheng SX, Galais P, Tsouderos Y, Crielaard JM, et al. Strontium ranelate increases cartilage matrix formation. J Bone Miner Res. 2001;16:299–308.
64. Pelletier JP, Kapoor M, Fahmi H, Lajeunesse D, Blesius A, Maillet J, et al. Strontium ranelate reduces the progression of experimental dog osteoarthritis by inhibiting the expression of key proteases in cartilage and of IL-1beta in the synovium. Ann Rheum Dis. 2013;72:250–7.
65. Bruyere O, Delferriere D, Roux C, Wark JD, Spector T, Devogelaer JP, et al. Effects of strontium ranelate on spinal osteoarthritis progression. Ann Rheum Dis. 2008;67:335–9.
66. Reginster JY, Badurski J, Bellamy N, Bensen W, Chapurlat R, Chevalier X, et al. Efficacy and safety of strontium ranelate in the treatment of knee osteoarthritis: results of a double-blind, randomised placebo-controlled trial. Ann Rheum Dis. 2013;72:179–86.
67. Bruyere O, Reginster JY, Bellamy N, Chapurlat R, Richette P, Cooper C, et al. Clinically meaningful effect of strontium ranelate on symptoms in knee osteoarthritis: a responder analysis. Rheumatology (Oxford). 2014;53:1457–64.
68. Pelletier JP, Roubille C, Raynauld JP, Abram F, Dorais M, Delorme P, et al. Disease-modifying effect of strontium ranelate in a subset of patients from the Phase III knee osteoarthritis study SEKOIA using quantitative MRI: reduction in bone marrow lesions protects against cartilage loss. Ann Rheum Dis. 2015;74(2):422–9.
69. Tat SK, Pelletier JP, Velasco CR, Padrines M, Martel-Pelletier J. New perspective in osteoarthritis: the OPG and RANKL system as a potential therapeutic target? Keio J Med. 2009;58:29–40.
70. Kwan Tat S, Pelletier JP, Lajeunesse D, Fahmi H, Lavigne M, Martel-Pelletier J. The differential expression of osteoprotegerin (OPG) and receptor activator of nuclear factor kappaB ligand (RANKL) in human osteoarthritic subchondral bone osteoblasts is an indicator of the metabolic state of these disease cells. Clin Exp Rheumatol. 2008;26:295–304.
71. Kwan Tat S, Amiable N, Pelletier JP, Boileau C, Lajeunesse D, Duval N, et al. Modulation of OPG, RANK and RANKL by human chondrocytes and their implication during osteoarthritis. Rheumatology (Oxford). 2009;48:1482–90.
72. Pilichou A, Papassotiriou I, Michalakakou K, Fessatou S, Fandridis E, Papachristou G, et al. High levels of synovial fluid osteoprotegerin (OPG) and increased serum ratio of receptor activator of nuclear factor-kappa B ligand (RANKL) to OPG correlate with disease severity in patients with primary knee osteoarthritis. Clin Biochem. 2008;41:746–9.
73. Kadri A, Ea HK, Bazille C, Hannouche D, Liote F, Cohen-Solal ME. Osteoprotegerin inhibits cartilage degradation through an effect on trabecular bone in murine experimental osteoarthritis. Arthritis Rheum. 2008;58:2379–86.
74. Josse R, Khan A, Ngui D, Shapiro M. Denosumab, a new pharmacotherapy option for postmenopausal osteoporosis. Curr Med Res Opin. 2013;29:205–16.
75. Cohen SB, Dore RK, Lane NE, Ory PA, Peterfy CG, Sharp JT, et al. Denosumab treatment effects on structural damage, bone mineral density, and bone turnover in rheumatoid arthritis: a twelve-month, multicenter, randomized, double-blind, placebo-controlled, phase II clinical trial. Arthritis Rheum. 2008;58:1299–309.

76. Hayami T, Zhuo Y, Wesolowski GA, Pickarski M, le Duong T. Inhibition of cathepsin K reduces cartilage degeneration in the anterior cruciate ligament transection rabbit and murine models of osteoarthritis. Bone. 2012;50:1250–9.
77. Sampson ER, Hilton MJ, Tian Y, Chen D, Schwarz EM, Mooney RA, et al. Teriparatide as a chondroregenerative therapy for injury-induced osteoarthritis. Sci Transl Med. 2011;3:101ra93.
78. Manicourt DH, Azria M, Mindeholm L, Thonar EJ, Devogelaer JP. Oral salmon calcitonin reduces Lequesne's algofunctional index scores and decreases urinary and serum levels of biomarkers of joint metabolism in knee osteoarthritis. Arthritis Rheum. 2006;54:3205–11.
79. Esenyel M, Icagasioglu A, Esenyel CZ. Effects of calcitonin on knee osteoarthritis and quality of life. Rheumatol Int. 2013;33:423–7.
80. Karsdal MA, Alexandersen P, John MR, Loeffler J, Arnold M, Azria M, et al. Oral calcitonin demonstrated symptom-modifying efficacy and increased cartilage volume: results from a 2-year Phase 3 trial in patients with osteoarthritis of the knee. Osteoarthritis Cartilage. 2011;19:S35.
81. Reginster JY, Pelousse F, Bruyere O. Safety concerns with the long-term management of osteoporosis. Expert Opin Drug Saf. 2013;12:507–22.
82. McAlindon T, LaValley M, Schneider E, Nuite M, Lee JY, Price LL, et al. Effect of vitamin D supplementation on progression of knee pain and cartilage volume loss in patients with symptomatic osteoarthritis: a randomized controlled trial. JAMA. 2013;309:155–62.
83. Cao Y, Jones G, Cicuttini F, Winzenberg T, Wluka A, Sharman J, et al. Vitamin D supplementation in the management of knee osteoarthritis: study protocol for a randomized controlled trial. Trials. 2012;13:131.
84. Kapoor M, Martel-Pelletier J, Lajeunesse D, Pelletier JP, Fahmi H. Role of proinflammatory cytokines in the pathophysiology of osteoarthritis. Nat Rev Rheumatol. 2011;7:33–42.
85. Wu X, Kondragunta V, Kornman KS, Wang H, Duff GW, Renner JB, et al. IL-1 receptor antagonist gene as a predictive biomarker of progression of knee osteoarthritis in a population cohort. Osteoarthritis Cartilage. 2013;21:930–8.
86. Caron JP, Fernandes JC, Martel-Pelletier J, Tardif G, Mineau F, Geng C, et al. Chondroprotective effect of intraarticular injections of interleukin-1 receptor antagonist in experimental osteoarthritis. Suppression of collagenase-1 expression. Arthritis Rheum. 1996;39:1535–44.
87. Chevalier X, Giraudeau B, Conrozier T, Marliere J, Kiefer P, Goupille P. Safety study of intraarticular injection of interleukin 1 receptor antagonist in patients with painful knee osteoarthritis: a multicenter study. J Rheumatol. 2005;32:1317–23.
88. Chevalier X, Goupille P, Beaulieu AD, Burch FX, Bensen WG, Conrozier T, et al. Intraarticular injection of anakinra in osteoarthritis of the knee: a multicenter, randomized, double-blind, placebo-controlled study. Arthritis Rheum. 2009;61:344–52.
89. Bacconnier L, Jorgensen C, Fabre S. Erosive osteoarthritis of the hand: clinical experience with anakinra. Ann Rheum Dis. 2009;68:1078–9.
90. Cohen SB, Proudman S, Kivitz AJ, Burch FX, Donohue JP, Burstein D, et al. A randomized, double-blind study of AMG 108 (a fully human monoclonal antibody to IL-1R1) in patients with osteoarthritis of the knee. Arthritis Res Ther. 2011;13:R125.
91. Chevalier X, Conrozier T, Richette P. Desperately looking for the right target in osteoarthritis: the anti-IL-1 strategy. Arthritis Res Ther. 2011;13:124.
92. Xoma to stop testing drug as arthritis treatment. Reuters Health. 2014. Available at: http://www.reuters.com/article/2014/03/05/us-xoma-arthritisdrug-idUSBREA241IP20140305. Accessed 25 May 2015.
93. Martel-Pelletier J, Pelletier JP. Osteoarthritis: a single injection of anakinra for treating knee OA? Nat Rev Rheumatol. 2009;5:363–4.
94. Yang KG, Raijmakers NJ, van Arkel ER, Caron JJ, Rijk PC, Willems WJ, et al. Autologous interleukin-1 receptor antagonist improves function and symptoms in osteoarthritis when compared to placebo in a prospective randomized controlled trial. Osteoarthritis Cartilage. 2008;16:498–505.

95. Baltzer AW, Moser C, Jansen SA, Krauspe R. Autologous conditioned serum (Orthokine) is an effective treatment for knee osteoarthritis. Osteoarthritis Cartilage. 2009;17:152–60.
96. Fioravanti A, Fabbroni M, Cerase A, Galeazzi M. Treatment of erosive osteoarthritis of the hands by intra-articular infliximab injections: a pilot study. Rheumatol Int. 2009;29:961–5.
97. Maksymowych WP, Russell AS, Chiu P, Yan A, Jones N, Clare T, et al. Targeting tumour necrosis factor alleviates signs and symptoms of inflammatory osteoarthritis of the knee. Arthritis Res Ther. 2012;14:R206.
98. Verbruggen G, Wittoek R, Vander Cruyssen B, Elewaut D. Tumour necrosis factor blockade for the treatment of erosive osteoarthritis of the interphalangeal finger joints: a double blind, randomised trial on structure modification. Ann Rheum Dis. 2012;71:891–8.
99. Magnano MD, Chakravarty EF, Broudy C, Chung L, Kelman A, Hillygus J, et al. A pilot study of tumor necrosis factor inhibition in erosive/inflammatory osteoarthritis of the hands. J Rheumatol. 2007;34:1323–7.
100. Chevalier X, Ravaud P, Maheu E, Baron G, Rialland A, Vergnaud P, et al. Adalimumab in patients with hand osteoarthritis refractory to analgesics and NSAIDs: a randomised, multicentre, double-blind, placebo-controlled trial. Ann Rheum Dis. 2014. doi:10.1136/annrheumdis-2014-205348.
101. Chevalier X, Eymard F, Richette P. Biologic agents in osteoarthritis: hopes and disappointments. Nat Rev Rheumatol. 2013;9:400–10.

Chapter 11
Safety Profile of Current OA Therapies: Evidence from Clinical Trials

Anthony V. Perruccio and Vinod Chandran

Key Points

- The pharmacologic management of osteoarthritis (OA) is primarily targeted at managing symptoms, and there are several classes of agents in current use. Many of these agents, though efficacious, are associated with adverse events.
- Over time, the complement of adverse events under investigation has broadened, expanding from gastrointestinal (GI) events to also include cardiovascular (CV) and neurological events.
- Pharmacologic management in OA is challenging, especially in older adults particularly due to comorbidities, different causes of pain, and a high rate of polypharmacy. In addition, while OA is treated as a homogeneous diagnostic category, there is evidence to suggest otherwise. This has implications for the pharmacologic management of OA and design of drug trials.

A.V. Perruccio, PhD (✉)
Arthritis Program and Toronto Western Research Institute, Toronto Western Hospital, University Health Network, 399 Bathurst St., East Wing, 1st Floor, Room 449, Toronto, ON M5T 2S8, Canada

Institute of Health Policy, Management and Evaluation, Dalla Lana School of Public Health, Toronto, ON, Canada

Department of Surgery, Faculty of Medicine, University of Toronto, Toronto, ON, Canada
e-mail: perrucci@uhnres.utoronto.ca

V. Chandran, MBBS, MD, DM, PhD
Division of Rheumatology, Department of Medicine, Faculty of Medicine, University of Toronto, Toronto, ON, Canada

Centre for Prognosis Studies in the Rheumatic Diseases, Toronto Western Research Institute, Toronto, ON, Canada

Institute of Medical Science, University of Toronto, Toronto, ON, Canada

M. Kapoor, N.N. Mahomed (eds.), *Osteoarthritis: Pathogenesis, Diagnosis, Available Treatments, Drug Safety, Regenerative and Precision Medicine*,
DOI 10.1007/978-3-319-19560-5_11

- There is significant adverse GI risk associated with nonselective NSAIDs and adverse CV risk associated with both nonselective and selective NSAIDs.
- While topical NSAIDs appear to have a better safety profile than oral NSAIDS, there can be some risk of GI and CVD adverse events associated with their use.
- Intra-articular treatment for knee OA is generally associated with risk of mild adverse events of limited duration. However, there is an identified need for studies of longer follow-up with this intervention. With respect to the use of platelet-rich plasma (PRP), it is suggested that the inclusion of leukocytes in the treatment of OA be avoided.
- Treatment with TNF blockers and IL-1β inhibition is generally well tolerated; majority of adverse events are graded as mild to moderate in severity. Further work with improved study designs is needed.
- Favorable safety profiles are critical from a clinical perspective. Pragmatic studies that include a wider range of people, including the older age groups with a greater burden of arthritis, are necessary to inform clinical practice.

Introduction

The pharmacologic management of OA is primarily targeted at managing symptoms such as pain and swelling, minimizing functional impairment, and preserving quality of life. Several classes of agents are currently in use. While many of these agents may be efficacious, many also are associated with adverse events, and thus there are safety concerns. Disease-modifying agents and novel drug formulations are currently under investigation.

There are a number of adverse events typically investigated in OA pharmacological studies, and over time the complement of adverse events under investigation has broadened. A recent systematic review by Wielage and colleagues traced the development of cost-effectiveness analyses (CEAs) for oral non-disease-altering treatments in OA [1]. Among a number of factors, adverse events appearing in each included CEA were extracted and organized by the authors. Thirty publications of 28 CEAs were identified and evaluated. The authors noted that developments in CEAs included an expanded set of comparators that broadened from nonsteroidal anti-inflammatory drugs (NSAIDs) only to NSAIDs plus gastroprotective agents, cyclooxygenase-2 inhibitors, and opioids. In turn, adverse events expanded from gastrointestinal (GI) events to also include cardiovascular (CV) and neurological events.

From their review, Wielage et al. found that in most models the principal differentiators of comparators were adverse events. GI events were modeled by all but one CEA, an analysis conducted alongside a clinical trial of opioids. All other CEAs considered GI adverse events, particularly GI events associated with treatment with NSAIDs. Starting with Maetzel et al. [2], CV events began to be modeled, with myocardial infarction (MI) modeled first. Schaefer et al. [3] was the first to add congestive heart failure (CHF), and Contreras-Hernandez et al. the first to add stroke [4]. Both Schaefer et al. and Contreras-Hernandez et al. also included renal failure as an event. Wielage et al. conclude that CEA developments have been in response to changes in treatments and the knowledge of their adverse events and that due to greater knowledge of CV events associated with NSAIDs, modeling techniques that incorporate longer time horizons have increasingly been used.

Several factors present challenges in pharmacologically managing OA, particularly in older adults, among whom the prevalence of OA is greatest, particularly due to the presence of multiple chronic conditions or causes of pain and a high rate of polypharmacy. Interestingly, for the first time, the latest guidelines released by the OA Research Society International (OARSI) for the nonsurgical management of knee OA provide treatment recommendations stratified into four clinical subphenotypes in order to enhance the specificity of the treatment recommendations for individuals with varying health profiles and OA burden [5]. The rationale for the stratifications was that comorbidities and the presence of OA in other joints might influence treatment choices.

This chapter presents the safety profile for some of the most commonly used therapeutic agents for OA. It begins with oral drugs, including acetaminophen, NSAIDs, opioids, and serotonin–norepinephrine reuptake inhibitors (SNRIs), for example, and continues with topical, intra-articular, and then biologic agents, such as anti-TNF therapy.

Oral

NSAIDS

Oral NSAIDs are associated with significant gastrointestinal, CV, and renal adverse events (AEs) [6–9]. GI side effects were the first adverse events to be recognized with the use of nonselective NSAIDS. COX-2 selective NSAIDS were developed to reduce GI risk but were subsequently found to be associated with higher CV side effects, after which nonselective NSAIDs also were suggested to be associated with higher event rates. Generally, there is an increase in the development of AEs with increasing NSAID dose [10], for which growing concern prompted the FDA in 2005 to release a Public Health Advisory, physician-education initiative, and class labeling template [11].

Oral NSAID-related GI complications comprise a significant proportion of all medication-related AEs [11, 12]. They are associated with a fivefold increased risk for incidence of peptic ulcer disease and peptic ulcer-related complications, including perforation and hemorrhage [13]. Though not without persistent risk, coadministration of gastroprotective agents can reduce GI adverse event rates [14].

Oral NSAIDs are also associated with small and large intestine disease development [15], and in addition, nonselective NSAIDs are associated with serious CV AEs (MI, stroke, exacerbation of chronic heart failure, hypertension, and CV death) [7, 16, 17]. In a Kaiser Permanente-conducted nested case–control study covering more than 2 million person-years, ibuprofen and naproxen were associated with an odds ratio of 1.26 and 1.36, respectively, for the development of MI [18]. Trelle et al. undertook a meta-analysis in which they identified CV mortality rate ratios of 2.39 and 2.07 for ibuprofen and celecoxib, respectively, compared with placebo [7]. In a retrospective analysis of close to 5,000 patients with stroke, the relative risk for the development of first stroke in patients receiving NSAIDs was 1.2 compared with non-NSAID users [19]. Schneider and colleagues matched >4,000 new NSAID users aged 65+ years with >80,000 controls [20]. Naproxen >750 mg was associated with a relative risk of 3.62 for acute renal failure hospitalizations. Finally, one prospective trial reported a relative risk of 1.26 for the development of chronic kidney failure in patients receiving high-dose (cumulative dose ≥90th percentile) NSAIDs [21].

The duration of NSAID exposure does not appear to be associated with related GI and CV AEs, which can occur at any time following administration [22–24]. Studies have documented that renal complications can develop within hours following NSAID administration, and GI complications within days [22, 23]. Schjerning and colleagues undertook a retrospective analysis for which they reported that duration of NSAID exposure was a poor predictor of CV risk [24], supported by a case–control study undertaken by Helin-Salmivaara and colleagues, where risk for MI was associated with both short- and long-term NSAID use [25].

Though not without persistent risk, the combination of NSAIDs with gastroprotective agents can reduce GI AE rates [14, 26–28].

While selective COX-2 inhibitors (selective for the cyclooxygenase-2 (COX-2) isoenzyme) were developed to reduce GI AE risk, they were associated with serious CV events. In fact, studies reporting increased CV risk with NSAID use initially were shown with COX-2-inhibitor drugs, including rofecoxib (Vioxx), valdecoxib (Bextra), and celecoxib (Celebrex). Both rofecoxib and valdecoxib were removed from the market as a consequence of this risk.

One study undertook systematic reviews of randomized control trials (RCTs) assessing the clinical effectiveness of COX-2 selective NSAIDs (etodolac, meloxicam, celecoxib, rofecoxib, etoricoxib, valdecoxib, and lumiracoxib) for OA and rheumatoid arthritis (RA) [29].

Etodolac was evaluated in 29 RCTs, comparing it to either placebo or nonselective NSAIDs. Compared with nonselective NSAIDs (naproxen, piroxicam, diclofenac, indomethacin, tenoxicam, ibuprofen, nabumetone, or nimesulide), etodolac showed the same or better GI tolerability. Pooled analysis showed no difference in complicated upper GI events (RR: 0.39, 95 % confidence limits: 0.12, 1.24), and significantly fewer clinical upper GI events (RR: 0.32, 95 % CL: 0.15, 0.71). MIs were not reported.

Meloxicam was assessed in 16 RCTs, comparing it with either placebo or nonselective NSAIDs. Compared with naproxen, diclofenac, nabumetone, or piroxicam, meloxicam was of better GI tolerability, associated with fewer clinical upper GI events (RR: 0.53, 95 % CL: 0.29, 0.97), and no difference was shown for complicated upper GI events. The review did not comment on MI risk as there were insufficient events.

Forty RCTs examined celecoxib, compared with placebo, nonselective NSAIDs, or other COX-2 selective NSAIDs. Compared with nonselective NSAIDs, celecoxib was associated with a reduced risk of clinical upper GI (RR: 0.55, 95 % CL: 0.40, 0.76) and complicated upper GI events (RR: 0.57, 95 % CL: 0.35, 0.95), but higher risk of MI (RR: 1.77, 95 % CL: 1.00, 3.11).

Seven RCT studies compared etoricoxib with either placebo or nonselective NSAIDs. Compared with naproxen, diclofenac, and ibuprofen, etoricoxib had equivalent or better GI tolerability. Significant differences in clinical and complicated upper GI events were not shown (RR, 0.23; 95 % CL, 0.05, 1.08; and RR, 0.46; 95 % CL, 0.07, 3.10, respectively). MI events were reported in one trial only (RR, 1.58; 95 % CL, 0.06, 38.66).

While the authors of the systematic review were careful to note that caution in interpretation was warranted as the meta-analysis results were based on small numbers of clinical GI and MI events across trials, the review concluded that COX-2 selective NSAIDs provided superior GI tolerability, although the magnitude of protection varied considerably across individual drugs. In addition, the increased risk of MI associated with COX-2 selective NSAIDs, compared to nonselective NSAIDs, also varied substantially across individual COX-2 NSAIDs [29].

Though rare, NSAID use has been linked to some central nervous system (CNS) side effects [30]. A longitudinal study looking at ibuprofen overdose noted that 30 % of patients experience CNS effects ranging from drowsiness to coma [31]. Aseptic meningitis also has been reported with NSAID use [30].

As a result of safety concerns associated with NSAID use, the American Geriatrics Society's clinical practice guidelines on the pharmacologic management of pain recommends the use of oral NSAIDs sparingly and "with extreme caution," [32] particularly as the increased risk of GI, CV, and renal AEs appears greater in the elderly patient population [33–38].

Acetaminophen

Where recommended, current Osteoarthritis Research Society International (OARSI), American Academy of Orthopaedic Surgeons (AAOS), National Institute for Health and Care Excellence (NICE), European League Against Rheumatism (EULAR), and American College of Rheumatology (ACR) guidelines indicate analgesia-based dose titrations of acetaminophen up to a maximum dose of 4 g/day [39–45]. This limit is principally derived from historical figures demonstrating hepatotoxicity at doses >4 g/day [46, 47]. Even so, when dosed at its recommended upper limit, its safety is not straightforward. Acetaminophen toxicity was the leading cause of acute liver failure in the United States from 1998 to 2003 [48].

Unintentional overdose is the leading cause of acetaminophen-induced hepatotoxicity, including over-the-counter drug polypharmacy [49, 50]; the vast majority of cases had taken acetaminophen to treat pain [48].

In January 2011, the Food and Drug Administration (FDA) instituted a boxed warning emphasizing the risk of liver failure with too much acetaminophen use [51]. Various medical organizations and the FDA have suggested limiting the maximum daily dose to 3 g/day. Investigations also suggest that acetaminophen, at elevated doses, may place patients at risk for upper GI complications. Garcia Rodriguez and Hernandez-Diaz, in a case–control study of nearly a million individuals receiving ≥2 g/day of acetaminophen, reported a relative risk (RR) of 3.6 for upper GI complications [52]. In patients receiving >3 g/day of acetaminophen, Rahme et al. reported elevated hospitalization rates for GI complications [53]. Acetaminophen also may be associated with an increased risk of CV complications. In a large prospective study, Chan et al. observed a dose-dependent relationship between acetaminophen and CV adverse events (MI, stroke, exacerbation of CHF, and CV-related deaths) [54]. Moreover, studies have shown that ongoing use of acetaminophen has a negative influence on blood pressure [55–57].

In addition, a large population-based retrospective cohort study found that older adults combining acetaminophen and NSAIDs had an increased risk of hospitalization for GI events compared with those using either acetaminophen or an NSAID alone [53]. The study was limited, however, by a lack of ability to account for over-the-counter analgesic use. It was such data that led to the aforementioned FDA's 2011 recommendations, with subsequent press releases, communications, and recommendations up to and including April 2014, that manufacturers cap the amount of acetaminophen in prescribed combination products, and that public awareness focus on the risk of acetaminophen-related liver injury [58].

Opioids

Opioids are strong analgesics usually given when other drug and nondrug interventions have failed. This class includes morphine, hydrocodone, oxycodone, hydromorphone, and fentanyl.

In a meta-analysis of 40 studies examining opioids in the treatment of chronic noncancer pain in older adults (predominantly OA of the hip or knee), Papaleontiou and colleagues reported that AEs were common and included constipation, nausea, and dizziness, prompting opioid discontinuation in about 25 % of cases [59]. In a 2007 meta-analysis by Avouac et al., including 18 RCTs comparing safety of opioids versus placebo or nonopioid analgesics in >4,000 OA patients, the most frequent AEs reported with opioids were nausea (30 %), constipation (23 %), dizziness (20 %), somnolence (18 %), and vomiting (13 %). The average treatment discontinuation rate for toxicity was 25 % (818/3,244) in the opioid group (516/1,650, 31 % for strong opioids and 302/1,594, 19 % for weak opioids) and 7 % (116/1,612) in the placebo group [60].

Using Medicare claims data (1995–2005), Solomon and colleagues examined the safety of opioids, COX-2-selective NSAIDS, and nonselective NSAIDs in older adults with arthritis, including >12,000 members after propensity score matching; >80 % in each category had OA [12]. Subjects receiving opioids had a higher risk for adverse CV outcomes compared with those receiving nonselective NSAIDs (hazard ratio: 1.77; 95 % CI: 1.39–2.24). No difference in GI tract bleeding risk was found between opioid and nonselective NSAID users. While both NSAID groups had similar fracture risks, increased risks of fracture were observed for opioid users (HR, 4.47; 95 % CI, 3.12–6.41), along with AEs requiring hospitalization (HR, 1.68; 95 % CI, 1.37–2.07), and all-cause mortality (HR, 1.87; 95 CI, 1.39–2.53), compared to nonselective NSAID users [12]. Solomon et al. conclude by noting that while opioid users experienced moderate risk early in treatment, the numbers needed to harm by 1 year were small and therefore clinically relevant.

Da Costa et al. undertook a review to determine the effects on pain, function, safety, and addiction of oral or transdermal opioids compared with placebo or no intervention in people with knee or hip OA [61]. They included randomized or quasi-randomized controlled trials; studies of tramadol were excluded. The authors reported a greater frequency of AEs among individuals receiving opioids compared with control, with a pooled risk ratio of 1.49 (95 % CL: 1.35, 1.63) for any AE (9 trials; 22 % among opioid users and 15 % among control experienced side effects). While high heterogeneity between different studies was reported, there was no evidence that risk ratios differed between different types of opioids (P-value for interaction: 0.47) or length of treatment duration (P value: 0.09). A risk ratio of 3.76 (95 % CL: 2.93, 4.82) was reported for drop outs due to AEs (19 trials; 6.4 % among opioid users and 1.7 % among placebo controls dropped out due to AEs). The highest pooled risk ratio was associated with oxycodone versus placebo (RR 5.55, 95 % CL: 3.47, 8.87, 9 trials) and the lowest for morphine versus placebo (RR 2.12, 95 % CL: 0.87, 5.15, 2 trials). While confidence limits were wide, the authors reported a nonsignificant test for interaction between type of opioids and relative risk of being withdrawn or dropping out because of AEs (P-value for interaction: 0.41). A risk ratio of 3.35 (95 % CL: 0.83, 13.56) was reported for serious AEs (2 trials; 1.3 % among opioid users and 0.4 % among controls experienced serious AEs). However, due to the low number of trials and events, an analysis of the association between treatment duration or equivalence dose and log relative risk for this outcome was not performed. Finally, withdrawal symptoms occurred more often in opioid compared with control treatment groups (odds ratio, 2.76; 95 % CL, 2.02, 3.77; 3 trials; 2.4 % of participants in opioid and 0.9 % of participants in control groups experienced withdrawal symptoms).

Finally, an often overlooked potential complication of chronic opioid therapy is its association with the development of opioid-induced hyperalgesia and tolerance, which can reduce analgesic efficacy over time and complicate pain management [62].

Generally, the prevalence of nausea, constipation, dizziness, vomiting, and drowsiness associated with opioid use has altered prescription practices, generally reducing opioid use, as has the potential risk for addiction associated with opioid use [60, 63, 64].

Serotonin–Norepinephrine Reuptake Inhibitors (SNRIs)

Tricyclic antidepressants and serotonin–norepinephrine reuptake inhibitors (SNRIs) have been investigated for use in OA [65–68]. Duloxetine is the only antidepressant currently approved by the FDA for the management of OA [69, 70].

There have been three large placebo-controlled RCTs assessing duloxetine as treatment for symptomatic knee OA [65, 66, 71]. In the initial study by Chappel et al. [65], patients were randomized to duloxetine beginning at a dose of 30 mg/day and increasing to 60 mg/day from week 2 to 6 or placebo. Those in the duloxetine group were subsequently further randomized to continue on 60 mg daily or increase to 120 mg daily at week 7. In the second trial by Chappel et al. [66], there was a slight difference in design, as only patients who did not have a predefined improvement in pain at week 7 had their dose increased to 120 mg daily in a blinded fashion. These two studies led to the FDA approval of duloxetine for the treatment of chronic knee pain due to OA. More duloxetine-treated patients compared with placebo-treated patients experienced ≥1 treatment-emergent AEs ($p=0.003$, number needed to harm = 8). Frakes et al. [71] found that duloxetine was superior to placebo when added to therapy with background NSAIDs in patients who continued to have moderate pain in their knee due to OA. All of these studies noted similar adverse effects of GI upset including nausea, constipation, and dry mouth as well as changes in appetite.

Though generally well tolerated, SNRIs have, in rare circumstances, been associated with hepatotoxicity and serotonin syndrome, a condition characterized by confusion, autonomic hyperactivity, and neuromuscular dysfunction [72–74]. Assessment of patient risk for AE development is important.

Topical Treatments

Topical NSAIDs (including gels, creams, and sprays [75]) appear to be safer than oral NSAIDs [76–79]. In some studies, these have demonstrated comparable analgesic efficacy to traditional oral NSAIDs [60, 75, 80, 81]. They directly deliver medication to the skin around the affected area [82, 83] and are associated with lower systemic absorption and lower incidence of GI (dyspepsia, abdominal pain, and diarrhea), renal, and CV AEs compared with traditional oral NSAIDs [81–87]. Nevertheless, one systematic review reported that about 20 % of patients receiving a prescription-strength topical NSAID reported a systemic adverse event such as GI problems and headache [85]. Since 2009, the FDA requires that topical NSAIDs carry the same box warning as oral NSAIDs regarding their potential for GI and CV AEs and hepatic function test abnormalities [88].

A recent study reviewed RCTs of topical capsaicin use in OA [89]. Five double-blind RCTs and one case-crossover trial of topical capsaicin use were identified, with formulations ranging from 0.025 to 0.075 % and trial durations from 4 to 12 weeks. Trials assessed OA of the knee ($n=3$), hand ($n=1$), and a mix of joints ($n=2$). Capsaicin treatment efficacy was evaluated vs. placebo. Capsaicin was reported as being safe and well tolerated, with no systemic toxicity. Mild application site burning affected 35–100 % of capsaicin-treated patients with a risk ratio of 4.22 (95 % CI 3.25–5.48, $n=5$ trials); incidence peaked at week 1 and declined over time. The authors concluded that topical capsaicin treatment four times daily is well tolerated.

Intra-articular Treatments

In a systematic review evaluating the efficacy and safety of intra-articular corticosteroids for treatment of knee OA, Bellamy et al. reported no statistically significant differences in total number of withdrawals overall or in the number of withdrawals due to lack of efficacy compared to placebo. Further, no statistically significant differences were detected in the number of patients reporting postinjection flare or in the number of patients reporting local discomfort when compared to placebo [90]. Similar safety findings were reported from studies assessing corticosteroid against hyaluronan or hylan, with no statistically significant differences in any of the extracted safety outcomes. Overall, most AEs from corticosteroid injection were rated as mild/moderate, and steroid injections were deemed to be safe [90–93].

A Cochrane review that synthesized results from 76 trials examining outcomes in those with knee OA found that when compared with placebo, treatment with hyaluronan and hylan derivatives (viscosupplements) noted no major safety issues, and in general, few AEs were reported in the hyaluronan/hylan trials included in their analyses [94]. Generally, typical AEs examined included total withdrawals overall, withdrawals due to inefficacy, AEs, number of patients affected, number of patients with nonserious AEs, and/or number of patients with serious AEs, as reported by included studies.

Rutjes and colleagues concluded that viscosupplementation for knee OA is associated with serious unexplained AEs [95]. They examined randomized trials that compared viscosupplementation with hyaluronic acid with sham or nonintervention control in adults with knee OA. The most frequent events were related to the GI system (2 events among viscosupplementation patients versus 8 events among control patients), CV system (5 versus 2 events), cancer (6 versus 0 events), and musculoskeletal system (4 versus 2 events). Though indicating that trial quality was generally low and safety data often not reported, Rutjes et al. concluded by discouraging the use of the intervention and suggested that an individual patient data meta-analysis would be needed to explore the issue of AEs further. An important need for using extreme caution in interpreting these findings was raised, however, as this conclusion was disputed by others who pointed out that the serious AEs attributed to the hyaluronic acid treatment in Rutjes et al.'s review had been reported as unrelated by primary study authors, noting also biological implausibility and lack of previous history of systemic toxicity affiliated with hyaluronic acid [96].

Miller and Block undertook a systematic review and meta-analysis of randomized saline-controlled trials to determine the safety and efficacy of US-approved intra-articular hyaluronic acid injections for symptomatic knee OA [97]. Twenty-nine studies with nearly 5,000 subjects (hyaluronic acid, 2,673; saline, 2,193) were included, with inclusion of different molecular weights of hyaluronic acid and different injection schedules. They reported no statistically significant differences between groups for any safety outcome, including serious AEs ($P=0.12$), treatment-related serious AEs ($P=1.0$), study withdrawal ($P=1.0$), and study withdrawal related to AEs ($P=0.46$). A critical assessment of this review, however, indicated that the limited duration of and size of trials meant that safety outcomes were imprecisely estimated, so the authors' conclusions on safety risk "may have confused lack of effect with lack of ability to detect effects" [98].

Recently, Bannaru and colleagues undertook a systematic review and meta-analysis examining intra-articular hyaluronic acid in comparison with oral NSAIDs for knee OA [99]. Five trials (712 participants) were included, with four different hyaluronic acid preparations used in these trials. GI AEs were more common in the NSAIDs group, and injection site pain was the most common adverse event reported in the hyaluronic acid group. Three serious AEs were reported among those receiving hyaluronic acid, though these events were reported as unrelated to the intervention. In the NSAIDs group, one related GI bleed was reported. Only two trials reported on withdrawals due to AEs by treatment group with no significant differences noted. While Bannaru et al. reported no safety concerns, follow-up length was short and adverse event reporting variable across trials, making definitive assessments of safety challenging, particularly as the study was unlikely to have captured the serious GI risk associated with longer NSAID use [7, 100–102].

One meta-analysis and systematic review explored the effectiveness and safety of hyaluronic acid administration for ankle OA [103]. Chang et al. reported that among the 285 participants undergoing the administration of intra-articular HA, 43 (15 %) participants had adverse effects. Transient postinjection pain was reported by 28 participants, with other AEs including inguinal lymph node enlargement ($n=1$), ankle effusion ($n=1$), and local pruritus ($n=1$). All adverse reactions resolved spontaneously without specific treatment. The authors conclude by noting that the side effects after intra-articular HA injection were mostly minor and self-limited. However, for postinjection pain, they found that the majority of such cases originated from studies that used hyaluronic acid (Synvisc), an HA product with a molecular weight of up to 6,000 kDa [104–108]. Although another trial that employed Synvisc did not report such AEs [109], the trial conductors administered HA arthroscopically rather than through conventional injection. Findings are in agreement with a recent meta-analysis indicating that the use of high-molecular-weight HA is associated with an increased risk of local adverse effects [110]. The authors recommend not using high-molecular-weight products in an attempt to lessen the likelihood of irritation resulting from extra-articular injection.

Following from their systematic reviews, Colen et al. [111, 112] concluded that well-designed RCTs assessing the effects (benefits and harms) of hyaluronic acid, incorporating longer duration of follow-up and larger samples, for treating knee and other OA are warranted.

Platelet-Rich Plasma (PRP)

Patel et al. [113], in a level 1 evidence study comparing PRP and saline solution, assessed 78 patients with bilateral knee OA (156 knees) graded 1 or 2. The sample was divided randomly into three groups: group 1, single injection of PRP; group 2, 2 injections 3 weeks apart; and group 3, single injection of normal saline. White blood cell (WBC)-filtered PRP (PRP type 4B) was used. Six patients (22.2 %) in group 1 and 11 patients (44 %) in group 2 had AEs at the time of injection, significant in comparison with group 3 which reported no AEs. Five patients (20 %) in the second group had AEs during the second injection, which variably included dizziness, syncope, nausea, headache, gastritis, sweating, and tachycardia, which were of short duration. Four patients in group 1 and 3 in group 2 had pain and stiffness after injection for 2 days. It was noted that the AE group had a significantly higher ($P = .02$) quantity of platelets injected compared with the group with no AEs.

Filardo et al. [114] undertook a randomized double-blind prospective trial assessing the efficacy of PRP compared to hyaluronic acid injections for the treatment of knee chondropathy or OA (Kellegren-Lawrence ≤ 3). One hundred nine patients received a cycle of 3 weekly injections administered blindly (54 treated with PRP, 55 with HA). Only minor AEs were detected in some patients, such as mild pain and effusion after the injections, in particular in the PRP group, where a significantly higher postinjective pain reaction was observed ($p = 0.039$), resolving within a few days.

Finally, in a systematic review [115] assessing safety and effectiveness, intra-articular injection of plasma rich in growth factors (PRGF) in the treatment of knee OA, Anitua et al. reviewed five studies comparing PRGF against a control group (HA or leukocyte-enriched PRP). Although all studies included a safety analysis of the treatments administered, only three listed the AEs [116–118]. Overall, no severe AEs were observed; they were generally mild and evenly distributed between the groups. Some of them, both related and unrelated to treatment, included nonspecific low-back pain, other knee surgery, febrile syndrome, abdominal pain, knee and hip pain, itching of both outer thighs, headache, dizziness, sciatica, cold, and pain after third injection.

In a double-blind multicenter clinical trial ($n = 173$) comparing efficacy and safety of PRGF-Endoret versus hyaluronic acid (3 injections on a weekly basis) as a short-term treatment for knee pain from OA, Sánchez et al. reported that AEs were mild and evenly distributed between groups [117]. Fifty AEs were reported in 50 patients, 26 in the PRGF-Endoret group and 24 in the HA group. They were generally mild and evenly distributed between the groups ($P = .811$). An excess of 90 % of these in each group was deemed unrelated to the type of treatment. The number of patients who withdrew because of AEs was similar between groups. Vaquerizo et al. reported 16 AEs in their study: 7 in the PRGF group and 9 in the control group [118]. All of the AEs in the PRGF group and 7 of 9 events in the control group were associated with the infiltration and were related to pain. In the study by Filardo et al. [116] both procedures showed a statistically significant difference in the number of AEs observed after the injections: both pain and swelling reaction were more frequent in the leukocyte-enriched PRP group than in the PRGF-treated group ($P<0.001$ for pain, $P=0.03$ for swelling). Brief comments about AEs were included by the two remaining studies, events which appeared related to the injection procedure, such as pain and swelling of short duration [119, 120]. Due to significant differences in the control group among the five studies and PRGF administration schedule differences, a formal meta-analysis could not be carried out.

It has been observed that the incidence of AEs related to pain and swelling increases in patients receiving PRP containing leukocytes. It is postulated that high concentrations of leukocytes can generate temporary inflammation, which in some instances may be reflected clinically [121]. Anitua et al. conclude that it is especially important to avoid the inclusion of leukocytes in the treatment of OA because their inclusion might not yield the optimal anabolic environment for OA treatment [115, 122–124].

Strontium Ranelate: Bone Turnover Agent Favoring Bone Formation

Reginster et al. recently reported from a large randomized placebo-controlled trial in which patients with knee OA (Kellgren–Lawrence grade 2 or 3, and joint space width 2.5–5 mm) were randomly allocated to strontium ranelate 1 g/day ($n=558$), 2 g/day ($n=566$) or placebo ($n=559$) [125]. Strontium ranelate was reported to be well tolerated. The rate of venous thromboembolic events was <1 % in all groups. The number of emergent AEs reported was similar across groups, 85.8%, 87.9%, and 86.5 % in the 1 g, 2 g, and placebo groups, as well as the number of serious emergent AEs, 17.0 %, 16.5 % and 17.4 %, respectively [126]. Diarrhea was reported by 3.3 %, 6.6 %, and 2.7 %, respectively; nausea by 2.0 %, 2.7 %, and 1.8 %, respectively; and headache by 1.6 % in each drug group and 0.7 % in the placebo group. Regarding cutaneous safety, 16.3 % of the patients reported skin disorders in the 2 g group compared to 12.4 % and 12.2 % in the 1 g group and in the placebo group, respectively. Creatine phosphokinase increased from baseline with treatment (11.7 ± 85.6 and 20.7 ± 104.4 IU/l with 1 and 2 g/day, respectively), but not placebo (-0.4 ± 68.1 IU/l) [125]. Eight patients (3, 1, and 4 in the 1 g/day, 2 g/day, and placebo groups, respectively) had values greater than five times the upper limit of normal. No cases of drug reaction with eosinophilia and systemic symptoms were reported. Concerns relating strontium ranelate use to CV events have been raised, and subsequent contraindications have been identified [127]. In a post hoc assessment of their data, where patients with contraindications were excluded, Reginster reported the number of MIs as comparable between the three treatment groups: 1 event in the 1 g group, 2 in the 2 g group, and 1 in the placebo group [126].

Tanezumab: NGF Blocker

There are currently no approved biological therapies for patients with OA. Tanezumab is a monoclonal antibody that inhibits nerve growth factor and is administered intravenously. Recent studies have shown mild to moderate AEs occurring with its use [128–131].

Lane et al. [128], in their proof-of-concept trial, randomly assigned 450 patients with knee OA to receive 10, 25, 50, 100, or 200 μg/kg body weight of tanezumab or placebo on days 1 and 56 administered intravenously. AE rates of 68 % and 55 % in the tanezumab and placebo groups, respectively, were reported. The most common among tanezumab-treated patients were headache (9 %), upper respiratory tract infection (7 %), and paresthesia (7 %). Treatment-related incidence of AEs was higher among patients treated with higher doses (28 % and 35 % in the groups receiving 100 μg and 200 μg/kg, respectively, vs. 11–18 % in the groups receiving lower doses). Peripheral sensory symptoms were reported in 14 % of the patients receiving tanezumab and 4 % among those receiving placebo. While the AEs were predominantly mild in 80 % of those receiving tanezumab, serious AEs were reported in 6 patients (2 %) receiving tanezumab (appendicitis, bacterial arthritis, cellulitis, spinal stenosis, breast cancer, and syncope) and in 1 patient (1 %) receiving placebo (noncardiac chest pain).

In several other phase III trials, tanezumab therapy was associated with rapid, progressive OA requiring total knee arthroplasty [132–134]. In June 2010, the US FDA placed all clinical trials of β-NGF antagonists on hold after cases of osteonecrosis were reported with the use of tanezumab in OA. Although investigations found that only 2 of 87 cases represented a drug-related side effect, 68 cases of progressive OA were associated with higher doses of tanezumab (10 mg) or its combination with NSAIDs [135]. Two key recommendations were to exclude tanezumab 10 mg from further investigation in OA and to exclude concomitant use of NSAIDs. β-NGF antagonists trials were allowed to subsequently resume. Even so, Seidel and Lane suggest that the cases of rapid progressive OA indicate a need for further investigation and great caution in monitoring and documenting adverse effects [132].

A multicenter phase II study by Schnitzer et al. using an open-label, multiple-dose extension of an earlier randomized clinical trial prioritized safety as the end point [130]. Minimal evidence of AEs with repeat injections was shown. Nagashima et al. [129] investigated the use of tanezumab in 83 patients with moderate and severe OA – all AEs were considered mild to moderate in severity. Overall, the use of tanezumab was considered safe and well tolerated.

In a phase III RCT, Brown et al. [133, 134] assessed NGF blockade by tanezumab versus placebo in hip and knee OA. The 690 knee and 621 hip patients received 1 of 3 intravenous doses of tanezumab (2.5 mg, 5 mg, or 10 mg) or placebo. Those who received tanezumab had a 55–60 % incidence of AEs, compared with 48 % in the placebo group, among the knee group, and a 55–58 % AE incidence, compared with 44 % in the placebo group, among the hip group. In general, the authors concluded that tanezumab was well tolerated, and reports of worsening OA and/or joint replacement were distributed equally among treatment groups. In both studies, the tanezumab OA clinical program was temporarily placed on hold because of AEs leading to joint replacement. Spierings et al. [131] investigated the efficacy and safety of tanezumab for hip and knee OA in a phase III RCT. Six hundred sixty patients were assigned to receive intravenous tanezumab (5 mg or 10 mg in 8-week intervals), oral controlled-release (CR) oxycodone (10–40 mg every 12 h), or placebo. AEs were more frequent with oxycodone (63.3 %) than tanezumab (41–45 %) or placebo (36 %). The more common AEs in the tanezumab group were nausea, headache, nasopharyngitis, arthralgia, and paresthesia. AEs of abnormal peripheral sensation were reported more frequently in the tanezumab groups than in the placebo or oxycodone CR groups, including paresthesia, and hypoesthesia. Categorization of final neurological consultations as suggestive of a new or worsened peripheral neuropathy was highest in the tanezumab 5-mg group (3.7 %) and lowest in the oxycodone CR group (0.6 %). The incidence of serious AEs was similar among treatment groups. Spierings et al. [136] concluded that the safety profile of tanezumab has not been thoroughly evaluated and agreed with Panzram and Schiltenwolf [137] that further studies are needed to identify which patients are at risk as well as to evaluate the optimal dose and duration of tanezumab treatment.

TNF Blockers

There have been trials evaluating tumor necrosis factor-alpha (TNF-α) inhibitors in OA [138, 139], with the majority involving the use of systemic TNF-α inhibitors in patients with erosive hand OA. Verbruggen et al. assessed the effects of adalimumab in controlling progression of structural damage in erosive hand OA [139]. Sixty patients with erosive hand OA received 40 mg adalimumab or placebo, subcutaneously, every 2 weeks during a 12-month randomized double-blind trial. No serious AEs or malignancies were reported, nor were significant differences in numbers of AEs between groups found. Magnano et al. [138] reported from an open-label pilot study of 12 patients with symptomatic erosive hand OA who received adalimumab 40 mg subcutaneously every 2 weeks, with safety assessed 4 weeks after the final dose. All AEs were graded as mild to moderate in severity; none required withdrawal from the study. The most commonly reported AEs were injection site reactions. A total of 6 mild infectious AEs were experienced by 4 patients; 3 required oral antibiotics. The study was limited, however, in that no comparator control group was included.

In an open-label study, Maksymowych and colleagues evaluated the use of adalimumab in 20 patients with knee OA and evidence of clinical effusion. Patients received subcutaneous injections of 40 mg adalimumab every other week over 12 weeks [140]. After 12 weeks, there were no safety concerns; AEs were minor with no serious events recorded. Treatment was well tolerated and completed by 17 patients with withdrawals unrelated to AEs.

The effects of adalimumab injections in patients with hand OA who were unresponsive to analgesics and NSAIDs have been examined in a randomized, placebo-controlled trial [141]. Patients ($n = 85$) were randomized to adalimumab 40 mg for two subcutaneous injections at a 15-day interval or placebo and monitored for 6 months. A similar adverse event rate was reported for both groups. Overall adverse event was 73.0 % (27/37) in the placebo group and 75.6 % (31/41) in the adalimumab group. Severe AEs were reported in 5.4 % (2/37) in the placebo group and 9.8 % (4/41) in the adalimumab group. No serious AEs related to subcutaneous injection of adalimumab were reported. Pain of mild or minor intensity associated with subcutaneous injection was observed in six patients: three in the treatment group and three in the placebo group.

IL-1β Inhibition

In 2005, Chevalier et al. showed in a phase II clinical trial that intra-articular administration of the IL-1Ra anakinra (up to 150 mg) was well tolerated and safe in patients with symptomatic knee OA [142]. Subsequently in 2009, they conducted a randomized, multicenter, double-blind, placebo-controlled trial, in which 160 patients with painful knee OA were allocated at random in a 2:2:1 ratio to single intra-articular injections of 150 mg or 50 mg of IL-1Ra or placebo [143]. The only adverse effect was an increased rate of upper respiratory infections in patients treated with 150 mg of IL-1Ra (6 %) compared with those in the placebo group (1 %). In a double-blind, placebo-controlled randomized trial, investigators evaluated the effect of treatment with AMG 108 in 159 patients with knee OA [144]. The study had two parts. In Part A, 64 patients were randomized 3:1 in each of four cohorts (12 active; four placebo) to receive AMG 108 subcutaneously (75 mg or 300 mg) or intravenously (100 mg or 300 mg) or placebo every 4 weeks for 12 weeks. In Part B, 160 patients were randomized 1:1 to receive 300 mg AMG 108 subcutaneously or placebo, using the same dosing schedule. The authors reported that AMG 108 was well tolerated. Most AEs, infectious AEs, serious AEs and infections, and withdrawals from study due to AEs occurred at similar rates in the AMG 108 and placebo groups [144]. The incidence of serious infections was similar between the two groups. However, the AMG 108 development program was stopped after the death of an 80-year-old man, in whom an indirect role for neutropenia was suspected.

Conclusions

Given the epidemiological profile of the OA population, and the reality of an aging population, the management of OA pain will require careful consideration of a number of age-related issues which can affect treatment safety. Aging brings about physiological changes which can affect the way drugs are absorbed, distributed, metabolized, and eliminated by the body [145–147]. These physiological changes occur at different rates, calling attention to the need for personalized treatment plans, particularly for older adults [148]. As well, medical comorbidities are common in OA [149–153], and investigators should give consideration to prevalent high-risk populations in OA drug trials. Favorable safety profiles are critical from a clinical perspective. Therefore, pragmatic studies that include a wider range of people, including the older age groups with a greater burden of arthritis, are requisite to inform clinical practice.

References

1. Wielage RC, Myers JA, Klein RW, Happich M. Cost-effectiveness analyses of osteoarthritis oral therapies: a systematic review. Appl Health Econ Health Policy. 2013;11(6):593–618.
2. Maetzel A, Krahn M, Naglie G. The cost effectiveness of rofecoxib and celecoxib in patients with osteoarthritis or rheumatoid arthritis. Arthritis Rheum. 2003;49(3):283–92.
3. Schaefer M, DeLattre M, Gao X, Stephens J, Botteman M, Morreale A. Assessing the cost-effectiveness of COX-2 specific inhibitors for arthritis in the Veterans Health Administration. Curr Med Res Opin. 2005;21(1):47–60.
4. Contreras-Hernandez I, Mould-Quevedo JF, Torres-Gonzalez R, Goycochea-Robles MV, Pacheco-Dominguez RL, Sanchez-Garcia S, et al. Cost-effectiveness analysis for joint pain treatment in patients with osteoarthritis treated at the Instituto Mexicano del Seguro Social (IMSS): comparison of nonsteroidal anti-inflammatory drugs (NSAIDs) vs. cyclooxygenase-2 selective inhibitors. Cost Eff Resour Alloc. 2008;6:21.
5. McAlindon TE, Bannuru RR, Sullivan MC, Arden NK, Berenbaum F, Bierma-Zeinstra SM, et al. OARSI guidelines for the non-surgical management of knee osteoarthritis. Osteoarthritis Cartilage. 2014;22(3):363–88.
6. Perez GS, Garcia Rodriguez LA, Raiford DS, Duque OA, Ris RJ. Nonsteroidal anti-inflammatory drugs and the risk of hospitalization for acute renal failure. Arch Intern Med. 1996;156(21):2433–9.
7. Trelle S, Reichenbach S, Wandel S, Hildebrand P, Tschannen B, Villiger PM, et al. Cardiovascular safety of non-steroidal anti-inflammatory drugs: network meta-analysis. BMJ. 2011;342:c7086.
8. Wolfe MM, Lichtenstein DR, Singh G. Gastrointestinal toxicity of nonsteroidal antiinflammatory drugs. N Engl J Med. 1999;340(24):1888–99.
9. Whelton A. Renal aspects of treatment with conventional nonsteroidal anti-inflammatory drugs versus cyclooxygenase-2-specific inhibitors. Am J Med. 2001;110(Suppl 3A):33S–42.
10. Hunt RH, Choquette D, Craig BN, De AC, Habal F, Fulthorpe G, et al. Approach to managing musculoskeletal pain: acetaminophen, cyclooxygenase-2 inhibitors, or traditional NSAIDs? Can Fam Physician. 2007;53(7):1177–84.
11. U.S. Food and Drug Administration. Public Health Advisory – FDA announces important changes and additional warnings for COX-2 selective and non-selective Non-Steroidal Anti-

Inflammatory Drugs (NSAIDs). U.S. Food and Drug Administration, U.S. Department of Health & Human Services, Silver Spring, MD; 2013.
12. Solomon DH, Rassen JA, Glynn RJ, Lee J, Levin R, Schneeweiss S. The comparative safety of analgesics in older adults with arthritis. Arch Intern Med. 2010;170(22):1968–76.
13. Hernandez-Diaz S, Rodriguez LA. Association between nonsteroidal anti-inflammatory drugs and upper gastrointestinal tract bleeding/perforation: an overview of epidemiologic studies published in the 1990s. Arch Intern Med. 2000;160(14):2093–9.
14. Leontiadis GI, Sreedharan A, Dorward S, Barton P, Delaney B, Howden CW, et al. Systematic reviews of the clinical effectiveness and cost-effectiveness of proton pump inhibitors in acute upper gastrointestinal bleeding. Health Technol Assess. 2007;11(51):iii–iv, 1–164.
15. Lanas A. A review of the gastrointestinal safety data – a gastroenterologist's perspective. Rheumatology (Oxford). 2010;49(Suppl 2):ii3–10.
16. Gislason GH, Jacobsen S, Rasmussen JN, Rasmussen S, Buch P, Friberg J, et al. Risk of death or reinfarction associated with the use of selective cyclooxygenase-2 inhibitors and non-selective nonsteroidal antiinflammatory drugs after acute myocardial infarction. Circulation. 2006;113(25):2906–13.
17. McGettigan P, Henry D. Cardiovascular risk with non-steroidal anti-inflammatory drugs: systematic review of population-based controlled observational studies. PLoS Med. 2011;8(9), e1001098.
18. Graham DJ, Campen D, Hui R, Spence M, Cheetham C, Levy G, et al. Risk of acute myocardial infarction and sudden cardiac death in patients treated with cyclo-oxygenase 2 selective and non-selective non-steroidal anti-inflammatory drugs: nested case-control study. Lancet. 2005;365(9458):475–81.
19. Bak S, Andersen M, Tsiropoulos I, Garcia Rodriguez LA, Hallas J, Christensen K, et al. Risk of stroke associated with nonsteroidal anti-inflammatory drugs: a nested case-control study. Stroke. 2003;34(2):379–86.
20. Schneider V, Levesque LE, Zhang B, Hutchinson T, Brophy JM. Association of selective and conventional nonsteroidal antiinflammatory drugs with acute renal failure: a population-based, nested case-control analysis. Am J Epidemiol. 2006;164(9):881–9.
21. Gooch K, Culleton BF, Manns BJ, Zhang J, Alfonso H, Tonelli M, et al. NSAID use and progression of chronic kidney disease. Am J Med. 2007;120(3):280–7.
22. Brater DC. Anti-inflammatory agents and renal function. Semin Arthritis Rheum. 2002;32(3 Suppl 1):33–42.
23. Richy F, Bruyere O, Ethgen O, Rabenda V, Bouvenot G, Audran M, et al. Time dependent risk of gastrointestinal complications induced by non-steroidal anti-inflammatory drug use: a consensus statement using a meta-analytic approach. Ann Rheum Dis. 2004;63(7):759–66.
24. Schjerning Olsen AM, Fosbol EL, Lindhardsen J, Folke F, Charlot M, Selmer C, et al. Duration of treatment with nonsteroidal anti-inflammatory drugs and impact on risk of death and recurrent myocardial infarction in patients with prior myocardial infarction: a nationwide cohort study. Circulation. 2011;123(20):2226–35.
25. Helin-Salmivaara A, Virtanen A, Vesalainen R, Gronroos JM, Klaukka T, Idanpaan-Heikkila JE, et al. NSAID use and the risk of hospitalization for first myocardial infarction in the general population: a nationwide case-control study from Finland. Eur Heart J. 2006;27(14):1657–63.
26. Gigante A, Tagarro I. Non-steroidal anti-inflammatory drugs and gastroprotection with proton pump inhibitors: a focus on ketoprofen/omeprazole. Clin Drug Investig. 2012;32(4):221–33.
27. Hochberg MC, Fort JG, Svensson O, Hwang C, Sostek M. Fixed-dose combination of enteric-coated naproxen and immediate-release esomeprazole has comparable efficacy to celecoxib for knee osteoarthritis: two randomized trials. Curr Med Res Opin. 2011;27(6):1243–53.
28. Laine L, Kivitz AJ, Bello AE, Grahn AY, Schiff MH, Taha AS. Double-blind randomized trials of single-tablet ibuprofen/high-dose famotidine vs. ibuprofen alone for reduction of gastric and duodenal ulcers. Am J Gastroenterol. 2012;107(3):379–86.
29. Chen YF, Jobanputra P, Barton P, Bryan S, Fry-Smith A, Harris G, et al. Cyclooxygenase-2 selective non-steroidal anti-inflammatory drugs (etodolac, meloxicam, celecoxib, rofecoxib,

etoricoxib, valdecoxib and lumiracoxib) for osteoarthritis and rheumatoid arthritis: a systematic review and economic evaluation. Health Technol Assess. 2008;12(11):1–278, iii.
30. Auriel E, Regev K, Korczyn AD. Nonsteroidal anti-inflammatory drugs exposure and the central nervous system. Handb Clin Neurol. 2014;119:577–84.
31. McElwee NE, Veltri JC, Bradford DC, Rollins DE. A prospective, population-based study of acute ibuprofen overdose: complications are rare and routine serum levels not warranted. Ann Emerg Med. 1990;19(6):657–62.
32. American Geriatrics Society Panel on Pharmacological Management of Persistent Pain in Older Persons. Pharmacological management of persistent pain in older persons. J Am Geriatr Soc. 2009;57(8):1331–46.
33. Cannon CP, Curtis SP, FitzGerald GA, Krum H, Kaur A, Bolognese JA, et al. Cardiovascular outcomes with etoricoxib and diclofenac in patients with osteoarthritis and rheumatoid arthritis in the Multinational Etoricoxib and Diclofenac Arthritis Long-term (MEDAL) programme: a randomised comparison. Lancet. 2006;368(9549):1771–81.
34. Hinz B, Dormann H, Brune K. More pronounced inhibition of cyclooxygenase 2, increase in blood pressure, and reduction of heart rate by treatment with diclofenac compared with celecoxib and rofecoxib. Arthritis Rheum. 2006;54(1):282–91.
35. Levesque LE, Brophy JM, Zhang B. The risk for myocardial infarction with cyclooxygenase-2 inhibitors: a population study of elderly adults. Ann Intern Med. 2005;142(7):481–9.
36. Roth SH, Bennett RE. Nonsteroidal anti-inflammatory drug gastropathy. Recognition and response. Arch Intern Med. 1987;147(12):2093–100.
37. Roth SH. Coming to terms with nonsteroidal anti-inflammatory drug gastropathy. Drugs. 2012;72(7):873–9.
38. Turajane T, Wongbunnak R, Patcharatrakul T, Ratansumawong K, Poigampetch Y, Songpatanasilp T. Gastrointestinal and cardiovascular risk of non-selective NSAIDs and COX-2 inhibitors in elderly patients with knee osteoarthritis. J Med Assoc Thai. 2009;92 Suppl 6:S19–26.
39. American Academy of Orthopaedic Surgeons (2013) Treatment of osteoarthritis of the knee evidence-based guideline. Am Acad Orthop Surg. 2. p. 343.
40. Jordan KM, Arden NK, Doherty M, Bannwarth B, Bijlsma JW, Dieppe P, et al. EULAR Recommendations 2003: an evidence based approach to the management of knee osteoarthritis: report of a Task Force of the Standing Committee for International Clinical Studies Including Therapeutic Trials (ESCISIT). Ann Rheum Dis. 2003;62(12):1145–55.
41. National Collaborating Centre for Chronic Conditions. Osteoarthritis: national clinical guideline for care and management in adults. London: Royal College of Physicians; 2008.
42. Zhang W, Doherty M, Arden N, Bannwarth B, Bijlsma J, Gunther KP, et al. EULAR evidence based recommendations for the management of hip osteoarthritis: report of a task force of the EULAR Standing Committee for International Clinical Studies Including Therapeutics (ESCISIT). Ann Rheum Dis. 2005;64(5):669–81.
43. Zhang W, Moskowitz RW, Nuki G, Abramson S, Altman RD, Arden N, et al. OARSI recommendations for the management of hip and knee osteoarthritis, part I: critical appraisal of existing treatment guidelines and systematic review of current research evidence. Osteoarthritis Cartilage. 2007;15(9):981–1000.
44. Zhang W, Moskowitz RW, Nuki G, Abramson S, Altman RD, Arden N, et al. OARSI recommendations for the management of hip and knee osteoarthritis, Part II: OARSI evidence-based, expert consensus guidelines. Osteoarthritis Cartilage. 2008;16(2):137–62.
45. Hochberg MC, Altman RD, April KT, Benkhalti M, Guyatt G, McGowan J, et al. American College of Rheumatology 2012 recommendations for the use of nonpharmacologic and pharmacologic therapies in osteoarthritis of the hand, hip, and knee. Arthritis Care Res (Hoboken). 2012;64(4):465–74.
46. James LP, Mayeux PR, Hinson JA. Acetaminophen-induced hepatotoxicity. Drug Metab Dispos. 2003;31(12):1499–506.
47. Zhang W, Nuki G, Moskowitz RW, Abramson S, Altman RD, Arden NK, et al. OARSI recommendations for the management of hip and knee osteoarthritis: part III: changes in evi-

dence following systematic cumulative update of research published through January 2009. Osteoarthritis Cartilage. 2010;18(4):476–99.
48. Larson AM, Polson J, Fontana RJ, Davern TJ, Lalani E, Hynan LS, et al. Acetaminophen-induced acute liver failure: results of a United States multicenter, prospective study. Hepatology. 2005;42(6):1364–72.
49. Gyamlani GG, Parikh CR. Acetaminophen toxicity: suicidal vs. accidental. Crit Care. 2002;6(2):155–9.
50. Schiodt FV, Rochling FA, Casey DL, Lee WM. Acetaminophen toxicity in an urban county hospital. N Engl J Med. 1997;337(16):1112–7.
51. U.S. Food and Drug Administration. FDA drug safety communication: prescription acetaminophen products to be limited to 325 mg per dosage unit; boxed warning will highlight potential for severe liver failure. U.S. Food and Drug Administration, U.S. Department of Health & Human Services, Silver Spring, MD; 2014.
52. Garcia Rodriguez LA, Hernandez-Diaz S. Relative risk of upper gastrointestinal complications among users of acetaminophen and nonsteroidal anti-inflammatory drugs. Epidemiology. 2001;12(5):570–6.
53. Rahme E, Barkun A, Nedjar H, Gaugris S, Watson D. Hospitalizations for upper and lower GI events associated with traditional NSAIDs and acetaminophen among the elderly in Quebec, Canada. Am J Gastroenterol. 2008;103(4):872–82.
54. Chan AT, Manson JE, Albert CM, Chae CU, Rexrode KM, Curhan GC, et al. Nonsteroidal antiinflammatory drugs, acetaminophen, and the risk of cardiovascular events. Circulation. 2006;113(12):1578–87.
55. Forman JP, Rimm EB, Curhan GC. Frequency of analgesic use and risk of hypertension among men. Arch Intern Med. 2007;167(4):394–9.
56. Curhan GC, Willett WC, Rosner B, Stampfer MJ. Frequency of analgesic use and risk of hypertension in younger women. Arch Intern Med. 2002;162(19):2204–8.
57. Dedier J, Stampfer MJ, Hankinson SE, Willett WC, Speizer FE, Curhan GC. Nonnarcotic analgesic use and the risk of hypertension in US women. Hypertension. 2002;40(5):604–8.
58. U.S. Food and Drug Administration. Limiting acetaminophen's strength in prescription medicines. U.S. Food and Drug Administration, U.S. Department of Health & Human Services, Silver Spring, MD; 2014.
59. Papaleontiou M, Henderson Jr CR, Turner BJ, Moore AA, Olkhovskaya Y, Amanfo L, et al. Outcomes associated with opioid use in the treatment of chronic noncancer pain in older adults: a systematic review and meta-analysis. J Am Geriatr Soc. 2010;58(7):1353–69.
60. Avouac J, Gossec L, Dougados M. Efficacy and safety of opioids for osteoarthritis: a meta-analysis of randomized controlled trials. Osteoarthritis Cartilage. 2007;15(8):957–65.
61. da Costa BR, Nuesch E, Kasteler R, Husni E, Welch V, Rutjes AW, et al. Oral or transdermal opioids for osteoarthritis of the knee or hip. Cochrane Database Syst Rev. 2014;9, CD003115.
62. Silverman SM. Opioid induced hyperalgesia: clinical implications for the pain practitioner. Pain Physician. 2009;12(3):679–84.
63. Furlan AD, Sandoval JA, Mailis-Gagnon A, Tunks E. Opioids for chronic noncancer pain: a meta-analysis of effectiveness and side effects. CMAJ. 2006;174(11):1589–94.
64. McCarberg BH. Pain management in primary care: strategies to mitigate opioid misuse, abuse, and diversion. Postgrad Med. 2011;123(2):119–30.
65. Chappell AS, Ossanna MJ, Liu-Seifert H, Iyengar S, Skljarevski V, Li LC, et al. Duloxetine, a centrally acting analgesic, in the treatment of patients with osteoarthritis knee pain: a 13-week, randomized, placebo-controlled trial. Pain. 2009;146(3):253–60.
66. Chappell AS, Desaiah D, Liu-Seifert H, Zhang S, Skljarevski V, Belenkov Y, et al. A double-blind, randomized, placebo-controlled study of the efficacy and safety of duloxetine for the treatment of chronic pain due to osteoarthritis of the knee. Pain Pract. 2011;11(1):33–41.
67. Sullivan M, Bentley S, Fan MY, Gardner G. A single-blind placebo run-in study of venlafaxine XR for activity-limiting osteoarthritis pain. Pain Med. 2009;10(5):806–12.
68. Sullivan MD, Bentley S, Fan MY, Gardner G. A single-blind, placebo run-in study of duloxetine for activity-limiting osteoarthritis pain. J Pain. 2009;10(2):208–13.

69. Conaghan PG, Dickson J, Grant RL. Care and management of osteoarthritis in adults: summary of NICE guidance. BMJ. 2008;336(7642):502–3.
70. U.S. Food and Drug Administration. FDA clears Cymbalta to treat chronic musculoskeletal pain. U.S. Food and Drug Administration, U.S. Department of Health & Human Services, Silver Spring, MD; 2013.
71. Frakes EP, Risser RC, Ball TD, Hochberg MC, Wohlreich MM. Duloxetine added to oral nonsteroidal anti-inflammatory drugs for treatment of knee pain due to osteoarthritis: results of a randomized, double-blind, placebo-controlled trial. Curr Med Res Opin. 2011;27(12):2361–72.
72. Boyer EW, Shannon M. The serotonin syndrome. N Engl J Med. 2005;352(11):1112–20.
73. Vuppalanchi R, Hayashi PH, Chalasani N, Fontana RJ, Bonkovsky H, Saxena R, et al. Duloxetine hepatotoxicity: a case-series from the drug-induced liver injury network. Aliment Pharmacol Ther. 2010;32(9):1174–83.
74. Kuehn BM. Serotonin syndrome update. JAMA. 2011;306(24):2661.
75. Arnstein PM. Evolution of topical NSAIDs in the guidelines for treatment of osteoarthritis in elderly patients. Drugs Aging. 2012;29(7):523–31.
76. Altman RD. New guidelines for topical NSAIDs in the osteoarthritis treatment paradigm. Curr Med Res Opin. 2010;26(12):2871–6.
77. Baraf HS, Gloth FM, Barthel HR, Gold MS, Altman RD. Safety and efficacy of topical diclofenac sodium gel for knee osteoarthritis in elderly and younger patients: pooled data from three randomized, double-blind, parallel-group, placebo-controlled, multicentre trials. Drugs Aging. 2011;28(1):27–40.
78. Haroutiunian S, Drennan DA, Lipman AG. Topical NSAID therapy for musculoskeletal pain. Pain Med. 2010;11(4):535–49.
79. Lin J, Zhang W, Jones A, Doherty M. Efficacy of topical non-steroidal anti-inflammatory drugs in the treatment of osteoarthritis: meta-analysis of randomised controlled trials. BMJ. 2004;329(7461):324.
80. Friedman PM, Mafong EA, Friedman ES, Geronemus RG. Topical anesthetics update: EMLA and beyond. Dermatol Surg. 2001;27(12):1019–26.
81. Tugwell PS, Wells GA, Shainhouse JZ. Equivalence study of a topical diclofenac solution (pennsaid) compared with oral diclofenac in symptomatic treatment of osteoarthritis of the knee: a randomized controlled trial. J Rheumatol. 2004;31(10):2002–12.
82. Heyneman CA, Lawless-Liday C, Wall GC. Oral versus topical NSAIDs in rheumatic diseases: a comparison. Drugs. 2000;60(3):555–74.
83. Jorge LL, Feres CC, Teles VE. Topical preparations for pain relief: efficacy and patient adherence. J Pain Res. 2011;4:11–24.
84. Altman RD, Barthel HR. Topical therapies for osteoarthritis. Drugs. 2011;71(10):1259–79.
85. Makris UE, Kohler MJ, Fraenkel L. Adverse effects of topical nonsteroidal antiinflammatory drugs in older adults with osteoarthritis: a systematic literature review. J Rheumatol. 2010;37(6):1236–43.
86. Roth SH, Fuller P. Diclofenac topical solution compared with oral diclofenac: a pooled safety analysis. J Pain Res. 2011;4:159–67.
87. Simon LS, Grierson LM, Naseer Z, Bookman AA, Zev SJ. Efficacy and safety of topical diclofenac containing dimethyl sulfoxide (DMSO) compared with those of topical placebo, DMSO vehicle and oral diclofenac for knee osteoarthritis. Pain. 2009;143(3):238–45.
88. U.S. Food and Drug Administration. Voltaren Gel (diclofenac sodium topical gel) 1% – hepatic effects labeling changes. U.S. Food and Drug Administration, U.S. Department of Health & Human Services, Silver Spring, MD; 2013.
89. Laslett LL, Jones G. Capsaicin for osteoarthritis pain. Prog Drug Res. 2014;68:277–91.
90. Bellamy N, Campbell J, Robinson V, Gee T, Bourne R, Wells G. Intraarticular corticosteroid for treatment of osteoarthritis of the knee. Cochrane Database Syst Rev. 2006;2, CD005328.
91. Atchia I, Kane D, Reed MR, Isaacs JD, Birrell F. Efficacy of a single ultrasound-guided injection for the treatment of hip osteoarthritis. Ann Rheum Dis. 2011;70(1):110–6.
92. Heyworth BE, Lee JH, Kim PD, Lipton CB, Strauch RJ, Rosenwasser MP. Hylan versus corticosteroid versus placebo for treatment of basal joint arthritis: a prospective, randomized, double-blinded clinical trial. J Hand Surg Am. 2008;33(1):40–8.

93. Shimizu M, Higuchi H, Takagishi K, Shinozaki T, Kobayashi T. Clinical and biochemical characteristics after intra-articular injection for the treatment of osteoarthritis of the knee: prospective randomized study of sodium hyaluronate and corticosteroid. J Orthop Sci. 2010;15(1):51–6.
94. Bellamy N, Campbell J, Robinson V, Gee T, Bourne R, Wells G. Viscosupplementation for the treatment of osteoarthritis of the knee. Cochrane Database Syst Rev. 2006;2, CD005321.
95. Rutjes AW, Juni P, da Costa BR, Trelle S, Nuesch E, Reichenbach S. Viscosupplementation for osteoarthritis of the knee: a systematic review and meta-analysis. Ann Intern Med. 2012;157(3):180–91.
96. McAlindon TE, Bannuru RR. Osteoarthritis: is viscosupplementation really so unsafe for knee OA? Nat Rev Rheumatol. 2012;8(11):635–6.
97. Miller LE, Block JE. US-approved intra-articular hyaluronic acid injections are safe and effective in patients with knee osteoarthritis: systematic review and meta-analysis of randomized, saline-controlled trials. Clin Med Insights Arthritis Musculoskelet Disord. 2013;6:57–63.
98. Database of Abstracts of Reviews of Effects (DARE): Quality-assessed Reviews. US-approved intra-articular hyaluronic acid injections are safe and effective in patients with knee osteoarthritis: systematic review and meta-analysis of randomized, saline-controlled trials. Centre for Reviews and Dissemination, University of York, UK; 2014.
99. Bannuru RR, Vaysbrot EE, Sullivan MC, McAlindon TE. Relative efficacy of hyaluronic acid in comparison with NSAIDs for knee osteoarthritis: a systematic review and meta-analysis. Semin Arthritis Rheum. 2014;43(5):593–9.
100. Garcia Rodriguez LA, Gonzalez-Perez A. Long-term use of non-steroidal anti-inflammatory drugs and the risk of myocardial infarction in the general population. BMC Med. 2005;3:17.
101. Kearney PM, Baigent C, Godwin J, Halls H, Emberson JR, Patrono C. Do selective cyclo-oxygenase-2 inhibitors and traditional non-steroidal anti-inflammatory drugs increase the risk of atherothrombosis? Meta-analysis of randomised trials. BMJ. 2006;332(7553):1302–8.
102. O'Neil CK, Hanlon JT, Marcum ZA. Adverse effects of analgesics commonly used by older adults with osteoarthritis: focus on non-opioid and opioid analgesics. Am J Geriatr Pharmacother. 2012;10(6):331–42.
103. Chang KV, Hsiao MY, Chen WS, Wang TG, Chien KL. Effectiveness of intra-articular hyaluronic acid for ankle osteoarthritis treatment: a systematic review and meta-analysis. Arch Phys Med Rehabil. 2013;94(5):951–60.
104. Cohen MM, Altman RD, Hollstrom R, Hollstrom C, Sun C, Gipson B. Safety and efficacy of intra-articular sodium hyaluronate (Hyalgan) in a randomized, double-blind study for osteoarthritis of the ankle. Foot Ankle Int. 2008;29(7):657–63.
105. DeGroot III H, Uzunishvili S, Weir R, Al-omari A, Gomes B. Intra-articular injection of hyaluronic acid is not superior to saline solution injection for ankle arthritis: a randomized, double-blind, placebo-controlled study. J Bone Joint Surg Am. 2012;94(1):2–8.
106. Luciani D, Cadossi M, Tesei F, Chiarello E, Giannini S. Viscosupplementation for grade II osteoarthritis of the ankle: a prospective study at 18 months' follow-up. Chir Organi Mov. 2008;92(3):155–60.
107. Salk RS, Chang TJ, D'Costa WF, Soomekh DJ, Grogan KA. Sodium hyaluronate in the treatment of osteoarthritis of the ankle: a controlled, randomized, double-blind pilot study. J Bone Joint Surg Am. 2006;88(2):295–302.
108. Witteveen AG, Giannini S, Guido G, Jerosch J, Lohrer H, Vannini F, et al. A prospective multi-centre, open study of the safety and efficacy of hylan G-F 20 (Synvisc) in patients with symptomatic ankle (talo-crural) osteoarthritis. Foot Ankle Surg. 2008;14(3):145–52.
109. Carpenter B, Motley T. The role of viscosupplementation in the ankle using hylan G-F 20. J Foot Ankle Surg. 2008;47(5):377–84.
110. Reichenbach S, Blank S, Rutjes AW, Shang A, King EA, Dieppe PA, et al. Hylan versus hyaluronic acid for osteoarthritis of the knee: a systematic review and meta-analysis. Arthritis Rheum. 2007;57(8):1410–8.

111. Colen S, van den Bekerom MP, Mulier M, Haverkamp D. Hyaluronic acid in the treatment of knee osteoarthritis: a systematic review and meta-analysis with emphasis on the efficacy of different products. BioDrugs. 2012;26(4):257–68.
112. Colen S, Haverkamp D, Mulier M, van den Bekerom MP. Hyaluronic acid for the treatment of osteoarthritis in all joints except the knee: what is the current evidence? BioDrugs. 2012;26(2):101–12.
113. Patel S, Dhillon MS, Aggarwal S, Marwaha N, Jain A. Treatment with platelet-rich plasma is more effective than placebo for knee osteoarthritis: a prospective, double-blind, randomized trial. Am J Sports Med. 2013;41(2):356–64.
114. Filardo G, Kon E, Di MA, Di MB, Merli ML, Cenacchi A, et al. Platelet-rich plasma vs hyaluronic acid to treat knee degenerative pathology: study design and preliminary results of a randomized controlled trial. BMC Musculoskelet Disord. 2012;13:229.
115. Anitua E, Sanchez M, Aguirre JJ, Prado R, Padilla S, Orive G. Efficacy and safety of plasma rich in growth factors intra-articular infiltrations in the treatment of knee osteoarthritis. Arthroscopy. 2014;30(8):1006–17.
116. Filardo G, Kon E, Pereira Ruiz MT, Vaccaro F, Guitaldi R, Di MA, et al. Platelet-rich plasma intra-articular injections for cartilage degeneration and osteoarthritis: single- versus double-spinning approach. Knee Surg Sports Traumatol Arthrosc. 2012;20(10):2082–91.
117. Sanchez M, Fiz N, Azofra J, Usabiaga J, Aduriz RE, Garcia GA, et al. A randomized clinical trial evaluating plasma rich in growth factors (PRGF-Endoret) versus hyaluronic acid in the short-term treatment of symptomatic knee osteoarthritis. Arthroscopy. 2012;28(8):1070–8.
118. Vaquerizo V, Plasencia MA, Arribas I, Seijas R, Padilla S, Orive G, et al. Comparison of intra-articular injections of plasma rich in growth factors (PRGF-Endoret) versus Durolane hyaluronic acid in the treatment of patients with symptomatic osteoarthritis: a randomized controlled trial. Arthroscopy. 2013;29(10):1635–43.
119. Sanchez M, Anitua E, Azofra J, Aguirre JJ, Andia I. Intra-articular injection of an autologous preparation rich in growth factors for the treatment of knee OA: a retrospective cohort study. Clin Exp Rheumatol. 2008;26(5):910–3.
120. Say F, Gurler D, Yener K, Bulbul M, Malkoc M. Platelet-rich plasma injection is more effective than hyaluronic acid in the treatment of knee osteoarthritis. Acta Chir Orthop Traumatol Cech. 2013;80(4):278–83.
121. Anitua E, Sanchez M, Prado R, Orive G. The type of platelet-rich plasma may influence the safety of the approach. Knee Surg Sports Traumatol Arthrosc. 2014;22(7):1708–9.
122. Anitua E, Sanchez M, Orive G, Padilla S. A biological therapy to osteoarthritis treatment using platelet-rich plasma. Expert Opin Biol Ther. 2013;13(8):1161–72.
123. McCarrel TM, Minas T, Fortier LA. Optimization of leukocyte concentration in platelet-rich plasma for the treatment of tendinopathy. J Bone Joint Surg Am. 2012;94(19):e143–8.
124. Sundman EA, Cole BJ, Fortier LA. Growth factor and catabolic cytokine concentrations are influenced by the cellular composition of platelet-rich plasma. Am J Sports Med. 2011;39(10):2135–40.
125. Reginster JY, Badurski J, Bellamy N, Bensen W, Chapurlat R, Chevalier X, et al. Efficacy and safety of strontium ranelate in the treatment of knee osteoarthritis: results of a double-blind, randomised placebo-controlled trial. Ann Rheum Dis. 2013;72(2):179–86.
126. Reginster JY. Response to Dr Bolland's eLetter: strontium and cardiovascular events. Ann Rheum Dis. 2014;73(2), e9.
127. European Medicines Agency. Recommendation to restrict the use of Protelos/Osseor (strontium ranelate). European Medicines Agency, London, UK; 2013.
128. Lane NE, Schnitzer TJ, Birbara CA, Mokhtarani M, Shelton DL, Smith MD, et al. Tanezumab for the treatment of pain from osteoarthritis of the knee. N Engl J Med. 2010;363(16):1521–31.
129. Nagashima H, Suzuki M, Araki S, Yamabe T, Muto C. Preliminary assessment of the safety and efficacy of tanezumab in Japanese patients with moderate to severe osteoarthritis of the knee: a randomized, double-blind, dose-escalation, placebo-controlled study. Osteoarthritis Cartilage. 2011;19(12):1405–12.

130. Schnitzer TJ, Lane NE, Birbara C, Smith MD, Simpson SL, Brown MT. Long-term open-label study of tanezumab for moderate to severe osteoarthritic knee pain. Osteoarthritis Cartilage. 2011;19(6):639–46.
131. Spierings EL, Fidelholtz J, Wolfram G, Smith MD, Brown MT, West CR. A phase III placebo- and oxycodone-controlled study of tanezumab in adults with osteoarthritis pain of the hip or knee. Pain. 2013;154(9):1603–12.
132. Seidel MF, Lane NE. Control of arthritis pain with anti-nerve-growth factor: risk and benefit. Curr Rheumatol Rep. 2012;14(6):583–8.
133. Brown MT, Murphy FT, Radin DM, Davignon I, Smith MD, West CR. Tanezumab reduces osteoarthritic knee pain: results of a randomized, double-blind, placebo-controlled phase III trial. J Pain. 2012;13(8):790–8.
134. Brown MT, Murphy FT, Radin DM, Davignon I, Smith MD, West CR. Tanezumab reduces osteoarthritic hip pain: results of a randomized, double-blind, placebo-controlled phase III trial. Arthritis Rheum. 2013;65(7):1795–803.
135. Pfizer Inc. Tanezumab Arthritis Advisory Committee briefing document. U.S. Food and Drug Administration, Silver Spring, MD; 2012.
136. Spierings EL, Fidelholtz J, Wolfram G, Smith MD, Brown MT, West CR. A phase III placebo- and oxycodone-controlled study of tanezumab in adults with osteoarthritis pain of the hip or knee: response to letter to the editor. Pain. 2014;155(11):2432–3.
137. Panzram B, Schiltenwolf M. Pain therapy with high risk: one-sided presentation of the results from the latest phase III study on tanezumab in osteoarthritis pain. Pain. 2014;155(11):2432.
138. Magnano MD, Chakravarty EF, Broudy C, Chung L, Kelman A, Hillygus J, et al. A pilot study of tumor necrosis factor inhibition in erosive/inflammatory osteoarthritis of the hands. J Rheumatol. 2007;34(6):1323–7.
139. Verbruggen G, Wittoek R, Vander CB, Elewaut D. Tumour necrosis factor blockade for the treatment of erosive osteoarthritis of the interphalangeal finger joints: a double blind, randomised trial on structure modification. Ann Rheum Dis. 2012;71(6):891–8.
140. Maksymowych WP, Russell AS, Chiu P, Yan A, Jones N, Clare T, et al. Targeting tumour necrosis factor alleviates signs and symptoms of inflammatory osteoarthritis of the knee. Arthritis Res Ther. 2012;14(5):R206.
141. Chevalier X, Ravaud P, Maheu E, Baron G, Rialland A, Vergnaud P, et al. Adalimumab in patients with hand osteoarthritis refractory to analgesics and NSAIDs: a randomised, multicentre, double-blind, placebo-controlled trial. Ann Rheum Dis. 2014. doi:10.1136/annrheumdis-2014-205348. [Epub ahead of print].
142. Chevalier X, Giraudeau B, Conrozier T, Marliere J, Kiefer P, Goupille P. Safety study of intraarticular injection of interleukin 1 receptor antagonist in patients with painful knee osteoarthritis: a multicenter study. J Rheumatol. 2005;32(7):1317–23.
143. Chevalier X, Goupille P, Beaulieu AD, Burch FX, Bensen WG, Conrozier T, et al. Intraarticular injection of anakinra in osteoarthritis of the knee: a multicenter, randomized, double-blind, placebo-controlled study. Arthritis Rheum. 2009;61(3):344–52.
144. Cohen SB, Proudman S, Kivitz AJ, Burch FX, Donohue JP, Burstein D, et al. A randomized, double-blind study of AMG 108 (a fully human monoclonal antibody to IL-1R1) in patients with osteoarthritis of the knee. Arthritis Res Ther. 2011;13(4):R125.
145. Perucca E. Age-related changes in pharmacokinetics: predictability and assessment methods. Int Rev Neurobiol. 2007;81:183–99.
146. Schmucker DL. Liver function and phase I drug metabolism in the elderly: a paradox. Drugs Aging. 2001;18(11):837–51.
147. Wynne H. Drug metabolism and ageing. J Br Menopause Soc. 2005;11(2):51–6.
148. Arnstein P. Balancing analgesic efficacy with safety concerns in the older patient. Pain Manag Nurs. 2010;11(2 Suppl):S11–22.
149. van Dijk GM, Veenhof C, Schellevis F, Hulsmans H, Bakker JP, Arwert H, et al. Comorbidity, limitations in activities and pain in patients with osteoarthritis of the hip or knee. BMC Musculoskelet Disord. 2008;9:95.
150. Kadam UT, Jordan K, Croft PR. Clinical comorbidity in patients with osteoarthritis: a case-control study of general practice consulters in England and Wales. Ann Rheum Dis. 2004;63(4):408–14.

151. Hoogeboom TJ, den Broeder AA, Swierstra BA, de Bie RA, van den Ende CH. Joint-pain comorbidity, health status, and medication use in hip and knee osteoarthritis: a cross-sectional study. Arthritis Care Res (Hoboken). 2012;64(1):54–8.
152. Perruccio AV, Power JD, Evans HM, Mahomed SR, Gandhi R, Mahomed NN, et al. Multiple joint involvement in total knee replacement for osteoarthritis: effects on patient-reported outcomes. Arthritis Care Res (Hoboken). 2012;64(6):838–46.
153. Slater M, Perruccio AV, Badley EM. Musculoskeletal comorbidities in cardiovascular disease, diabetes and respiratory disease: the impact on activity limitations; a representative population-based study. BMC Public Health. 2011;11:77.

Chapter 12
Regenerative Medicine Approaches for Treatment of Osteoarthritis

Sowmya Viswanathan, Jesse Wolfstadt, Jaskarndip Chahal, and Alejandro Gómez-Aristizábal

Key Points

- To be effective, regenerative medicine-based treatment strategies for osteoarthritis (OA) should address multiple aspects of OA – which involves inflammation, loss of chondrocytes, remodeling of subchondral bone and endochondral ossification.
- Biologics involving growth factors to trigger appropriate chondrocyte proliferation, anti-inflammatory cytokines to combat inflammation, and the use of cartilage transcription factors are being considered in clinical investigations for the treatment of OA.
- Cellular therapy, including autologous chondrocytes, allogeneic cadaveric chondrocytes, mesenchymal stromal cells, and pluripotent stem cell-derived chondrocytes, is also being investigated for their ability to directly or indirectly replace the loss of chondrocytes.

S. Viswanathan, PhD (✉)
Cell Therapy Program, University Health Network, Toronto, ON, Canada

Arthritis Program, University Health Network, Toronto, ON, Canada

Institute of Biomaterials and Biomedical Engineering, University of Toronto, 620 University Avenue, Suite 8-105, Toronto, ON M5G 1Z6, Canada
e-mail: Sowmya.viswanathan@uhnresearch.ca

J. Wolfstadt, MD • A. Gómez-Aristizábal, PhD
Arthritis Program, University Health Network, Toronto, ON, Canada

J. Chahal, MD, MSc, FRCSC
Arthritis Program, University Health Network, Toronto, ON, Canada

University of Toronto Orthopaedic Sports Medicine Program, Toronto, ON, Canada

Women's College Hospital, Toronto, ON, Canada

M. Kapoor, N.N. Mahomed (eds.), *Osteoarthritis: Pathogenesis, Diagnosis, Available Treatments, Drug Safety, Regenerative and Precision Medicine*,
DOI 10.1007/978-3-319-19560-5_12

- As part of treatment strategies for OA, natural and synthetic biomaterials are used to mimic the biomechanical properties and function of cartilage, which could be key to providing functional repair of degenerative OA.

Introduction

Regenerative medicine offers the potential for disease modification and thereby offers more than symptomatic treatment for OA patients. While regenerative medicine applications have begun to make inroads in other complex indications including cardiac diseases, graft-versus-host disease, and even treatment of cancer, treatment options for OA have been relatively limited. ChondroCelect, a cell-based medicinal product based on autologous chondrocyte implantation, was approved in Europe in 2009 [1]; Carticel, a Food and Drug Administration (FDA)-approved product, was launched in 1997 [2]; neither is approved for treatment of general OA [3]. MEDIPOST Inc. received approval in S. Korea for CARTISTEM™ for treating cartilage defects in the OA knee (ICRS Grade IV).

The relative paucity of regenerative medicine solutions is largely due to the avascular nature of cartilage, which when damaged is unable to mount a sufficiently robust innate healing response. There is limited access to nutrients, which are largely obtained through perfusion by the synovial fluid, and to progenitor cells to help heal cartilage injuries. The challenge is even more pronounced moving from treating a small cartilage defect, in an otherwise healthy cartilage to treating a cartilage defect in a severely degraded arthritic joint. OA is a multifaceted disease involving inflammatory processes [4–6], loss of chondrocytes due to apoptosis [7], remodeling of subchondral bone and endochondral ossification; therefore, treatment strategies for OA must approach it as a disease of the entire joint [8].

To facilitate endogenous repair of articular cartilage and induce anti-inflammatory effects in the context of OA, a number of biological agents which can either stimulate chondrocyte progenitors such as fibroblast growth factor (FGF-18) [9] or block inflammatory processes such as interleukin-1 receptor antagonist (IL-1RA) are being considered, although results have not been compelling to date [10]. Autologous serum that is enriched for anti-inflammatory cytokines (Orthokin® and Onoccomed®) [11] and autologous platelet-rich plasma (PRP) that contain various growth factors [12] are also being investigated. In this chapter, we discuss some of the biologics that are being investigated for OA as well as novel strategies including the use of interfering RNAs (iRNAs), use of viral vectors to deliver SOX9, a cartilage transcription factor [13], or genetically modified cells to provide sustained delivery of therapeutic factors such as IL-1RA and IL-10 [14].

One currently used treatment approach for articular cartilage damage includes stimulation of bone marrow by microfracture to provoke release of bone marrow progenitor cells to induce repair [15]. The use of exogenously manipulated cells such as autologous chondrocytes that are expanded in culture, allogeneic chondrocytes from cadaveric donors, and mesenchymal stromal cell (MSCs) from various sources are being intensely investigated for their regenerative potential to replace degraded cartilage. However, long-term maintenance of the chondrocyte phenotype has proven to be elusive with the chondrocytes tending toward either a fibrocartilage phenotype or a hypertrophic phenotype, neither of which can provide the required mechanical strength. In this chapter, we review the different types of cells used and proposed, and discuss the advantages and disadvantages of each cell type.

The need to have biomechanical support, one of the inherent features of cartilage, has spawned considerable research into developing supportive scaffolds which can mimic, to some extent the dichotomous properties of joint cartilage (load bearing, yet flexible, a low coefficient of friction, sufficient tensile modulus strength, ability to maintain rounded chondrocyte morphology and phenotype, biocompatible, and biodegradable). The hierarchical organization of articular cartilage into three zones, a superficial zone (collagen II rich), a deep zone (cartilage-bone interface area), and middle zone (proteoglycan rich), helps achieve tensile and compression-resistance properties of native cartilage – this level of engineering is really needed to produce biomaterials that can mimic the properties of native cartilage [16]. In this chapter, we review the different approaches to generating scaffolds and engineering them to have suitable biocompatible, biomechanical, and in some cases bioactive properties that are conducive to cartilage tissue repair and regeneration.

In the sections below, we will highlight the importance of using biologics, cell and scaffolds. While each section is presented separately, it is likely that a true solution for managing OA from a regenerative medicine perspective will involve an integration and synthesis of more than one of these concepts (Table 12.1).

Biologics

Hyaluronic Acid and Platelet-Rich Plasma

Hyaluronic acid (HA) and platelet-rich plasma (PRP) represent two popular nonoperative treatments for patients with OA. While HA has been studied extensively and has been used clinically for up to two decades, PRP has seen a relative recent increase in both lay and scientific popularity. Both are considered to be "biological" interventions and should be considered as part of the existing treatment armamentarium for knee OA.

Hyaluronan is a polyanionic, unbranched glycosaminoglycan polymer composed of disaccharide subunits [17]. HA is endogenously produced by synoviocytes, fibroblasts, chondrocytes, and MSCs, and is a major constituent of synovial fluid. Its functions include providing viscoelastic properties to achieve boundary

Table 12.1 Summary of current and predicted regenerative medicine approaches for OA

	Therapy		Advantages	Disadvantages
Biologics	Platelet-rich plasma (PRP)		Multiple growth factors Anti-inflammatory effects	Regenerative effectiveness unknown
	Hyaluronic acid (HA)		Anti-inflammatory and antinociceptive effects	Controversial data regarding efficacy
	IL-1RA		Autologous conditioned serum has high concentration of IL-RA Excellent preliminary outcomes	Further study required to be accepted as a standard of care Considered as a device and not available in North America
	Antibodies to nerve growth factor		Superior to placebo and oxycodone in a phase III study	Possibly more adverse events than placebo
	Small interfering RNA		Upstream strategy to block production of proinflammatory mediators	Transient effects Transcripts with high turnover difficult to silence Off-target effect
	Gene therapy:	Ex vivo	Continuous delivery of high levels of therapeutic factors High control over cells to be delivered	Needs carrier cells for delivery
		In vivo	Stronger modifications of the environment Easy delivery Need for few doses	Lacks control over cells that get modified Possible immunological rejection
Cells	Autologous chondrocyte transplantation		Perfect HLA matching Partial repair	Donor morbidity High cost and technically tedious Chondrocyte dedifferentiation Cannot treat severe OA
	Particulated cartilage		Lower cost Less ex vivo manipulation Chondrocyte in native state Reparative potential	Allografts: need of HLA matching? Cannot treat severe OA Definite effectiveness unknown Autologous: limited cartilage
	Bone marrow mononuclear cells		Perfect HLA matching Cheap and easy to generate	Effectiveness unknown
	Adipose stromal vascular fraction		Perfect HLA matching Low cost	Effectiveness unknown
	MSCs		Reparative potential Anti-inflammatory Antifibrotic Large number of cells Readily available	Effectiveness unknown Expensive production
	ESC/iPSC-chondrocytes		Unlimited cell number	Teratogenic and/or tumorigenic Differentiation not yet well defined

(continued)

Table 12.1 (continued)

	Therapy	Advantages	Disadvantages
Scaffolds	Fibrin	Easily harvested Widely available commercially Excellent biocompatibility	Poor mechanical strength
	Collagen	Good biocompatibility and biodegradability Low immunogenic response	Poor mechanical strength
	Modified HA	May be engineered to release growth factors May be augmented with structural proteins	Poor mechanical strength Impurities
	Synthetics	Highly porous Can be engineered with desired mechanical strength, shape, and biodegradable properties	Poor biocompatibility Potential for immunogenic response Toxic breakdown products
	Hybrid/composite	Harness the attractive properties of natural and synthetic biomaterials	Cost

lubrication and hence low friction levels in the synovial joint [17]. High molecular weight (HMW) HA has also shown to be immunosuppressive, anti-inflammatory, and anti-angiogenic and is potentially more therapeutic than the low molecular weight (LMW) varieties [18, 19]. In OA, the concentration and molecular weight of HA decreases [20, 21]. It is likely that smaller HA fragments become proinflammatory and pro-angiogenic by engaging toll-like receptors 2 and 4 in macrophages and chondrocytes [22]. Furthermore, the viscosity of the synovial fluid decreases which in turn results in an increase in mechanical stress to cartilage [17]. From a therapeutic standpoint, HA is hypothesized to be an anti-inflammatory agent and also involved in direct analgesia [17], in part by stimulating the κ-opiod receptor (KOP) having direct action on synovial nerve endings [23].

With respect to the clinical evidence for HA, the results in the literature, to date, have been controversial, with support for and against the routine use of HA. Miller et al. conducted a systematic review of US-approved intra-articular HA injections which were studied in the context of randomized, saline-controlled trials. Using data from 29 trials and 4,866 patients, the authors concluded that HA is safe for intra-articular administration and efficacious compared to control treatments with respect to pain and function restoration [24]. In contrast, Rutjes et al. performed a meta-analysis of 89 trials with 12,677 patients. In this study, 71 of 89 trials showed that HA reduced pain. However, when looking only at blinded trials with a minimum of 100 patients in each treatment arm, the results were nonsignificant. Furthermore, there were more adverse effects in the HA group in the latter studies [25]. In general, however, greater benefits have been observed with low-grade OA when using HA. Moreover, the studies in the literature have a large degree of variability with regard to HA dosing, number of injections, the use of HMW versus LMW HA, as well as variable outcome measures and follow-up periods [17].

In comparison to HA, the use of PRP represents a shift in our approach to treating OA in the context of biological treatment strategies [17]. Specifically, there has been a shift from a single molecule approach to an idea of co-delivering multiple bioactive factors which in turn, theoretically, is more apt to mimic the complex intra-articular environment [17]. PRP has mostly been defined as a sample of autologous blood with concentrations of platelets above baseline values [26]. The main growth factors in PRP are transforming growth factor beta-1 (TGF-β), platelet-derived growth factor (PDGF), vascular endothelial growth factor (VEGF), hepatocyte growth factor (HGF), and insulin-like growth factor 1 (IGF-1) [26]. These growth factors are found in the alpha-granules of platelets and released upon platelet activation [27]. In vitro studies of PRP have shown increases in chondrocyte viability, proliferation, and synthetic capability, as well as an inhibitory effect on the inflammatory cascade. In vivo studies have shown that PRP improves both cartilage stiffness and the histological appearance of cartilage repair tissue, specifically increased proteoglycan and type II collagen content [27]. Possible mechanisms by which PRP may exert reparative effects include creating a gradient of growth factors which is a stimulus for cell migration (i.e., mesenchymal progenitors, chondrocytes), stimulation of endogenous production of HA, stimulation of MSC proliferation and increased chondrogenic differentiation [17].

Despite the increasing use of PRP, there are several variables that require further study. At the present time, there is no agreement regarding the ideal platelet concentration, the presence or absence of white blood cells (the former may be related to a proinflammatory response), the use of anticoagulants and platelet activators, injection frequency, and the concomitant use of local anesthetics [28]. If an anticoagulant is used, then platelet activation becomes important since clot formation is pivotal to sustained release of growth factors in a gradient-dependent fashion [28]. Sundman et al. [29] have also demonstrated that growth factor and catabolic cytokine concentrations were influenced by the cellular composition of PRP. Platelets increased anabolic signaling, while leukocytes increased catabolic signaling molecules. Thus, PRP products should be analyzed for their platelet and leukocyte content, as both can influence the biologic effects of PRP [29].

In a recent study by Sundman et al. [30], synovium and cartilage were harvested from patients undergoing total knee arthroplasty, and the tissues were co-cultured in HA, PRP, or control medium. In both HA and PRP conditions, the tumor necrosis factor alpha (TNF-α) concentration was decreased compared to control. Additionally, in PRP co-cultures, synoviocytes downregulated the expression of matrix metalloproteinase (MMP)-13 expression while upregulating hyaluronic acid synthase-2. Co-cultures with HA had lower levels of interleukin (IL)-6, relative to controls. These results demonstrated that while PRP and HA treatment of OA joint tissues resulted in decreased inflammation (via different mechanisms), PRP treatment also has the ability to enhance endogenous HA production and decrease cartilage catabolism. This study was unique because it looked at an ex vivo culture system of cartilage and synovium in different media conditions, which is more likely to represent the complex intra-articular environment in OA compared to a single tissue culture system [30].

A recent systematic review and meta-analysis by Khoshbin et al. [27] reviewed six level I and II studies which compared PRP with either HA or saline. Pooled results demonstrated that disease-specific functional outcomes were superior in patients treated with multiple sequential PRP injections compared with other treatment groups at a follow-up period of six months. However, there was a slightly higher rate of nonspecific knee-related adverse events in the PRP group.

Andia et al. [17] have suggested that due to the overlapping yet distinct mechanism which underlies the basis of PRP and HA, combination therapy has the potential to create a synergistic effect for symptom control and disease modification. Certainly, further studies from a clinical and basic science perspective are required to corroborate this.

IL-1 and TNF-α Blockade

Interleukin 1 (IL-1) appears to be one of the most important mediators of cartilage loss [11]. The naturally occurring inhibitor of IL-1 is called the IL-1RA which has been shown to be therapeutic when delivered via intra-articular injection in canine models of OA as well as other large animal models [10, 11, 31]. Autologous conditioned serum (ACS) was developed in the mid-1990s in an attempt to generate an injectable material enriched in IL-1RA. Meijer et al. [32] demonstrated that when whole blood is exposed to medical-grade glass beads and cultured for 24 h at 37 °C, there is a rapid increase in the synthesis of several anti-inflammatory cytokines including IL-1RA, IL-4, IL-10 and others to a lesser degree [33]. Baltzer et al. have conducted a three-arm parallel-group randomized trial and demonstrated superiority of ACS, compared with HA and saline controls, up to 2 years following treatment in patients with low- to medium-grade OA [11]. At the present time, ACS (Orthokine™) is approved in Europe, Australia, and some Asian countries. The Orthokine™ (specifically the syringe with the glass beads) method is approved as a medical device; the ACS itself is considered to be within the physician scope of practice, and this aspect of the procedure does not require drug approval [33]. Nevertheless, more studies with Orthokine™ are required before it can be considered a first-line biological treatment for OA.

IL-1 and TNF-α are proinflammatory cytokines produced in response to injury and animal models support the dominant role of IL-1 early in the development of arthritis [34]. There is therefore an increased focus on the use of cytokine blockade immediately following acute joint injury in order to determine whether such an intervention can prevent downstream chondral damage. Certainly in a canine ACL transection model, Caron et al. [35] have shown that IL-RA administration is chondroprotective. Similar effects have been shown with TNF-α inhibition in a rat ACL transection model [36]. Ongoing clinical trials in humans will determine whether such an approach has merit and ultimately efficacy from a disease prevention perspective.

Antibodies Against Nerve Growth Factor

Another recent approach to treating OA is related to the use of humanized IgG2 antibodies (Tanezumab) that targets nerve growth factor (NGF). In adults, NGF is essential in raising awareness of the nociceptor function of neurons with the onset of pain and hyperalgesia in chronic pain [37]. NGF becomes important in injury and inflammation even in the context of the OA environment. Lane et al. conducted a proof of concept study in 450 patients and demonstrated that tanezumab resulted in an overall reduction in joint pain and improvement in function, yet a higher rate of mild to moderate adverse events compared to placebo [38]. Subsequent trials, including phase III superiority trial, have demonstrated similar levels of efficacy without any notable differences in adverse event rates [39, 40].

Small Interfering RNAs

In the setting of mechanical stress, nuclear factor kappa beta (NFkB) transcription factors are activated and are associated with the production of proinflammatory cytokines [37]. Biological inhibitors and the use of highly specific drugs and small interfering RNAs (siRNAs) is one strategy to inhibit such proinflammatory actions. At the present time, the use of siRNAs remains investigational. Akagi et al. [41] injected chemically modified siRNAs into knee joints of mice with surgically induced OA in order to create a matrix metalloproteinase-13 (MMP-13) knockdown. Injections took place 1 week postmedial meniscus destabilization. The authors noted a significant improvement in histological scores in the treatment versus control group 8 weeks after the surgery. Thus, an effective knockdown of MMP-13 expression resulted in delayed cartilage degradation. It was also determined that uptake of the siRNAs was predominantly in the synovium and that blockade of MMP-13 expression was likely present for at least 2 weeks. Such genetic upstream approaches appear promising, but it will take time for such treatment options to be available for clinical use.

Gene Therapy

With gene therapy, one can deliver cells that have been genetically modified (ex vivo) or deliver the genes without any vehicles directly to the OA joint tissue (in vivo). While the ex vivo technique allows more control over the cells that will be delivered, it is also more labor, time, and resource intensive than the in vivo delivery, which only requires the infusion of the vector into the joint. The main targets for the in vivo approach are chondrocytes and cells of the synovium in the OA joint, while chondrocytes, synoviocytes, and MSCs are candidate vehicles for the ex vivo approach. Cell modifications could include insertion of genes coding for anti-inflammatory, anti-apoptotic, and pro-chondrogenic factors [42]. Both viral and nonviral vectors are appropriate modes of delivery for both ex vivo and in vivo approaches, although adeno-associated viral (AAV) vectors are preferred for in vivo delivery, as they have low immunogenicity and have been shown to efficiently modify synovial cells without insertion into their genomic DNA [42, 43].

To date, only safety has been proven for the ex vivo delivery of cells modified to express IL-1RA (anti-inflammatory factor) or TGF-β (pro-chondrogenic factor) [43]; efficacy in humans remains to be proven although both genes demonstrated efficacy in mitigating OA progression in animal models.

Cells for OA Therapy

Chondrocytes

Autologous chondrocyte transplantation (ACT) has been developed to aid chondral defect regeneration: briefly, a piece of healthy cartilage is first removed from the affected joint, to be later digested to acquire the contained chondrocytes. These chondrocytes are expanded in monolayer culture and reimplanted into the cartilage defect [44]. Since this technique has been used for at least two decades, there is convincing data showing that ACT does improve the condition of patients with cartilage defects [45, 46]. Furthermore, ACT, overall, has shown better clinical outcomes than microfracture in the long term (3–5 years) [47].

Despite the success of ACT, it is not yet a technique that can be applied to treat severe OA [48], because of underlying disease which affects subchondral bone. However, early OA treated with ACT can delay OA degeneration [49], and because chondral defects are associated with the onset of OA, healing these defects can delay OA incidence [46]. Since the development of ACT in 1987 [44], it continues evolving as a high-cost procedure ranging from US $33–$67 thousand (depending on the country of execution) [50]. However, it is labor-intensive and patient-specific and may not provide optimal outcomes. A study showed that after 5–11 years of ACT treatment, repaired cartilage was typically hyaline cartilage, although 25 % of the cases had fibrous cartilage [51]. Chondrocytes expanded in monolayer culture tend to dedifferentiate, losing their mature hyaline chondrocyte phenotype; thus, continued effort has been aimed at improving culture conditions [44]. While the use of autologous chondrocytes reduces the risk of immune rejection and disease transmission, it also increases the costs. Thus, it is important to find alternative chondrocyte sources, such as allogeneic cells or stem cell-derived chondrocytes.

One alternative technique for chondrocyte implantation is the use of particulated cartilage autografts and allografts. Unlike ACT, these particles are minimally manipulated as they are simply minced cartilage, and thus, the chondrocytes contained within them are in their native state. Additionally, due to lower manipulation, the technical tediousness of ACT is greatly diminished. Upon implantation, the chondrocytes contained within the cartilage particles are able to contribute to the repair of the affected area. To date, not much data regarding the effectiveness of the autologous or allogeneic approach in humans has been generated, although one small study has shown that autologous cartilage particles outperform microfractures at 12, 18, and 24 months post-treatment [52]. Similarly, juvenile particulated cartilage allografts have shown improvement of the symptoms after 12 months in four patients with apparent defect filling, as judged by MRI [52]. The particulates thus appear to present a viable alternative, although to decipher their real potential, larger trials are still needed. Specifically for the allografts, a randomized or controlled study has not yet been performed, leaving many questions unanswered.

Bone Marrow Mononuclear Cells (BM-MNCs)

BM-MNCs are a highly heterogeneous population of cells acquired by eliminating erythrocytes and granulocytes from whole bone marrow (BM). As such, BM-MNCs contain monocytes, lymphocytes, mature and immature hematopoietic progenitors, hematopoietic stem cells, MSCs, endothelial progenitors, and other subpopulations [53]. In a sheep study, BM-MNCs improved cartilage repair, but their effect was significantly lower than that of BM-MSCs [54]. It is thus likely that the positive effects of BM-MNCs mainly come from MSCs, although the effects of other subpopulations cannot be ignored [55]. To date, there have been no randomized human trials using BM-MNCs, and thus no conclusions can be reached with regard to their efficacy. Despite this, BM-MNC treatments are quite prevalent for OA [50] as they do not require much processing, equipment, or time; the whole procedure from aspiration to generating a concentrated solution of BM-MNCs takes less than 4 hours.

Adipose Stromal Vascular Fraction (A-SVF)

A-SVF isolation is a slightly more complex procedure than BM aspiration, but it is still a short procedure compared to isolation and longer-term expansion of purified cell types (on the order of weeks). Lipoaspirates are enzymatically digested and adipocytes removed by density separation from the A-SVF. Thus, A-SVF contains all cells from adipose tissue except mature adipocytes and includes 28 % blood-derived cells (CD45+), 29 % adipose stromal cells (ASC) (CD45−CD31−CD34+), 13 % endothelial cells (CD45-CD31+CD34+), and other cells (CD45−CD34−) [56].

A cartilage defect model in sheep has shown that A-SVF has good effects that definitely outperform the vehicle [57]. It is thought the MSC fraction in A-SVF is primarily responsible for its benefits, yet A-SVF can outperform MSCs [57], indicating that other components of A-SVF may have therapeutic properties for cartilage regeneration.

As with BM-MNCs, A-SVF treatment of cartilage defects is clinically offered all over the world, and while clinical studies have shown benefits in OA patients [50], the only study comparing it to a placebo control failed to show improved efficacy [58].

Mesenchymal Stromal Cells (MSCs)

MSCs were originally isolated from the BM, and it has been found that they are present almost ubiquitously all over the body. They can be isolated from the BM, adipose tissue, placenta, the umbilical cord and its blood, synovium, other tissues, and even synovial fluid from OA joints [59–62]. MSCs have been described, by the International Society for Cellular Therapy, as cells that are plastic-adherent; positive for CD105, CD73, and CD90; negative for hematopoietic-specific surface molecules; and that can at least differentiate in vitro into bone, cartilage, and fat cells [63]. MSCs may also decrease inflammation and provide support to other cell types, thus promoting angiogenesis, cell survival, cell differentiation, and inhibiting fibrosis [64]. Thus, MSCs are ideal cells for OA therapy, as they could potentially decrease inflammation, while contributing to cartilage regeneration both directly and indirectly and diminishing synovial fibrosis.

MSCs have indeed shown reparative effects in various animal models of OA and human OA, yet controlled, randomized, large trials are needed for humans, as most of the benefits seen in humans have not been compared to proper controls [50, 65–71].

The main disadvantage for all sources of MSCs is the incapacity to predetermine the quality of the MSC products, as there are no definitive markers for MSCs or predictive in vitro assays. Global efforts, led by us and other groups, are thus looking for strategies to develop reference materials for MSCs to standardize their characterization [72]. Systematic studies to address inter- and intra-donor variability, effect of culture conditions, and tissue sources need to be undertaken to get a handle on this variability.

Stem Cell-Derived Chondrocytes and Directed Transdifferentiation

Currently, chondrocyte-like cells can be derived from stem cells from different sources including MSCs [73], embryonic stem cells (ESCs) [73, 74], and induced pluripotent stem cells (iPSCs) [75]. While MSCs can be implanted safely as they are not known to be teratogenic or tumorigenic, it has not been definitively shown that they can replace endogenous cartilage in clinical trials. ESCs are pluripotent and proliferate indefinitely allowing for the production of a virtually infinite number of differentiated chondrocytes from one cell, although induction of mature chondrocytes still remains under investigation [73, 74]. ESCs being a virtually limitless source of cells allow for automatized production and lower production costs: a number of human leukocyte antigen (HLA)-matched banks could be created to facilitate major HLA matching of a high percentage of the population and thus diminish the risks of allorejection. On the other hand, their infinite proliferative capacity and pluripotency comes with the high risks of tumorigenicity; thus, any chondrocytes produced would have to be fully committed to that lineage, and growth-arrested, with perhaps mechanisms to kill off aberrant cells [76]. In addition, ESCs raise ethical issues that limit their use considerably. iPSCs have no such ethical constraints, as they are derived by modifying virtually any somatic cell and have similar behavior to ESCs [75]. Since iPSCs can be produced from adult cells, they present an alternative autologous product, although this would greatly increase costs. A strategy for creation of HLA-matched banks for allotherapies would be more efficient [77], although it would require putting patients on immunosuppressants, which carry their own risks.

Another approach for the production of chondrocyte-like cells would be the directed transdifferentiation of cells [78], which would direct cells to chondrocytes without first dedifferentiating them to a primitive ESC-like stage. The main advantage of this technique would be that tumorigenicity could be avoided and the process to get chondrocytes could be potentially shorter compared to iPSCs. However, one would be limited by cell supply, and thus, this approach would be similar to MSC-derived chondrocytes. Still, it is an interesting potential source of chondrocytes which is just starting to be investigated.

Scaffolds for Cartilage Regeneration

The optimal route of administering biologics to treat OA remains unanswered. Biologics may be administered with a scaffold or in a suspension intra-articularly [50]. While some newer studies have investigated the use of scaffold-less tissues [79], the majority of research focusing on cell therapies and their use for bioengineering hyaline cartilage has utilized scaffolds [80].

The overarching role of scaffolds is to mimic the extracellular matrix of the native tissue [81]. Scaffolds improve cell survival and optimize the environment for cells to function at the site of cartilage loss. Scaffolds function by providing mechanical support for implanted cells and chemotaxis to induce the formation of new hyaline cartilage [82]. The mechanical strength of the scaffold must be balanced with its porosity, which allows for transport of nutrients, growth factors, and metabolites within the developing extracellular matrix (ECM) [83]. A scaffold should be biocompatible and allow for cell adhesion, proliferation, and matrix synthesis, ensuring that cells are incorporated into the host tissue [84, 85]. The scaffold must mimic the natural environment of chondrocytes and ideally should be bioactive, biomimetic, biodegradable, and bioresponsive [16, 86]. It is essential that the scaffolds are resorbable, ensuring that over time the scaffold degrades and is replaced by new hyaline cartilage [87]. The scaffolds may be enhanced by peptides or cytokines, which provide spatial and temporal signals to promote cells to differentiate into chondrocytic phenotypes, minimize the degradation of implanted cells, and improve cell viability. Historically, scaffolds have been produced in the form of solid implants. However, more recently, scaffolds have been developed in the form of a liquid or paste form [88].

Scaffold Biomaterials

There are three main categories of scaffold biomaterials used for cartilage regeneration [89]: natural, synthetic, and hybrid/composite.

Natural Biomaterial Scaffolds

Natural biomaterials, such as collagen type I or III, are the most commonly used materials for bioengineering articular cartilage [16]. Natural scaffolds utilize materials that typically occur in a healthy joint [83]. In general, the advantages of natural biomaterials are high biocompatibility, ample sources for procurement, and excellent bioactivity. However, they can be immunogenic when they are harvested from allogeneic or xenogeneic sources [83, 90]. Natural biomaterials can be further subdivided into proteins and polysaccharides [85].

Collagen is the most common protein used in scaffolds [91]. One of the earliest investigations of MSCs used a collagen gel to regenerate cartilage defects in rabbits [92]. Not only can it be harvested from multiple sources such as skin, tendon, and bone [93], but also demonstrates good biocompatibility, biodegradability, and low immunogenicity. However, collagen has poor mechanical strength compared to other natural scaffolds. Typically, porcine or bovine type I/III collagen has been used as scaffold material. While these sources are abundant in nature, the use of animal tissues in humans raises concerns about the risks of transmitting infectious agents or inducing immune reactions. Moreover, animal tissues are harvested from a heterogeneous mixture with high variability in tissue quality. More recently, investigators have utilized recombinant human type II collagen [94]. Recombinant human tissues are more expensive than porcine or bovine sources, but have demonstrated good biocompatibility and safety [95]. Recombinant tissues can also be customized to exact specifications and come from a homogeneous source [96].

Silk is a natural protein [97] with high mechanical strength that can be engineered into many different shapes and structures. The most common source of silk is the silkworm *B. Mori,* but silk may also be harvested from spiders such as *N. clavipes* or artificially engineered [98]. Naturally occurring silk can be harvested easily, in large amounts, and at a low cost. The scaffolds have slow degradation rates with excellent biocompatibility and biomechanical properties.

Fibrin is a protein involved in the blood-clotting cascade that can be easily harvested from human or animal sources and is widely available commercially [99]. It has many advantages as a biological scaffold: it can be injected arthroscopically and be molded into many shapes, can act as a plug to seal cartilage defects and has excellent biocompatibility. However, fibrin-based scaffolds have poor mechanical properties, rendering them unable to support high mechanical loads [100].

HA, a naturally occurring polysaccharide mentioned in the biologics section, as one of the main components of the natural extracellular matrix in healthy joint tissue [86], can also serve as a scaffold. Researchers have augmented HA-based scaffolds with structural proteins like fibrin or collagen to improve their poor mechanical strength [16]. HA scaffolds may also be engineered to release growth factors such as TGF-β1 [101]. Recently, investigators have engineered a HA hydrogel that is liquid at room temperature and solidifies at body temperature, allowing the scaffold to fill the defect before solidifying [102]. Other polysaccharides that may be used include gelatin, alginate, agarose, and chitosan [103]. They are often used in formulations with synthetic biomaterials such as poly(L-lactide-co-caprolactone) (PLCL) [104] and poly(lactic acid) (PLA) [105], with varying results.

Synthetic Biomaterial Scaffolds

Synthetic biomaterials, the most common alternative to natural biomaterials, allow for the diffusion of nutrients and cells within the scaffold as they are highly porous [89]. They can be woven into three-dimensional shapes, mirroring the shape and mechanical properties of the normal joint. The scaffolds may be individualized to each patient based on their anatomy and can allow for immediate load bearing, followed by cartilage regeneration over time. The scaffolds can also be engineered with desired mechanical strength, shape, and biodegradable properties. The major advantage over natural biomaterials is the ability to tailor the degradation rate of the scaffold. Synthetic biomaterials can be augmented with matrix metalloproteinase-sensitive peptides, which help direct MSCs to differentiate into chondrocytes [106].

They have two major disadvantages. The first is poor biocompatibility due to a lack of sites for cell adhesion, resulting in synthetic polymers often failing to maintain the chondrocytic phenotype [81]. Secondly, synthetic scaffolds can elicit an immune response and the breakdown products can be toxic to host tissues. One of the main goals of biologic therapy is to decrease the inflammatory state of an arthritic joint, making this is a particularly troublesome drawback of synthetic biomaterials.

PLA is a frequently used synthetic biomaterial that demonstrates good mechanical strength and a modifiable degradation rate [107]. However, it typically has a stronger inflammatory response than natural polymers because of the breakdown products. Other examples of synthetic biomaterials are polyglycolic acid (PGA)

[108], poly(ethylene glycol) (PEG) [106], poly(lactic-co-glycolic acid) (PLGA) [109], polyurethane, and polycaprolactone (PCL).

Hybrid/Composite Biomaterial Scaffolds

More recently, composite scaffolds have been developed which harness the attractive properties of various natural and synthetic biomaterials. These include hyaluronan-collagen, gelatin-hyaluronan, PEG-hyaluronan, and PGA-fibrin hybrids, which can be manufactured into three-dimensional cartilage-scaffold constructs unique to individual defects and the contour of the affected joint [16]. Since healthy articular cartilage is highly hydrated and comprised mostly of collagen, hyaluronan-collagen composites may offer the ideal combination for arthritic joints. Even magnets have been investigated as a scaffold for implanting mesenchymal stem cells into a degenerative joint [110].

Scaffold Architecture

Scaffolds can be implanted as a hydrogel, devitalized ECM from donor tissue, as cell sheets that secrete ECM, or pre-made porous scaffolds [83]. They can take the form of gels, foams, sponges, or solid woven polymers, which can be placed in areas of damaged articular cartilage [111]. The architecture of the scaffold is a delicate balance between porosity and strength – larger pore sizes increase the extension of ECM, whereas smaller pore sizes ensure that implanted cells differentiate into chondrocytic phenotypes. It is important that the scaffold architecture is strong enough to withstand the mechanical load of the joint surface. If the scaffold is too soft, breakdown products will be produced which can cause degeneration in surrounding healthy articular cartilage. Moreover, the scaffold should help recreate the natural structure of healthy cartilage. The superficial layer of healthy cartilage is composed of collagen fibrils aligned tangentially to the articular surface, whereas collagen fibrils in the deep zone are oriented radially [112]. Self-assembling scaffolds have the potential to repair multiple different layers within damaged articular cartilage and mimic healthy tissue.

Hydrogels are biphasic materials with properties similar to articular cartilage and are innately hydrated structures with unique biocompatibility similar to native ECM [16]. They are viscoelastic, exhibiting cartilage-like flexibility, and can form stable and highly ordered scaffolds on which biologics can be implanted [86]. The main pitfall of hydrogels is their low mechanical strength, which may be as low as 10 % of natural cartilage compression moduli [85].

Sponges are highly porous, whereas woven scaffolds have poorer porosity. Gradient structures can combine different porosities to maximize the extension of ECM and chondrocyte differentiation.

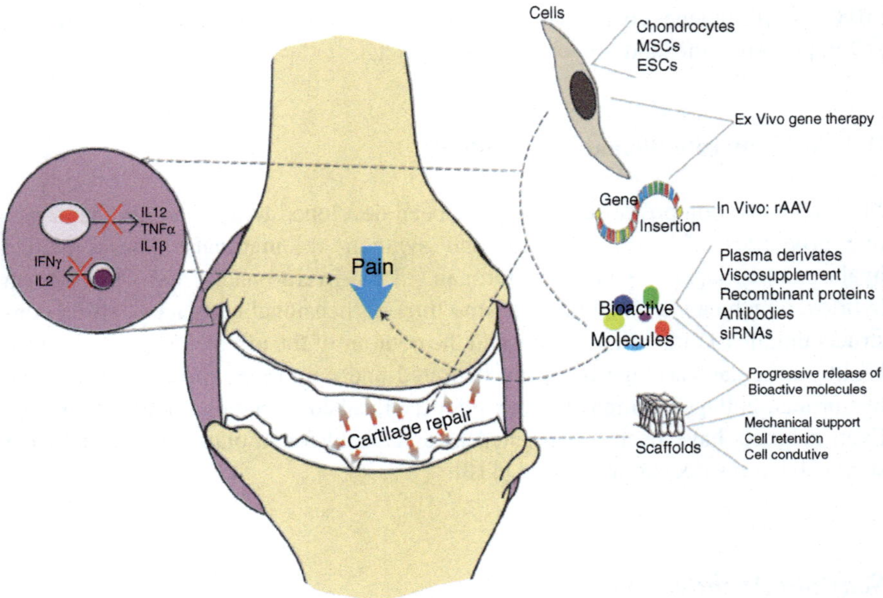

Fig. 12.1 Schematic for potential regenerative medicine approaches to treating OA. OA is a multifactorial disease which comprises chronic inflammation, cartilage degradation, osteophyte formation, and synovial fibrosis. Regenerative medicine currently aims to address the main factors that are thought to sustain OA, inflammation, and cartilage degradation. Cell- and gene-based therapies are both being designed so that they can address either inflammation or cartilage repair or both. Bioactive molecules have been mainly thought as means to reduce inflammation, although some of them could be helpful on promoting cartilage repair or at least decrease the degradation rate. Scaffolds have been designed in order to provide a helpful environment that can promote cartilage and sometimes bone regeneration from surrounding progenitors or from exogenous cells while also integrating with cartilage

Future Research for Scaffolds

The optimal scaffold architecture and biomaterial for regeneration of articular cartilage remains elusive. Some researchers have suggested that cartilage engineering should focus on scaffold-less techniques because of the various limitations of scaffold biomaterials [113]. The ideal scaffold is likely a composite, self-assembling scaffold that mimics the properties of the four distinct regions of articular cartilage (superficial, middle, deep, and calcified zone). A summary of emerging and existing scaffolds can be found in our recent review [50].

Conclusion

Regenerative medicine approaches which include cell-based therapies, the use of anti-inflammatory cytokines and/or supportive growth factors, and tissue-engineered scaffolds offer the potential to combat the multiple modalities of OA progression and degradation. The combination of various individual regenerative therapies may indeed be required to attenuate the destructive inflammatory process and provide the accompanying structural changes to be truly disease modifying. The emerging conceptual and technical solutions outlined in this chapter are becoming increasingly sophisticated as they evolve and offer the potential for achieving this goal (Fig. 12.1).

References

1. Gerlier L, et al. The cost utility of autologous chondrocytes implantation using ChondroCelect® in symptomatic knee cartilage lesions in Belgium. Pharmacoeconomics. 2010;28(12):1129–46.
2. Carticel. About CARTICEL. http://www.carticel.com/patients/about.aspx. Accessed Sept 2014.
3. MEDIPOST. The future of biotechnology, MEDIPOST. http://www.medi-post.com/sp_5_1.asp. Accessed Sept 2014.
4. Dhinsa BS, Adesida AB. Current clinical therapies for cartilage repair, their limitation and the role of stem cells. Curr Stem Cell Res Ther. 2012;7(2):143–8.
5. Kapoor M, et al. Role of proinflammatory cytokines in the pathophysiology of osteoarthritis. Nat Rev Rheumatol. 2011;7(1):33–42.
6. Goldring MB, Otero M. Inflammation in osteoarthritis. Curr Opin Rheumatol. 2011;23(5):471–8.
7. Zamli Z, Sharif M. Chondrocyte apoptosis: a cause or consequence of osteoarthritis? Int J Rheum Dis. 2011;14(2):159–66.
8. Loeser RF, et al. Osteoarthritis: a disease of the joint as an organ. Arthritis Rheum. 2012;64(6):1697–707.
9. Beyer C, Schett G. Pharmacotherapy: concepts of pathogenesis and emerging treatments. Novel targets in bone and cartilage. Best Pract Res Clin Rheumatol. 2010;24(4):489–96.
10. Chevalier X, et al. Safety study of intraarticular injection of interleukin 1 receptor antagonist in patients with painful knee osteoarthritis: a multicenter study. J Rheumatol. 2005;32(7):1317–23.
11. Baltzer AW, et al. Autologous conditioned serum (Orthokine) is an effective treatment for knee osteoarthritis. Osteoarthritis Cartilage. 2009;17(2):152–60.
12. Kon E, et al. Platelet-rich plasma intra-articular injection versus hyaluronic acid viscosupplementation as treatments for cartilage pathology: from early degeneration to osteoarthritis. Arthroscopy. 2011;27(11):1490–501.
13. Cao L, et al. The promotion of cartilage defect repair using adenovirus mediated Sox9 gene transfer of rabbit bone marrow mesenchymal stem cells. Biomaterials. 2011;32(16):3910–20.
14. Zhang X, Mao Z, Yu C. Suppression of early experimental osteoarthritis by gene transfer of interleukin-1 receptor antagonist and interleukin-10. J Orthop Res. 2004;22(4):742–50.
15. Steadman JR, et al. Outcomes of microfracture for traumatic chondral defects of the knee: average 11-year follow-up. Arthroscopy. 2003;19(5):477–84.
16. Johnstone B, et al. Tissue engineering for articular cartilage repair–the state of the art. Eur Cell Mater. 2013;25:248–67.
17. Andia I, Abate M. Knee osteoarthritis: hyaluronic acid, platelet-rich plasma or both in association? Expert Opin Biol Ther. 2014;14(5):635–49.
18. Bollyky PL, et al. Intact extracellular matrix and the maintenance of immune tolerance: high molecular weight hyaluronan promotes persistence of induced CD4+CD25+ regulatory T cells. J Leukoc Biol. 2009;86(3):567–72.
19. Muto J, et al. Engagement of CD44 by hyaluronan suppresses TLR4 signaling and the septic response to LPS. Mol Immunol. 2009;47(2–3):449–56.
20. Takahashi T, et al. A decrease in the molecular weight of hyaluronic acid in synovial fluid from patients with temporomandibular disorders. J Oral Pathol Medicine (Official Publication of the

International Association of Oral Pathologists and the American Academy of Oral Pathology). 2004;33(4):224–9.
21. Dahl LB, et al. Concentration and molecular weight of sodium hyaluronate in synovial fluid from patients with rheumatoid arthritis and other arthropathies. Ann Rheum Dis. 1985;44(12):817–22.
22. Scheibner KA, et al. Hyaluronan fragments act as an endogenous danger signal by engaging TLR2. J Immunol. 2006;177(2):1272–81.
23. Zavan B, et al. Hyaluronic acid induces activation of the kappa-opioid receptor. PLoS One. 2013;8(1), e55510.
24. Miller LE, Block JE. US-approved intra-articular hyaluronic acid injections are safe and effective in patients with knee osteoarthritis: systematic review and meta-analysis of randomized, saline-controlled trials. Clin Med Insights Arthritis Musculoskelet Disord. 2013;6:57–63.
25. Rutjes AW, et al. Viscosupplementation for osteoarthritis of the knee: a systematic review and meta-analysis. Ann Intern Med. 2012;157(3):180–91.
26. Chahal J, et al. The role of platelet-rich plasma in arthroscopic rotator cuff repair: a systematic review with quantitative synthesis. Arthroscopy. 2012;28(11):1718–27.
27. Khoshbin A, et al. The efficacy of platelet-rich plasma in the treatment of symptomatic knee osteoarthritis: a systematic review with quantitative synthesis. Arthroscopy. 2013;29(12):2037–48.
28. Pourcho AM, et al. Intraarticular platelet-rich plasma injection in the treatment of knee osteoarthritis: review and recommendations. Am J Phys Med Rehabil. 2014;93(11 Suppl 3):S108–21.
29. Sundman EA, Cole BJ, Fortier LA. Growth factor and catabolic cytokine concentrations are influenced by the cellular composition of platelet-rich plasma. Am J Sports Med. 2011;39(10):2135–40.
30. Sundman EA, et al. The anti-inflammatory and matrix restorative mechanisms of platelet-rich plasma in osteoarthritis. Am J Sports Med. 2014;42(1):35–41.
31. Chevalier X, Conrozier T. Biological markers for osteoarthritis: an update. Joint Bone Spine. 2005;72(2):106–9.
32. Meijer H, et al. The production of anti-inflammatory cytokines in whole blood by physico-chemical induction. Inflamm Res. 2003;52(10):404–7.
33. Fox BA, Stephens MM. Treatment of knee osteoarthritis with Orthokine-derived autologous conditioned serum. Expert Rev Clin Immunol. 2010;6(3):335–45.
34. Lawrence JT, Birmingham J, Toth AP. Emerging ideas: prevention of posttraumatic arthritis through interleukin-1 and tumor necrosis factor-alpha inhibition. Clin Orthop Relat Res. 2011;469(12):3522–6.
35. Caron JP, et al. Chondroprotective effect of intraarticular injections of interleukin-1 receptor antagonist in experimental osteoarthritis. Suppression of collagenase-1 expression. Arthritis Rheum. 1996;39(9):1535–44.
36. Elsaid KA, et al. The impact of anterior cruciate ligament injury on lubricin metabolism and the effect of inhibiting tumor necrosis factor alpha on chondroprotection in an animal model. Arthritis Rheum. 2009;60(10):2997–3006.
37. Pintan GF, et al. Update on biological therapies for knee injuries: osteoarthritis. Curr Rev Musculoskelet Med. 2014;7(3):263–9.
38. Lane NE, et al. Tanezumab for the treatment of pain from osteoarthritis of the knee. N Engl J Med. 2010;363(16):1521–31.
39. Brown MT, et al. Tanezumab reduces osteoarthritic knee pain: results of a randomized, double-blind, placebo-controlled phase III trial. J Pain. 2012;13(8):790–8.
40. Spierings EL, et al. A phase III placebo- and oxycodone-controlled study of tanezumab in adults with osteoarthritis pain of the hip or knee. Pain. 2013;154(9):1603–12.
41. Akagi R, et al. Effective knock down of matrix metalloproteinase-13 by an intra-articular injection of small interfering RNA (siRNA) in a murine surgically-induced osteoarthritis model. J Orthop Res. 2014;32(9):1175–80.
42. Madry H, Cucchiarini M. Advances and challenges in gene-based approaches for osteoarthritis. J Gene Med. 2013;15(10):343–55.

43. Evans CH, Ghivizzani SC, Robbins PD. Arthritis gene therapy and its tortuous path into the clinic. Transl Res (The Journal of Laboratory and Clinical Medicine). 2013;161(4):205–16.
44. Demoor M, et al. Cartilage tissue engineering: Molecular control of chondrocyte differentiation for proper cartilage matrix reconstruction. Biochimica Et Biophysica Acta. 2014;1840(8):2414–40.
45. Peterson L, et al. Autologous chondrocyte implantation: a long-term follow-up. Am J Sports Med. 2010;38(6):1117–24.
46. Nawaz SZ, et al. Autologous chondrocyte implantation in the knee: mid-term to long-term results. J Bone Joint Surg Am. 2014;96(10):824–30.
47. Harris JD, et al. Autologous chondrocyte implantation: a systematic review. J Bone Joint Surg Am. 2010;92(12):2220–33.
48. Brittberg M. Autologous chondrocyte implantation–technique and long-term follow-up. Injury. 2008;39 Suppl 1:S40–9.
49. Minas T, et al. Autologous chondrocyte implantation for joint preservation in patients with early osteoarthritis. Clin Orthop Relat Res. 2010;468(1):147–57.
50. Viswanathan S, Gomez-Aristizabal A. Review of patents and commercial opportunities involving Mesenchymal Stromal Cells (MSCs) therapies in osteoarthritis. Recent Pat Regen Med. 2014;4(1):1–15.
51. Peterson L, et al. Autologous chondrocyte transplantation. Biomechanics and long-term durability. Am J Sports Med. 2002;30(1):2–12.
52. Farr J, et al. Particulated articular cartilage: CAIS and DeNovo NT. J Knee Surg. 2012;25(1):23–9.
53. Cuende N, Rico L, Herrera C. Concise review: bone marrow mononuclear cells for the treatment of ischemic syndromes: medicinal product or cell transplantation? Stem Cells Transl Med. 2012;1(5):403–8.
54. Song F, et al. Comparison of the efficacy of bone marrow mononuclear cells and bone mesenchymal stem cells in the treatment of osteoarthritis in a sheep model. Int J Clin Exp Pathol. 2014;7(4):1415–26.
55. Deng M-W, et al. Cell therapy with G-CSF-mobilized stem cells in a rat osteoarthritis model. Cell Transplant. 2014. [Epub ahead of print]
56. Dong Z, et al. The survival condition and immunoregulatory function of adipose Stromal Vascular Fraction (SVF) in the early stage of nonvascularized adipose transplantation. PLoS One. 2013;8(11), e80364.
57. Jurgens WJFM, et al. One-step surgical procedure for the treatment of osteochondral defects with adipose-derived stem cells in a caprine knee defect: a pilot study. BioRes Open Access. 2013;2(4):315–25.
58. HiQcell. Australian world first placebo-controlled clinical study of HiQCell. Available from: http://www.imaginelessjointpain.com.au/about-hiqcell-treatment/clinical-studies/. Accessed 27 July 2014.
59. Erices A, Conget P, Minguell JJ. Mesenchymal progenitor cells in human umbilical cord blood. Br J Haematol. 2000;109(1):235–42.
60. Zuk PA, et al. Multilineage cells from human adipose tissue: implications for cell-based therapies. Tissue Eng. 2001;7(2):211–28.
61. Hass R, et al. Different populations and sources of human mesenchymal stem cells (MSC): a comparison of adult and neonatal tissue-derived MSC. Cell Commun Signal. 2011;9:12.
62. Lee DH, et al. Synovial fluid CD34–CD44+ CD90+ mesenchymal stem cell levels are associated with the severity of primary knee osteoarthritis. Osteoarthritis Cartilage (OARS, Osteoarthritis Research Society). 2012;20(2):106–9.
63. Dominici M, et al. Minimal criteria for defining multipotent mesenchymal stromal cells. The International Society for Cellular Therapy position statement. Cytotherapy. 2006;8(4):315–7.
64. Singer NG, Caplan AI. Mesenchymal stem cells: mechanisms of inflammation. Annu Rev Pathol. 2011;6:457–78.
65. Vangsness Jr CT, et al. Adult human mesenchymal stem cells delivered via intra-articular injection to the knee following partial medial meniscectomy: a randomized, double-blind, controlled study. J Bone Joint Surg Am. 2014;96(2):90–8.

66. Orozco L, et al. Treatment of knee osteoarthritis with autologous mesenchymal stem cells: a pilot study. Transplantation. 2013;95(12):1535–41.
67. Wakitani S, et al. Human autologous culture expanded bone marrow mesenchymal cell transplantation for repair of cartilage defects in osteoarthritic knees. Osteoarthritis Cartilage. 2002;10(3):199–206.
68. Centeno CJ, et al. Increased knee cartilage volume in degenerative joint disease using percutaneously implanted, autologous mesenchymal stem cells. Pain Physician. 2008;11(3):343–53.
69. Davatchi F, et al. Mesenchymal stem cell therapy for knee osteoarthritis. Preliminary report of four patients. Int J Rheum Dis. 2011;14(2):211–5.
70. Emadedin M, et al. Intra-articular injection of autologous mesenchymal stem cells in six patients with knee osteoarthritis. Arch Iran Med. 2012;15(7):422–8.
71. Koh Y-G, et al. Mesenchymal stem cell injections improve symptoms of knee osteoarthritis. Arthroscopy (The Journal of Arthroscopic & Related Surgery: Official Publication of the Arthroscopy Association of North America and the International Arthroscopy Association). 2013;29(4):748–55.
72. Viswanathan S, et al. Soliciting strategies for developing cell-based reference materials to advance mesenchymal stromal cell research and clinical translation. Stem Cells Dev. 2014;23(11):1157–67.
73. Oldershaw RA. Cell sources for the regeneration of articular cartilage: the past, the horizon and the future. Int J Exp Pathol. 2012;93(6):389–400.
74. Craft AM, et al. Specification of chondrocytes and cartilage tissues from embryonic stem cells. Development. 2013;140(12):2597–610.
75. Diekman BO, et al. Cartilage tissue engineering using differentiated and purified induced pluripotent stem cells. Proc Natl Acad Sci U S A. 2012;109(47):19172–7.
76. Sato T, et al. The engineered thymidylate kinase (TMPK)/AZT enzyme-prodrug axis offers efficient bystander cell killing for suicide gene therapy of cancer. PLoS One. 2013;8(10), e78711.
77. Taylor CJ, et al. Banking on human embryonic stem cells: estimating the number of donor cell lines needed for HLA matching. Lancet. 2005;366(9502):2019–25.
78. Ishii R, et al. Placenta to cartilage: direct conversion of human placenta to chondrocytes with transformation by defined factors. Mol Biol Cell. 2012;23(18):3511–21.
79. Anz AW, et al. Application of biologics in the treatment of the rotator cuff, meniscus, cartilage, and osteoarthritis. J Am Acad Orthop Surg. 2014;22(2):68–79.
80. Filardo G, et al. Scaffold-based repair for cartilage healing: a systematic review and technical note. Arthroscopy. 2013;29(1):174–86.
81. Kock L, van Donkelaar CC, Ito K. Tissue engineering of functional articular cartilage: the current status. Cell Tissue Res. 2012;347(3):613–27.
82. Myers KR, Sgaglione NA, Grande DA. Trends in biological joint resurfacing. Bone Joint Res. 2013;2(9):193–9.
83. Chan BP, Leong KW. Scaffolding in tissue engineering: general approaches and tissue-specific considerations. Eur Spine J. 2008;17 Suppl 4:467–79.
84. Childs A, et al. Novel biologically-inspired rosette nanotube PLLA scaffolds for improving human mesenchymal stem cell chondrogenic differentiation. Biomed Mater. 2013;8(6):065003.
85. Izadifar Z, Chen X, Kulyk W. Strategic design and fabrication of engineered scaffolds for articular cartilage repair. J Funct Biomater. 2012;3(4):799–838.
86. Musumeci G, et al. New perspectives for articular cartilage repair treatment through tissue engineering: a contemporary review. World J Orthop. 2014;5(2):80–8.
87. Hollister SJ. Porous scaffold design for tissue engineering. Nat Mater. 2005;4(7):518–24.
88. Evans CH. Advances in regenerative orthopedics. Mayo Clin Proc. 2013;88(11):1323–39.
89. Willerth SM, Sakiyama-Elbert SE. Combining stem cells and biomaterial scaffolds for constructing tissues and cell delivery. In StemBook. Massachusetts General Hospital. Cambridge, MA; 2008.
90. Bacakova L, Novotna K, Parizek M. Polysaccharides as cell carriers for tissue engineering: the use of cellulose in vascular wall reconstruction. Physiol Res. 2014;63 Suppl 1:S29–47.
91. Kwon H, et al. The influence of scaffold material on chondrocytes under inflammatory conditions. Acta Biomater. 2013;9(5):6563–75.

92. Wakitani S, et al. Mesenchymal cell-based repair of large, full-thickness defects of articular cartilage. J Bone Joint Surg Am. 1994;76(4):579–92.
93. Sumanasinghe RD, Bernacki SH, Loboa EG. Osteogenic differentiation of human mesenchymal stem cells in collagen matrices: effect of uniaxial cyclic tensile strain on bone morphogenetic protein (BMP-2) mRNA expression. Tissue Eng. 2006;12(12):3459–65.
94. Pulkkinen HJ, et al. Engineering of cartilage in recombinant human type II collagen gel in nude mouse model in vivo. Osteoarthritis Cartilage. 2010;18(8):1077–87.
95. Pulkkinen HJ, et al. Repair of osteochondral defects with recombinant human type II collagen gel and autologous chondrocytes in rabbit. Osteoarthritis Cartilage. 2013;21(3):481–90.
96. Yang C, et al. The application of recombinant human collagen in tissue engineering. BioDrugs. 2004;18(2):103–19.
97. Meinel L, et al. Engineering cartilage-like tissue using human mesenchymal stem cells and silk protein scaffolds. Biotechnol Bioeng. 2004;88(3):379–91.
98. Sofia S, et al. Functionalized silk-based biomaterials for bone formation. J Biomed Mater Res. 2001;54(1):139–48.
99. Worster AA, et al. Chondrocytic differentiation of mesenchymal stem cells sequentially exposed to transforming growth factor-beta1 in monolayer and insulin-like growth factor-I in a three-dimensional matrix. J Orthop Res. 2001;19(4):738–49.
100. Bulman SE, et al. Enhancing the mesenchymal stem cell therapeutic response: cell localization and support for cartilage repair. Tissue Eng Part B Rev. 2013;19(1):58–68.
101. Erickson IE, et al. High mesenchymal stem cell seeding densities in hyaluronic acid hydrogels produce engineered cartilage with native tissue properties. Acta Biomater. 2012;8(8):3027–34.
102. Mortisen D, et al. Tailoring thermoreversible hyaluronan hydrogels by "click" chemistry and RAFT polymerization for cell and drug therapy. Biomacromolecules. 2010;11(5):1261–72.
103. Stanish WD, et al. Novel scaffold-based BST-CarGel treatment results in superior cartilage repair compared with microfracture in a randomized controlled trial. J Bone Joint Surg Am. 2013;95(18):1640–50.
104. Yang Z, et al. Improved mesenchymal stem cells attachment and in vitro cartilage tissue formation on chitosan-modified poly(L-lactide-co-epsilon-caprolactone) scaffold. Tissue Eng Part A. 2012;18(3–4):242–51.
105. Haaparanta AM, et al. Preparation and characterization of collagen/PLA, chitosan/PLA, and collagen/chitosan/PLA hybrid scaffolds for cartilage tissue engineering. J Mater Sci Mater Med. 2014;25(4):1129–36.
106. Nguyen LH, et al. Engineering articular cartilage with spatially-varying matrix composition and mechanical properties from a single stem cell population using a multi-layered hydrogel. Biomaterials. 2011;32(29):6946–52.
107. Chung C, Burdick JA. Engineering cartilage tissue. Adv Drug Deliv Rev. 2008;60(2):243–62.
108. Varghese S, et al. Chondroitin sulfate based niches for chondrogenic differentiation of mesenchymal stem cells. Matrix Biol. 2008;27(1):12–21.
109. Uematsu K, et al. Cartilage regeneration using mesenchymal stem cells and a three-dimensional poly-lactic-glycolic acid (PLGA) scaffold. Biomaterials. 2005;26(20):4273–9.
110. Hori J, et al. Articular cartilage repair using an intra-articular magnet and synovium-derived cells. J Orthop Res. 2011;29(4):531–8.
111. Freed LE, et al. Advanced material strategies for tissue engineering scaffolds. Adv Mater. 2009;21(32–33):3410–8.
112. O'Connell GD, et al. Toward engineering a biological joint replacement. J Knee Surg. 2012;25(3):187–96.
113. Huey DJ, Hu JC, Athanasiou KA. Unlike bone, cartilage regeneration remains elusive. Science. 2012;338(6109):917–21.

Chapter 13
Precision Medicine for Osteoarthritis

Christian J.H. Veillette and Igor Jurisica

Key Points

1. Precision medicine, or what patients and the media often call personalized medicine, aims to utilize molecular profiles of patient biospecimens and increasingly precise outcome metrics from diverse biosensors to more accurately diagnose a disease, tailor the therapy a patient receives, and monitor response.
2. In order to accomplish the goals of precision medicine in osteoarthritis, several key components of biomedical research (target identification, marker identification, molecular mechanisms) and clinical medicine (treatment, diagnosis, health outcomes) must be seamlessly integrated across several data repositories (clinical records, biospecimen, -omics databases) and analyzed using integrative data mining and iterative learning strategies.
3. A clinically meaningful and feasible strategy is required for identifying OA phenotypes for targeted treatment.
4. The OA Data Integration Platform (OADIP) provides comprehensive, expert curated clinical and molecular data repository across OA. Advances in molecular profiling, interoperability, integration, and exchange of data

C.J.H. Veillette, MD, MSc, FRCSC (✉)
Division of Orthopaedic Surgery, Department of Surgery, Toronto Western Hospital, University Health Network, 399 Bathurst Street, East Wing Rm 1-440, Toronto, ON M5T 2S8, Canada

University of Toronto, Toronto, ON, Canada
e-mail: christian.veillette@uhn.ca

I. Jurisica, PhD
Princess Margaret Cancer Centre, University Health Network, IBM Life Sciences Discovery Centre, Toronto, ON, Canada

M. Kapoor, N.N. Mahomed (eds.), *Osteoarthritis: Pathogenesis, Diagnosis, Available Treatments, Drug Safety, Regenerative and Precision Medicine*,
DOI 10.1007/978-3-319-19560-5_13

combined with machine learning techniques will enable comprehensive signatures for OA subtypes to be identified and targeted for treatment and discovery.
5. The feasibility and reality of precision medicine for OA are on the horizon as we strive to provide the right care to the right patient at the right time.

Introduction

While evidence-based medicine has long influenced the way patients are treated, a coming revolution questions whether undertaking larger studies to refine the evidence is the path to better patient outcomes. Importantly, the aim is to move medicine closer to data science and through integrative analyses from current "reactive" to preventive medicine. Precision medicine, or what patients and the media often call personalized medicine, aims to utilize molecular profiles of patient biospecimens (genes, proteins, microRNAs, metabolites, etc.) and increasingly precise outcome metrics from diverse biosensors to more accurately diagnose a disease, tailor the therapy a patient receives, and monitor response [1, 2]. The goal is to integrate molecular and biosensor information to provide a more precise classification of disease of a given individual patient, compared to past when we could not discriminate between patient subgroups. While personalized medicine might say, "patient X with disease Y should get drug Z," precision medicine says, "patient X has a subtype of disease Y – actually, disease Y3, not disease Y1, Y2, or Y4 – and patients with subtype Y3 tend to respond more favorably to treatment A not treatment Z" [1]. This approach aims to transform the paradigm from trial-and-error-based medicine with therapies directed toward broad patient segments to drugs or surgeries targeted at small segments defined by molecular profiles and biometrics to provide the best possible therapeutic outcome with minimal adverse events. This is particularly important in high-stakes medical decisions such as oncology and surgery. Topol has highlighted that the typical number needed to treat (NNT) accepted in large trials means that a majority of patients take therapies to benefit one, often at astronomical cost and with a risk of adverse events [3].

In the field of OA, the identification of the optimal treatment for each individual patient is a pressing concern for all stakeholders (patients, physicians, healthcare payers, pharmaceutical, and device industry), due to the heterogeneity of the disease and the very large number of individuals affected [4]. Over the past several decades, there has been a lack of progress in identifying structure modifying treatments for OA, and therefore it is even more important to identify the optimal patient population in which to test a given treatment. The lack of efficacy of OA drugs and therapies highlights the need for precision medicine for OA. OA drugs have been shown to be ineffective in up to 50 % of a patient population and rank second only to cancer drugs and Alzheimer's drugs [5]. Even the response and satisfaction to joint replacement surgery have been shown to be poor in up to 30 % of patients undergoing knee replacement for OA [6, 7]. This is highly reminiscent of examples of successful precision medicine approaches for non-small cell lung cancer where initial clinical trials had failed but when drugs were targeted to patients with specific molecular profiles were highly effective [8, 9]. This paradigm shift in our current traditional evidence-based strategies needs to be kept in mind when evaluating treatments – just because a medication or treatment is not effective for everyone does not mean it will not be effective for anyone. The task is to identify the biomarkers or subtypes of disease that predicts response – whether the treatment is a medication, psychosocial intervention, or surgical procedure.

Why Is OA an Optimal Candidate for Precision Medicine?

The majority of examples of successful precision medicine is currently derived from oncology and, in comparison to a polygenic disease like OA, represents a relatively simple stratification of treatment based on targeting a specific activated pathway in an oligogenic disease [2, 4, 10]. However, it seems likely that specific polygenic diseases with epigenetic influences and certain therapeutic situations may prove better suited to the application of precision medicine than others [11]. OA is an optimal candidate disease for precision medicine because it is characterized by a highly heterogeneous patient population, low response rates to treatments, increased risk of significant adverse events, and large economic burden due to high-cost therapies from a trial-and-error approach which typifies our current management [12].

Karsdel et al. have identified four major drivers of precision medicine: (1) identification of patients that are in the greatest need of treatment, (2) identification of patients whom may respond optimally with the highest efficacy and lowest safety concerns to a given treatment, (3) development strategy for a selected subpopulation of patients, and (4) efficient use of healthcare resources [4]. The interplay of these four drivers dictates the overall economic and ethical benefits of a precision medicine strategy and is a key requirement for improving OA care.

It has become increasingly evident from failures of clinical trials that OA is not one disease but has different phenotypes [12]. Although there are currently no effective treatments to validate this hypothesis, several subtypes and proposed treatment strategies have been identified [13–19]. Five subtypes have received the most attention in the current literature: metabolic OA (including obesity) [20–23], posttraumatic OA (including malalignment) [24, 25], inflammation driven OA [26–29], subchondral bone turnover driven OA [30–33], and genetic-based OA [11, 34, 35]. Consideration of just these basic subtypes alone and the different pathological processes involved highlights why the response rate for a particular therapy will be low in the absence of patient selection for a subset of patients with a specific OA phenotype. The disappointing results of initially promising clinical treatments for OA such as iNOS, strontium ranelate, calcitonin, MMP inhibitors, cathepsin K inhibitors, and bisphosphonates are likely due to applying these therapies to nonselected or poorly phenotyped patient populations [36–40].

How Do We Get to Precision Medicine in OA?

In order to accomplish the goals of precision medicine in OA, several key components of biomedical research (target identification, marker identification, molecular mechanisms) and clinical medicine (treatment, diagnosis, health outcomes) must be seamlessly integrated across several data repositories (clinical records, biospecimen, -omics databases) and analyzed using integrative data mining and iterative learning strategies [2]. Although this is a formidable task, evolving technologies that improve interoperability and exchange of data combined with machine learning techniques are enabling the potential to be realized.

Biomarkers Central to Precision Medicine in OA

Biomarkers are central to the concept of precision medicine in OA. A biomarker is defined as a characteristic that is objectively measured and evaluated as an indicator of normal biological processes, pathological processes, or pharmacologic responses to a therapeutic intervention [41–43]. Biomarkers are often only thought of as molecular markers from blood, urine, or joint fluid; however, current classifications of biomarkers recognize the importance of both soluble or wet biomarkers such as RNA, DNA, miRNA, peptides, proteins, and metabolites and dry biomarkers such as clinical factors, imaging (X-ray, MRI, US), and health outcomes (WOOS, painDETECT). The properties of an ideal biomarker include being readily available for acquisition and testing, being stable in storage, and being an accurate surrogate for a specific disease pathogenesis or treatment goal. At present, very few tests function well enough to meet these basic requirements; however, there is emerging evidence to consider multiple biomarkers as valuable assets in caring for patients with OA [44], leading to prognostic and predictive signatures.

Bauer et al. have outlined a classification of OA biomarkers (burden of disease, investigative, prognosis, efficacy, and diagnosis – BIPED) to provide a logical structure for the characterization of markers according to specific functions [45]. For example, one marker such as sCOMP might measure aspects of burden of disease (B) while also aiding in diagnosis (D). Specific combinations of biomarkers such as DNA or proteins ("signature") may be associated with OA subtypes, indicate a patient's risk of OA progression, or indicate probability of patient's response to specific treatment. Importantly, it has been shown that signatures far outperform individual markers [9, 46, 47].

Identifying Clear OA Phenotypes for Targeting Treatment

A clinically meaningful and feasible strategy is required for identifying OA phenotypes for targeted treatment. OA is a progressive heterogeneous disease with different clinical phenotypes that change and evolve over the course of the disease leading

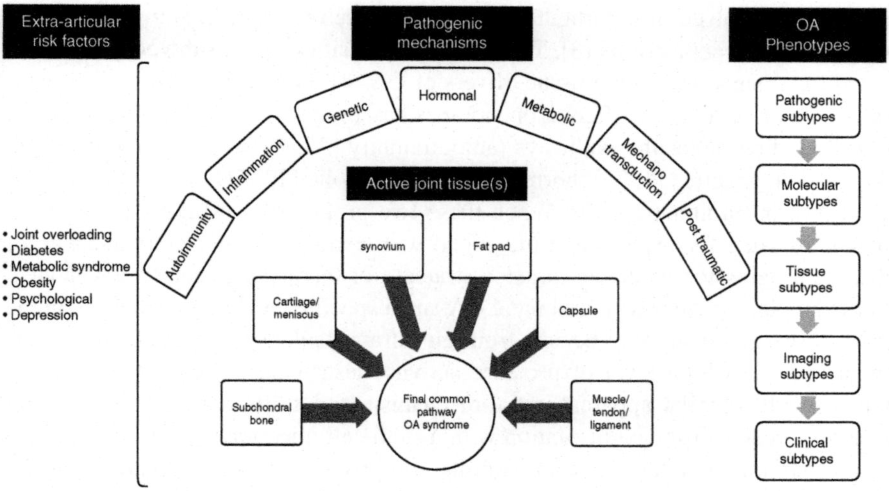

Fig. 13.1 A comprehensive view of the complexity of OA phenotypes and their relationships to pathogenic mechanisms and predominately active joint tissue(s) at a given stage of the disease and modification by extra-articular risk factors and comorbidities

to common clinical manifestations [12, 14]. The clinical presentation of a specific phenotype at a point in time depends on the most active joint tissue (bone, cartilage, synovium, fat pad, capsule, ligaments/muscles) and the predominant underlying pathogenic mechanisms (autoimmunity, inflammation, genetic, hormonal, metabolic, mechanotransduction, ageing, posttraumatic). In addition, OA needs to be considered as a joint disease with other comorbidities and extra-articular risk factors (joint overloading, diabetes, metabolic syndrome, obesity, psychosocial, depression) that often overlap and modulate the OA process. All of these factors, the overlap of several pathogenic processes and the various tissues that are dominant at different stages of the disease progression, have led to the difficulties in identifying clear OA phenotypes (Fig. 13.1).

Knoop et al. have identified five clinical phenotypes in a population with OA of the knees based on four clinically relevant patient characteristics: severity of radiographic OA, lower extremity muscle strength, body mass index (BMI), and depression [17]. The proposed phenotypes of knee OA patients include (1) minimal joint disease phenotype, (2) strong muscle phenotype, (3) nonobese and weak muscle phenotype, (4) obese and weak muscle phenotype, and (5) depressive phenotype. Higher pain levels and activity limitations occurred in patients with depressive and obese and weak muscle phenotypes. Although this identification of these phenotypes can be readily applied in a clinical practice and helpful in prediction of clinical outcomes, it does not incorporate underlying pathogenic mechanisms that most likely determine these end-stage clinical expressions. Importantly, such characteristics are not yet readily measured as accurately as expression of molecular markers. However, wearable technologies are revolutionizing this field.

OA can be divided into at least six different subtypes based on the predominant joint tissue (subchondral bone, cartilage, synovium, fat pad, capsule, muscle/tendon/

ligaments) involved at a particular stage of disease or the most active tissue in a specific patient population [18]. This proposed classification of subtypes allows targeted treatments toward the tissue drivers of OA [4]. In addition, OA can be separated into at least seven different phenotypes based on pathogenic mechanisms and corresponding molecular pathways (autoimmunity [27, 48, 49], inflammation [26, 34, 48, 50], genetic [11, 35], hormonal [20], metabolic [22, 51], mechanotransduction [24], posttraumatic [25]). When these two proposed classifications are combined, adjusted for overlap and integrated with extra-articular factors and rate of disease progression, a clearer targeted strategy for therapeutics can be envisioned. For example, a patient with traumatic OA and a specific molecular signature, in the early disease course, may benefit from an intra-articular protease inhibitor treatment, due to a high level of protease activity destroying the cartilage. Another patient with a similar apparent initial mechanism and a different molecular signature may benefit from augmentation with a stem cell injection to recalibrate a dysfunctional inflammatory cascade. Similar proposed treatment scenarios can be envisioned for a patient with generalized OA with a molecular signature for high bone turnover, where an antiresorptive treatment would be best indicated to help regulate subchondral bone turnover at a specific stage of the disease.

Recently, Zhang et al. have proposed a classification of OA phenotypes by metabolomic analysis of synovial fluid from hip and knee joints with OA [52]. They demonstrated that their OA cohort comprised at least three metabolically distinct subgroups due primarily to differences in carnitine, lipid, and collagen metabolism. A targeted metabolomics approach may enable improved understanding and profiling of the biological response of cellular processes to the complex interplay of genotypic and environmental influences that occur in the joint.

Building an OA Data Integration Platform

In 2011, the National Academy of Sciences established a committee and published a report entitled "*Toward Precision Medicine: Building a Knowledge Network for Biomedical Research and a New Taxonomy of Disease*" [2]. The report recommends the development of a knowledge management system, or Information Commons, structured similar to a layered geographical information system used for applications like Google Maps. Instead of being organized by geographical positioning, the Information Commons would be organized around individual patients as the bottom layer of all the overlays. This multilayered system would collect a broad range of health data including demographics, sign and symptoms, patient outcomes, genome, microbiome, epigenome, and exposome through a vast knowledge network integrated into observational studies during the normal course of clinical care. Rather than considering research efforts as separate from health care, the report suggests we collect standardized clinical, molecular, and exposure data useful for research as part of routine health care. The "new taxonomy" that

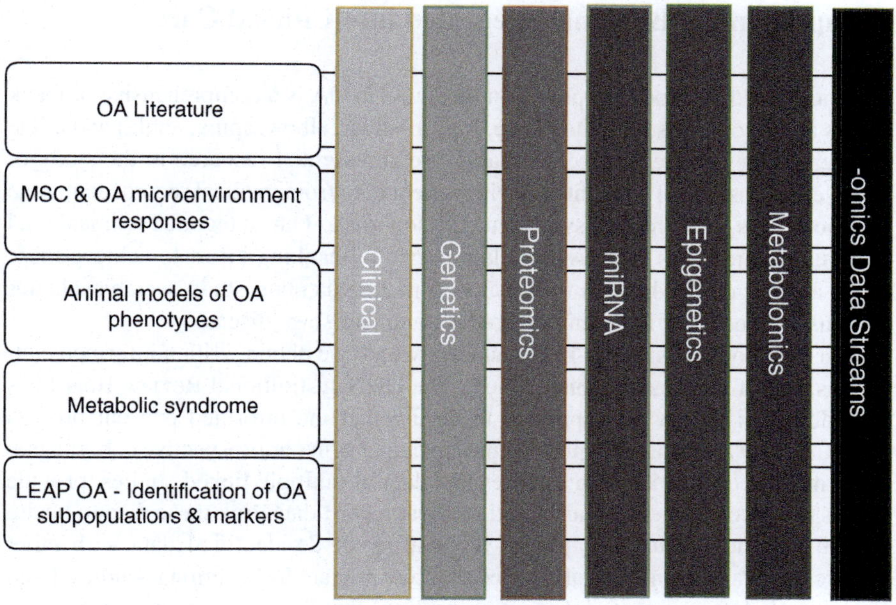

Fig. 13.2 Osteoarthritis Data Integration Portal (OADIP). The OADIP is analogous to a layered geographical information system (GIS). The OADIP connects data from (1) curated clinical and molecular literature published on OA and our internal core research programs including (2) mesenchymal stem cells (MSC) and OA microenvironment responses, (3) animal models of OA phenotypes, (4) metabolic syndrome, and an (5) observational cohort of OA patients (LEAP OA) across clinical and molecular data sources

emerges would define diseases by their underlying molecular causes and other factors in addition to their traditional physical signs and symptoms through intralayer clusters and interlayer connections. In the context of OA, the individual patterns emerging from this multilayered data would define specific OA subtypes or phenotypes that are clinically relevant.

Our group has been building a translational framework for precision medicine in OA that shares similarities in concepts and vision despite being conceived prior to 2011. The OA Data Integration Platform (OADIP) provides comprehensive, expert curated clinical and molecular data repository across OA and can be compared with similar efforts in rheumatoid arthritis and psoriatic arthritis (Fig. 13.2). Multiple experimental platforms are included such as mRNA microarray, aCGH, SNP, microRNA, proteomics, methylation, and different histologies. One can search based on studies, gene expression, chromosomal aberrations, SNPs, or pathways. OADIP facilitates connection and integration of individual cores of our research program and ultimately enables us to determine the most biologically relevant and clinically useful candidates for precision medicine therapies and methods to augment a personalized therapy strategy. The platform will ultimately provide the most cost-effective and fastest approach to move from research discoveries to cures.

Comprehensive Biobank Integrated into Clinical Care

A critical building block for precision medicine in OA is a comprehensive biobank across all major joints with OA (knee, hip, shoulder, elbow, spine, ankle) and at the different stages of the disease. Biobanks are an essential resource in the study of complex diseases [53] when linked with patient data from medical records, outcome questionnaires, and health system utilization data. Our integrated clinical and research program has established a large-scale biobanking effort to achieve these needs and has embedded this within an observational cohort study, which evaluates response to treatment including early-stage and late-stage disease.

Our OA biobank is an opt-in biobank for which we obtain written informed consent as part of our observational cohort. The UHN Institutional Review Board has provided final review and approval to ensure that the informed consent process meets all legal and ethical requirements. Participants in our prospective cohort agree to permit use of biospecimen samples and data in multiple linked studies, provide access to outcome questionnaires and medical record data, link these data to health system utilization data, and permit the sharing of de-identified data with other researchers. Participants can also agree to future contact for additional studies. Each linked study has a separate information package that discusses privacy protections and risks involved in participating.

Patients assessed within the UHN Arthritis Program who are 18 years or older are able to communicate in English, have mental capacity to consent, and are eligible for the OA Biobank. Currently, focus has been placed on individuals with late-stage disease undergoing joint replacement or early- to mid-stage disease being treated with arthroscopic or other joint-preserving procedures, but the framework is in place to include specific target populations or nonoperative treatments. The baseline questionnaire was developed after a systematic review of the literature and meetings with an academic advisory board. The final questionnaire includes general health questions from the 12-Item Short Form Health Survey, joint-specific outcome measures, demographics, comorbidities, medications, painDETECT, Patient Health Questionnaire-9 (PHQ-9), Pain Catastrophizing Scale (PCS), and response to treatment. Questionnaires are completed by participants on a tablet using the DADOS Electronic Data Capture Platform with real-time reports integrated into the clinical care. All questionnaires can also be completed using a paper-based version and can be validated by a research assistant and scanned into the secure centralized database. Participants are asked to provide blood and urine samples at baseline and during follow-up over the course of 1 year. Tissue biospecimens including synovial fluid, cartilage, synovium, subchondral bone, and capsule are obtained from standardized locations for each joint. Specimen metadata such as aliquot amount, size, and time from harvest to freeze in liquid nitrogen are recorded during processing in the OA Biospecimen Management database. Unique identifiers and 2D bar-coded labels are attached to each individual container used for storage. Custom searches and reports can be generated based on any demographic, clinical data, or outcome questionnaire scores with the end goal to link to our -omics data repositories.

The Arthritis Program Biobank Governance Committee reviews all requests from investigators who wish to access OA Biobank samples and data. Only internal requests are currently considered; however, our future goal is to consider all requests including both academic and commercial.

Big Data Analytics and Machine Learning in OA

Understanding OA and advancing more personalized treatment regimens require access to the full spectrum of bioclinical data for the individual and for large cohorts. Regardless of whether these data are being used in mechanistic research or in the pursuit of biomarker-based clinical decision strategies, we need to integrate diverse, multimodal information (clinical, imaging, treatment, and tissue-derived data) in a quantitative manner to generate biological insight and provide specific clinical predictions and decision support that has clinical relevance. Identifying the key signals or groups of signals can only be achieved through integrative data mining and machine learning approaches. Conventional learning methods are not capable of extracting simple correlations from these large datasets let alone including prior probabilities ("priors") associated with our biological or clinical understanding. Machine learning methods and integrative computational biology are central to advancing our understanding of OA. Many within the OA research community are realizing that unimodal statistical or learning activities suffer from a variety of confounders that reflect the complexity of the disease, the patient, and our interventions [54].

To make a clinical impact, we must discover specific groups of markers (signatures) that can be used to significantly improve detection, diagnosis, prognosis, and treatment of OA. An integrative computational analysis and comprehensive computational and biological validation of putative markers identified from prospective OA cohorts and molecular profiles of samples from patients with early-to-moderate OA and end-stage OA is required [55]. The road to mapping OA markers focuses on three goals: (1) identify signatures to detect patients with high risk of developing subtypes of OA and increase the possibility of early detection; (2) identify signatures for predicting patient's response to specific treatments (this would help make the treatment more personalized and could guide the development of customized therapeutic treatments for that patient and the respective subgroup); and (3) develop more efficient computational methods for discovering relevant patterns of markers and create a public resource for OA research.

Two essential technologies are needed to enable scalable and effective data integration, annotation, and analysis: (1) IBM Watson system to process vast volumes of unstructured information and (2) IBM InfoSphere Streams to provide real-time data analytics for our World Community Grid Mapping Markers project [56]. Combined, this will enable us to significantly increase breadth and depth of integrative analyses, organize knowledge sources based on evidence, and implement effectively a prioritized ranking and recommending system.

Specifically, integrative data mining approaches that utilize state-of-the-art machine learning techniques are required that in addition to clinical data can analyze integrated networks of physical protein interactions, microRNA-gene networks, transcriptional regulatory networks, and metabolic networks [54, 55, 57, 58]. This process needs to be combined with expert clinical opinion as to which of the identified machine-generated risk factors can be feasibly determined at the clinical level or used to identify the need for further investigation (e.g., MRI or blood tests).

Briefly, a proposed strategy can be considered where clinical data from health records is combined with patient-reported outcomes, assessment data, and molecular profiles, in three steps. First, machine-generated phenotypes are determined using only sociodemographic, patient-reported outcomes, and clinical data obtained at baseline. Here, the IBM Watson system is used primarily. Second, iterative addition of more quantitative activity data, patient healthcare utilization, and molecular profiles is used to assess the impact on phenotypes (i.e., which quantitative factor(s) increases or decreases the association with high risk of persistent pain) determined from the first step. Importantly, association-mining algorithm (with direction for clinical experts and physicians) is used to optimize the clinical and molecular factors used. Case-based reasoning system is used to provide decision support and relevant evidence for risk assessment. In the third step, clinical input from clinical experts is used to ensure relevance and clinical usability of the computational output regarding the specific risk factors and frequency of combined risk factors to determine phenotypes (including low-risk scenarios) with consensus-based (i.e., Delhi method) association of the risk factor(s) individually or in combinations to known evidence-based treatment (simple or complex multidisciplinary management) that has been shown to be effective. The application of traditional methods, e.g., stratified analyses, multilevel regressions, or recursive partitioning, to assess for advantages or disadvantages of the machine learning strategies is important for clinical and analytical internal validation. During this process, the existing evidence-based interventions are assembled, and regionally appropriate recommendations for implementation from clinicians and knowledge users with integrated patient feedback are developed. The results of this iterative process will lead to a web-based risk-stratification tool and evidence-based, computational decision support system for patients with OA. Signaling networks will serve as an integration platform to build hypotheses and models for further functional studies of disease mechanisms and for clinical validation of optimized interventions for the identified risk stratified phenotypes [54].

Despite the obvious opportunity such a "big data" approach provides in the diagnosis, treatment, and particularly prevention of OA, there are several obstacles preventing the widespread adoption of this novel paradigm of care. Although infrastructure investments are decreasing in terms of the equipment necessary to determine genetic profiles since the emergence of companies such as 23andMe [59, 60] and others, developing the data analysis and informatics function within a clinical practice is time consuming and expensive. As a result of the complexity of the data streams, it is not possible to simply glance at raw data and determine a treatment directly. Also, seamless access to data recorded by different services such as consumer-based genetic analyses, activity trackers [61], and third-party data mining enterprises is often not available given the value of the information. In addition, when applying consumer products within the medical system, concerns related to the protection of privacy, accuracy, and reliability of measurements will need to be addressed.

Conclusion

The failure to date of most traditional evidence-based approaches in the management of patients with OA highlights that treatments need to be targeted to specific OA subgroups using the proposed precision medicine framework. Advances in molecular profiling, interoperability, integration, and exchange of data combined with machine learning techniques will enable comprehensive signatures for OA subtypes to be identified and targeted for treatment and discovery. The feasibility and reality of precision medicine for OA are on the horizon as we strive to provide the right care to the right patient at the right time.

References

1. Katsnelson A. Momentum grows to make "personalized" medicine more "precise". Nat Med. 2013;19(3):249.
2. National Research Council (US) Committee on a Framework for Developing a New Taxonomy of Disease. Toward Precision Medicine: Building a Knowledge Network for Biomedical Research and a New Taxonomy of Disease [Internet]. Washington, DC: National Academies Press (US); 2011. http://www.ncbi.nlm.nih.gov/books/NBK91503/. Cited 6 Mar 2015.
3. Topol EJ. The creative destruction of medicine: how the digital revolution will create better health care. New York: Basic Books; 2012. 322 p.
4. Karsdal MA, Christiansen C, Ladel C, Henriksen K, Kraus VB, Bay-Jensen AC. Osteoarthritis–a case for personalized health care? Osteoarthr Cartil OARS Osteoarthr Res Soc. 2014;22(1):7–16.
5. Spear BB, Heath-Chiozzi M, Huff J. Clinical application of pharmacogenetics. Trends Mol Med. 2001;7(5):201–4.
6. Baumann C, Rat A-C, Mainard D, Cuny C, Guillemin F. Importance of patient satisfaction with care in predicting osteoarthritis-specific health-related quality of life one year after total joint arthroplasty. Qual Life Res Int J Qual Life Asp Treat Care Rehabil. 2011;20(10):1581–8.
7. Becker R, Döring C, Denecke A, Brosz M. Expectation, satisfaction and clinical outcome of patients after total knee arthroplasty. Knee Surg Sports Traumatol Arthrosc Off J ESSKA. 2011;19(9):1433–41.
8. Pao W, Hutchinson KE. Chipping away at the lung cancer genome. Nat Med. 2012;18(3):349–51.
9. Zhu C-Q, Pintilie M, John T, Strumpf D, Shepherd FA, Der SD, et al. Understanding prognostic gene expression signatures in lung cancer. Clin Lung Cancer. 2009;10(5):331–40.
10. Sawitzke AD. Personalized medicine for osteoarthritis: where are we now? Ther Adv Musculoskelet Dis. 2013;5(2):67–75.
11. Reynard LN, Loughlin J. Genetics and epigenetics of osteoarthritis. Maturitas. 2012;71(3):200–4.

12. Bijlsma JWJ, Berenbaum F, Lafeber FPJG. Osteoarthritis: an update with relevance for clinical practice. Lancet. 2011;377(9783):2115–26.
13. Carroll GJ, Breidahl WH, Jazayeri J. Confirmation of two major polyarticular osteoarthritis (POA) phenotypes–differentiation on the basis of joint topography. Osteoarthr Cartil OARS Osteoarthr Res Soc. 2009;17(7):891–5.
14. Castañeda S, Roman-Blas JA, Largo R, Herrero-Beaumont G. Osteoarthritis: a progressive disease with changing phenotypes. Rheumatol Oxf Engl. 2014;53(1):1–3.
15. Herrero-Beaumont G, Roman-Blas JA, Castañeda S, Jimenez SA. Primary osteoarthritis no longer primary: three subsets with distinct etiological, clinical, and therapeutic characteristics. Semin Arthritis Rheum. 2009;39(2):71–80.
16. Karsdal MA, Bihlet A, Byrjalsen I, Alexandersen P, Ladel C, Michaels M, et al. OA phenotypes, rather than disease stage, drive structural progression – identification of structural progressors from 2 phase III randomized clinical studies with symptomatic knee OA. Osteoarthr Cartil OARS Osteoarthr Res Soc. 2015;23(4):550–8.
17. Knoop J, van der Leeden M, Thorstensson CA, Roorda LD, Lems WF, Knol DL, et al. Identification of phenotypes with different clinical outcomes in knee osteoarthritis: data from the Osteoarthritis Initiative. Arthritis Care Res. 2011;63(11):1535–42.
18. McGonagle D, Tan AL, Carey J, Benjamin M. The anatomical basis for a novel classification of osteoarthritis and allied disorders. J Anat. 2010;216(3):279–91.
19. Van Spil WE, Jansen NWD, Bijlsma JWJ, Reijman M, DeGroot J, Welsing PMJ, et al. Clusters within a wide spectrum of biochemical markers for osteoarthritis: data from CHECK, a large cohort of individuals with very early symptomatic osteoarthritis. Osteoarthr Cartil OARS Osteoarthr Res Soc. 2012;20(7):745–54.
20. Bay-Jensen AC, Slagboom E, Chen-An P, Alexandersen P, Qvist P, Christiansen C, et al. Role of hormones in cartilage and joint metabolism: understanding an unhealthy metabolic phenotype in osteoarthritis. Menopause N Y N. 2013;20(5):578–86.
21. Bos SD, Beekman M, Maier AB, Karsdal MA, Kwok W-Y, Bay-Jensen AC, et al. Metabolic health in families enriched for longevity is associated with low prevalence of hand osteoarthritis and influences OA biomarker profiles. Ann Rheum Dis. 2013;72(10):1669–74.
22. Gandhi R, Razak F, Davey JR, Mahomed NN. Metabolic syndrome and the functional outcomes of hip and knee arthroplasty. J Rheumatol. 2010;37(9):1917–22.
23. Zhuo Q, Yang W, Chen J, Wang Y. Metabolic syndrome meets osteoarthritis. Nat Rev Rheumatol. 2012;8(12):729–37.
24. Gelber AC, Hochberg MC, Mead LA, Wang NY, Wigley FM, Klag MJ. Body mass index in young men and the risk of subsequent knee and hip osteoarthritis. Am J Med. 1999;107(6):542–8.
25. Gelber AC, Hochberg MC, Mead LA, Wang NY, Wigley FM, Klag MJ. Joint injury in young adults and risk for subsequent knee and hip osteoarthritis. Ann Intern Med. 2000;133(5):321–8.
26. Attur M, Belitskaya-Lévy I, Oh C, Krasnokutsky S, Greenberg J, Samuels J, et al. Increased interleukin-1β gene expression in peripheral blood leukocytes is associated with increased pain and predicts risk for progression of symptomatic knee osteoarthritis. Arthritis Rheum. 2011;63(7):1908–17.
27. Dolzani P, Assirelli E, Pulsatelli L, Addimanda O, Mancarella L, Peri G, et al. Systemic inflammation and antibodies to citrullinated peptides in hand osteoarthritis. Clin Exp Rheumatol. 2011;29(6):1006–9.
28. Goldring MB, Berenbaum F. The regulation of chondrocyte function by proinflammatory mediators: prostaglandins and nitric oxide. Clin Orthop. 2004;(427 Suppl):S37–46.
29. Scanzello CR, Umoh E, Pessler F, Diaz-Torne C, Miles T, Dicarlo E, et al. Local cytokine profiles in knee osteoarthritis: elevated synovial fluid interleukin-15 differentiates early from end-stage disease. Osteoarthr Cartil OARS Osteoarthr Res Soc. 2009;17(8):1040–8.
30. Henriksen K, Karsdal MA, Martin TJ. Osteoclast-derived coupling factors in bone remodeling. Calcif Tissue Int. 2014;94(1):88–97.
31. Henriksen K, Neutzsky-Wulff AV, Bonewald LF, Karsdal MA. Local communication on and within bone controls bone remodeling. Bone. 2009;44(6):1026–33.

32. Karsdal MA, Leeming DJ, Dam EB, Henriksen K, Alexandersen P, Pastoureau P, et al. Should subchondral bone turnover be targeted when treating osteoarthritis? Osteoarthr Cartil OARS Osteoarthr Res Soc. 2008;16(6):638–46.
33. Karsdal MA, Nielsen MJ, Sand JM, Henriksen K, Genovese F, Bay-Jensen A-C, et al. Extracellular matrix remodeling: the common denominator in connective tissue diseases. Possibilities for evaluation and current understanding of the matrix as more than a passive architecture, but a key player in tissue failure. Assay Drug Dev Technol. 2013;11(2):70–92.
34. Attur M, Wang H-Y, Kraus VB, Bukowski JF, Aziz N, Krasnokutsky S, et al. Radiographic severity of knee osteoarthritis is conditional on interleukin 1 receptor antagonist gene variations. Ann Rheum Dis. 2010;69(5):856–61.
35. Dodd AW, Syddall CM, Loughlin J. A rare variant in the osteoarthritis-associated locus GDF5 is functional and reveals a site that can be manipulated to modulate GDF5 expression. Eur J Hum Genet EJHG. 2013;21(5):517–21.
36. Alexandersen P, Karsdal MA, Byrjalsen I, Christiansen C. Strontium ranelate effect in postmenopausal women with different clinical levels of osteoarthritis. Climacteric J Int Menopause Soc. 2011;14(2):236–43.
37. Karsdal MA, Byrjalsen I, Henriksen K, Riis BJ, Lau EM, Arnold M, et al. The effect of oral salmon calcitonin delivered with 5-CNAC on bone and cartilage degradation in osteoarthritic patients: a 14-day randomized study. Osteoarthr Cartil OARS Osteoarthr Res Soc. 2010;18(2):150–9.
38. Reginster J-Y, Beaudart C, Neuprez A, Bruyère O. Strontium ranelate in the treatment of knee osteoarthritis: new insights and emerging clinical evidence. Ther Adv Musculoskelet Dis. 2013;5(5):268–76.
39. Reginster J-Y. Efficacy and safety of strontium ranelate in the treatment of knee osteoarthritis: results of a double-blind randomised, placebo-controlled trial. Ann Rheum Dis. 2014;73(2):e8.
40. Spector TD, Conaghan PG, Buckland-Wright JC, Garnero P, Cline GA, Beary JF, et al. Effect of risedronate on joint structure and symptoms of knee osteoarthritis: results of the BRISK randomized, controlled trial [ISRCTN01928173]. Arthritis Res Ther. 2005;7(3):R625–33.
41. Biomarkers Definitions Working Group. Biomarkers and surrogate endpoints: preferred definitions and conceptual framework. Clin Pharmacol Ther. 2001;69(3):89–95.
42. Kraus VB, Burnett B, Coindreau J, Cottrell S, Eyre D, Gendreau M, et al. Application of biomarkers in the development of drugs intended for the treatment of osteoarthritis. Osteoarthr Cartil OARS Osteoarthr Res Soc. 2011;19(5):515–42.
43. Lotz M, Martel-Pelletier J, Christiansen C, Brandi M-L, Bruyère O, Chapurlat R, et al. Value of biomarkers in osteoarthritis: current status and perspectives. Ann Rheum Dis. 2013;72(11):1756–63.
44. Van Spil WE, DeGroot J, Lems WF, Oostveen JCM, Lafeber FPJG. Serum and urinary biochemical markers for knee and hip-osteoarthritis: a systematic review applying the consensus BIPED criteria. Osteoarthr Cartil OARS Osteoarthr Res Soc. 2010;18(5):605–12.
45. Bauer DC, Hunter DJ, Abramson SB, Attur M, Corr M, Felson D, et al. Classification of osteoarthritis biomarkers: a proposed approach. Osteoarthr Cartil OARS Osteoarthr Res Soc. 2006;14(8):723–7.
46. Jurisica I. Integrative cancer informatics for the identification of prognostic and predictive biomarkers. BMC Proc. 2013;7(Suppl 2 Sao Paulo Advanced School of Comparative Oncology: AbstractsClaudia Aparecida Rainho, Patricia Pintor dos Reis and Silvia Regina RogattoPublication of this supplement was funded by the Sao Paulo Research Foundation (FAPESP)):K7.
47. Zhu C-Q, Ding K, Strumpf D, Weir BA, Meyerson M, Pennell N, et al. Prognostic and predictive gene signature for adjuvant chemotherapy in resected non-small-cell lung cancer. J Clin Oncol Off J Am Soc Clin Oncol. 2010;28(29):4417–24.
48. Frisenda S, Perricone C, Valesini G. Cartilage as a target of autoimmunity: a thin layer. Autoimmun Rev. 2013;12(5):591–8.
49. Nishioka K. Autoimmune response in cartilage-delivered peptides in a patient with osteoarthritis. Arthritis Res Ther. 2004;6(1):6–7.

50. Cooke TD. Significance of immune complex deposits in osteoarthritic cartilage. J Rheumatol. 1987;14 Spec No:77–9.
51. Gandhi R, Tsvetkov D, Dhottar H, Davey JR, Mahomed NN. Quantifying the pain experience in hip and knee osteoarthritis. Pain Res Manag J Can Pain Soc J Société Can Pour Trait Douleur. 2010;15(4):224–8.
52. Zhang W, Likhodii S, Zhang Y, Aref-Eshghi E, Harper PE, Randell E, et al. Classification of osteoarthritis phenotypes by metabolomics analysis. BMJ Open. 2014;4(11), e006286.
53. Gaskell G, Gottweis H. Biobanks need publicity. Nature. 2011;471(7337):159–60.
54. Holzinger A, Dehmer M, Jurisica I. Knowledge discovery and interactive data mining in bioinformatics–state-of-the-art, future challenges and research directions. BMC Bioinformatics. 2014;15(Suppl 6):I1.
55. Fortney K, Jurisica I. Integrative computational biology for cancer research. Hum Genet. 2011;130(4):465–81.
56. Jurisica I. Mapping cancer markers – towards precision medicine [Internet]. http://www.cs.toronto.edu/~juris/MCM.htm. Cited 5 Apr 2015.
57. Starmans MH, Pintilie M, John T, Der SD, Shepherd FA, Jurisica I, et al. Exploiting the noise: improving biomarkers with ensembles of data analysis methodologies. Genome Med. 2012;4(11):84.
58. Pastrello C, Pasini E, Kotlyar M, Otasek D, Wong S, Sangrar W, et al. Integration, visualization and analysis of human interactome. Biochem Biophys Res Commun. 2014;445(4):757–73.
59. Mullard A. 23andMe sets sights on UK/Canada, signs up Genentech. Nat Biotechnol. 2015;33(2):119.
60. Yim S-H, Chung Y-J. Reflections on the US FDA's warning on direct-to-consumer genetic testing. Genomics Inform. 2014;12(4):151–5.
61. Slade Shantz JA, Veillette CJH. The application of wearable technology in surgery: ensuring the positive impact of the wearable revolution on surgical patients. Front Surg. 2014;1:39.

Index

M. Kapoor, N.N. Mahomed (eds.), *Osteoarthritis: Pathogenesis, Diagnosis, Available Treatments, Drug Safety, Regenerative and Precision Medicine*,
DOI 10.1007/978-3-319-19560-5

Printed by Printforce, the Netherlands